MAKING ROUNDS

MAKING ROUNDS

Love, Loss, and Lessons Learned from an Indomitable Woman in Medicine

Sharon L. Hostler, MD

UNIVERSITY OF VIRGINIA PRESS
Charlottesville and London

The University of Virginia Press is situated on the traditional lands of the Monacan Nation, and the Commonwealth of Virginia was and is home to many other Indigenous people. We pay our respect to all of them, past and present. We also honor the enslaved African and African American people who built the University of Virginia, and we recognize their descendants. We commit to fostering voices from these communities through our publications and to deepening our collective understanding of their histories and contributions.

University of Virginia Press

Printed in the United States of America on acid-free paper

First published 2026

9 8 7 6 5 4 3 2 1

LIBRARY OF CONGRESS CATALOGING-IN-PUBLICATION DATA

Names: Hostler, Sharon L. author
Title: Making rounds : love, loss, and lessons learned from an indomitable woman in medicine / Sharon L. Hostler, MD.
Description: Charlottesville : University of Virginia Press, 2026.
Identifiers: LCCN 2026013685 (print) | LCCN 2026013686 (ebook) | ISBN 9780813955827 hardback | ISBN 9780813955834 ebook
Subjects: LCSH: Hostler, Sharon L. | Physicians—Virginia | Women physicians—Virginia | Pediatricians—Virginia | Women pediatricians—Virginia | Sex discrimination in medicine—Virginia | University of Virginia. School of Medicine | LCGFT: Autobiographies
Classification: LCC R154.H6677 A3 2026 (print) | LCC R154.H6677 (ebook)
LC record available at https://lccn.loc.gov/2026013685
LC ebook record available at https://lccn.loc.gov/2026013686

Unless otherwise noted, images in the photo gallery are from the author's collection.

Cover photo © Dan Grogan
Cover design by Joel W. Coggins

For Kaki and Dylan

· CONTENTS ·

· FOREWORD ·

When Sharon Hostler embarked on a career in medicine in the early 1960s, American medicine and the healthcare system were being transformed. After decades of marginalization, structural and cultural barriers to women's participation in medicine were breaking down. In 1961, when Dr. Hostler enrolled in medical school at the University of Vermont, just 6 percent of physicians were women. Despite being in the midst of a physician shortage, medical educators were deeply ambivalent toward women in medicine, contending that women physicians were not as productive as men physicians nor as reliable, assuming they would leave full-time medical practice to marry and raise children. At that time, the majority of women physicians specialized in pediatrics, internal medicine, psychiatry, or obstetrics-gynecology—specialties that had since the late nineteenth century been more open to women physicians but were also associated with less prestige and lower pay. By the early 1970s, the legal victories of the civil rights and women's movements had reduced women's barriers to pursuing careers in medicine, and significantly greater numbers of women were applying to and being admitted to medical school. However, women physicians continued to experience discrimination in medicine in the form of sexual harassment, pay inequities, and discrimination in hiring and promotion. And the structure of medical education, training, and practice at best deterred and at worst punished women who wanted to have children as well as a career in medicine. Even as the percentage of women in medicine increased during the 1970s and 1980s, their representation in the highest ranks of academic medicine and in leadership positions remained disproportionately low. By 1995, for example, women comprised 25 percent of full-time faculty in medical schools but only 10 percent of full professors.

The system of segregated healthcare was also being dismantled, albeit slowly. When Hostler arrived in Charlottesville in 1965 to begin her internship and residency in pediatrics at the University of Virginia Hospital, the hospital was in the process of desegregating. Since its founding in 1901, UVA Hospital had been a segregated institution, providing separate and unequal care to Black patients and relegating Black employees to the lowest-paid, lowest-status positions in the hospital. Although the 1963 Supreme Court decision *Simkins v. Cone* and the 1964 Civil Rights Act had mandated hospital desegregation, and the passage of Medicare in 1965 meant the federal government could withhold Medicare funds from hospitals that refused to desegregate, hospitals throughout the South were generally slow to comply. In 1965, for example, the local chapter of the NAACP filed a complaint with the secretary of Health, Education, and Welfare alleging ongoing civil rights violations and discrimination at UVA Hospital. At the time, no Black physicians worked at the hospital, and only 5 percent of the hospital's registered nurses were Black.

The field of pediatrics, as well as young people's access to and experience of healthcare, were also being transformed. As part of President Lyndon B. Johnson's War on Poverty, the federal government provided funds to establish programs affording comprehensive education and comprehensive healthcare to low-income children and their families, and their healthcare access was also bolstered by the introduction of Medicaid in 1965. Meanwhile, the introduction of neonatal intensive care units, prenatal and newborn screening for genetic disorders, and new childhood vaccines, as well as other medical innovations, were transforming pediatric care and the health of children and adolescents. Hostler's experience as a young pediatrician coming of age during the late 1960s and 1970s provides a window to these changes and so much more.

Sharon Hostler's memoir is a deeply personal reflection of her life, from growing up in difficult circumstances in Vermont, through her journey in academic medicine, first at the University of Vermont as a medical student and then at UVA, where she completed her training in pediatrics and subsequently joined the faculty of the Department of Pediatrics. Hostler shares her experiences navigating professional opportunities, family responsibilities, personal loss and grief, and a sexist and elitist Southern medical culture. Along the way, we are given a view of the social, political, economic, and cultural factors that shaped UVA and academic medicine during the 1960s and 1970s, as well as insights into how the intersections of race, gender, and class in Virginia shaped different people's access to and experiences of healthcare in the Commonwealth. Ultimately, this is a powerful story of one woman physician's efforts to pursue both family and career on her own terms during a period of profound sexism and misogyny, not only in American medicine but also in American society more generally.

Dominique Tobbell, PhD
Centennial Distinguished Professor
Director, Bjoring Center for Nursing Historical Inquiry
University of Virginia School of Nursing

MAKING ROUNDS

· 1 ·

Escaping the Harness

1939–1953

Nellie had been a Miss America contestant, dreaming of a life in the lights, when she met my father at a dance marathon. Hop, a swaggering athlete who started serial seasons of college football without completing a single semester, was reeling from the death of his fiancé. Nellie and Hop married in January 1939. Nellie said she married the Holy Trinity—Hop; Hop's father, Pa Hostler; and the kitchen at 72 Library Avenue in Rutland, Vermont. I was born that October.

Nellie liked to tell people my birth story. It opened with Hop swigging whiskey from a brown paper bag and hollering, "Bear down, Nellie!" with each contraction. And when Nellie crested, he'd cheered, "Bring him on, my All-American!" Hop stormed out when Nellie failed to deliver a future football star. The nurse entered the name Sharon Lee on the birth certificate from the detective novel she was reading so that Nellie and the baby could be discharged.

Nellie ended the story when Hop refused to come pick us up at the hospital and Pa brought us home in a cab. It was Pa who told the story of the screaming baby who refused the bottle and refused to sleep. And he included the tirades Hop directed at Nellie.

Pa was twice a widower. His first wife died delivering Hop, and then his second wife, Hop's stepmother, died not long before Hop met Nellie at the dance marathon. For different reasons, both Pa and Hop needed a woman in the house.

Pa was the janitor at Rutland High School across the street from their home on Library Avenue. He wore gray overalls to work, carried a huge ring with keys to all the locks, and knew the physical plant inside and out. Pa had worked at the high school since he immigrated from Quebec as a young man. He was respected by all the teachers and the coaches and revered by a generation of students for whom he had held the morning bell. Pa was delighted to have Nellie in the kitchen to prepare Sunday dinner, even if it was chicken fricassee or tripe. There was no beef or pork during wartime.

Nellie worked as a cocktail waitress. Hop drove a cab, but his real gig was running the black market by night train from Montreal. His specialties were cigarettes, butter, and Canadian bacon. Nellie and Hop partied, argued, and worked on getting Hop his football player.

By the time I was four, Nellie had miscarried twice and delivered one stillborn, all boys. Hop was disgusted with Nellie and said so, sometimes even ranting during Pa's noontime *News of the War* on the radio. One day, Hop showed up with a three-year-old boy from somewhere, but that didn't last long. He wasn't toilet-trained, and he bit both Nellie and Hop.

Nellie wasn't cut out for motherhood. And, she told anyone who would listen, from Pa to the maiden sisters and their mother who lived next door, I didn't make her job any easier. I could talk, but I wouldn't talk, and I ended up having my tonsils taken out. I failed ballet and tap lessons, skills critical to my future as a successful beauty queen.

Most days, Nellie had had it with me by midmorning. She said I gave her a headache. She said she had no choice. *She had to put me in the harness.*

Nellie attached the harness to my sunsuit straps, front and back, then hooked a link from the harness to one end of a rope and clipped the other end to the clothesline. My range of freedom was between the two poles.

Day after day, I tried to escape. One day, I did.

I wiggled my way out of the sunsuit and out of the yard before Nellie spotted me. I was naked except for my white sandals.

I headed out of the yard and around the corner from Library Avenue to Grove Street and sat on the synagogue steps, waving to the cars. Some slowed down. A few blew their horns. Mostly, they laughed and waved.

I walked along Grove all the way to Williams Street, looking at the fancy houses and flower gardens. People were out on their porches or mowing lawns. Nobody paid any attention to me, but I did meet Susan Smith, still a friend eight decades later, and her mother picking flowers in one of those yards.

I turned left onto Williams Street and again onto Chestnut Avenue. That's when I spotted him. A little boy, acting like he owned the place.

He was riding his tricycle on the sidewalk, decked out in a navy-blue sailor suit complete with little anchors on the cuffs of his socks. I ran up and pushed him off the trike. I didn't know why. He fell on the grass and lay there, crying like a baby. I laughed, got on his trike, and started to pedal home.

He chased after me and managed to knock me off the trike, and all the time hollered, "Stupid, naked girl. Buck naked except for shoes."

I spit at him and tore at the collar of his sailor shirt. We struggled on the grass until I pulled off his shoe and tossed it down the storm drain. He knelt at the edge of the road by the sewer and howled.

I ran home and I waited, cross-legged and naked under the clothesline. I didn't wait long.

Nellie was hot. "What'd you do to that crying kid?" She tried to stuff me back into the sunsuit, but it was tangled up in the harness. "Hop's going to hear about this."

She yanked me one way, then another, as we headed into the house. "Pa will be fit to be tied. This is Pa's neighborhood, and that was Dr. Leyton's son." She shoved me into the kitchen. "Stay the hell out of my sight."

She got a beer, lit a cigarette—one of Hop's Camels—and sat on the front stoop to wait for Hop.

It wasn't until the next day that the grown-ups understood that I had thrown the kid's leather shoe down the sewer. I watched from the corner as Pa, Hop, and Dr. Leyton, in his seersucker suit and white bucks, tried to retrieve the shoe.

At supper, Hop grabbed the back of my chair and jerked it around. I sat very still. "Why the hell, Sharon?" he asked. "Why throw just one shoe down the sewer?"

He said it as if that was the only part that didn't make sense. *Why only one shoe?*

But I had other questions. Why did I escape from the harness? Why did I push the kid down?

Then, I was aware of only one reason: He was too smug, that kid on the bike with anchors on the cuffs of his socks.

Now, decades later, I can think of lots of reasons. I would never be Nellie's Miss America. I couldn't be an All-American quarterback. A girl had to be tough to survive. It would be decades later in my professional life before I finally understood that bullying was not an effective strategy.

Another two years went by with no babies, but lots of drinking, arguments about Hop playing the horses, and Nellie turning the house upside down searching for where he'd hid his track winnings.

In September 1945, I started first grade at Lincoln Elementary School. Mrs. Smith walked with Susan and me for the first week, but then we were on our own—going and coming. I loved school.

But then, that Christmas Eve, Hop and Nellie were in a car crash—drunk and driving Hop's work cab.

When I woke up Christmas morning, the goose was still strung up by its neck on the back stoop. Celery stuffed with cream cheese and parsley was on a tray in the refrigerator. A doll with eyes that opened and shut sat under the Christmas tree. The house was empty.

I played with the doll, ate some celery, and found the fancy cookies Nellie had hidden. It was dark outside by the time Pa came home. He sat on the couch, still in his overcoat and scarf, and started to cry. He said that Nellie might lose her legs and Hop was still in the hospital. Pa lay back on the couch, rolled away from me, and faced the wall.

"I'll figure out what to do with you later."

Pa had a lot to figure out over the next few weeks. Nellie had smashed legs, and Hop lost his job driving the cab. When Nellie finally came home from the hospital, she couldn't even stand up on her own.

Hattie, Nellie's mother, showed up to take care of Nellie and, I guess, me too. Hattie introduced random fainting spells, morning farting contests, and after-school lice searches in my scalp. Hop was rarely around. Hattie and Nellie shared the bed, so Hop slept on the couch when he managed to stagger in. But once their laughter and their farts started in the morning, he'd slam out of the house. Pa followed. I met Susan for school.

Pa shopped at the butcher once a week. He was proud that he got good cuts of beef. "No more eating tripe like during the war," he said. "No pretending rabbit is fricasseed chicken." But Hattie burned everything. She even charred a fancy roast for Sunday. No one except Pa went to Mass, but Sunday dinner was still a special meal. Pa insisted I go to Catechism with the nuns, but after Nellie's accident there was no one to take me. When I didn't make my First Communion, the neighbor ladies next door started taking me with them to the Episcopal church.

Sometimes, during that spring of first grade, Nellie and Hattie played dolls with me after school, but mostly I went home with Susan. Hattie complained about me being underfoot. I liked to be home when, once a week, Dr. Ryan checked on Nellie's progress. He always asked about school. It was six months, almost summer, before Dr. Ryan finally allowed Nellie out of bed. And then she had to learn to walk again.

Not long after that, Hop moved permanently from the living room couch to Rosalie-the-other-woman's bed. When Nellie and Hop cursed and threw the lamps at each other, Pa would take me over to the high school. We watched the tennis teams practice, the crowning of the Homecoming King and Queen, and sometimes even visited the classrooms. Pa loved the geography room with its globes and bulletin boards. He pointed out London, Berlin, and Hiroshima on the maps and talked about "the bomb." But when Hattie's son by her third cousin came to visit, not even Pa paid attention to his visits to my room in the middle of the night.

"Touch it," he said as he leaned with his penis on the edge of my bed. "Watch it dance. Go ahead, touch it." I didn't dare tell anyone but Susan. Susan and I decided the best course was to pretend to be asleep and ignore him. And that's what I did, night after night. I would report to Susan at school the next morning.

When Pa wasn't around, Hop ragged at Nellie. "Miss America, my ass. Not with those beat-up legs."

It took almost a year, but by Christmas in the middle of second grade, Pa had figured out what to do. He sent Hattie packing and bought a house for Hop and Nellie. I never thought of Pa as old, but he was retiring. With his janitor's pension, Pa made the down payment on the eight-thousand-dollar house at 15 Vernon Street.

Hop bought a player piano for the new house, and Nellie started me taking piano lessons, more talent preparation for the Miss America contest in my future. I'd already failed tap and ballet. Hop didn't keep up the payments. The piano was gone one day after school, but Nellie sent me to lessons anyway until the teacher figured out that I had no piano to practice on. The piano was like the encyclopedias that Hop bought at the grocery store. We only had volumes ABC and DEF. We had no books around until Pa started the Book-of-the-Month Club for Nellie.

Hop promised Pa he would live with us on Vernon Street. But Hop didn't move. He stayed with Rosalie.

But Hop visited when Uncle Tom died from diabetes and was laid out in the living room. Aunt Hilda was Hop's half sister and a nurse, the one who intervened when I didn't gain weight as a baby and later when Nellie had a miscarriage. Hop wouldn't want Hilda to know about Rosalie.

Pa was getting weaker. By the fall of fourth grade, Dr. Ryan had hung a pee bag by Pa's bed. Harry Ryan had played ball with Hop before he went to medical school, and when he came back to practice in Rutland, he saw us in his office, made home visits, and never sent a bill.

By the time I'd get home from school, the air in Pa's bedroom stank of old man, tobacco, and pee. He fussed if I dillydallied with Susan on the way home. Nellie left early to catch the city bus for her night shift waitressing. It took me awhile to realize that Pa was lonely all by himself in the new house far away from the high school.

"Tobbacky, young lady, the tobbacky." That was how Pa greeted me every day when I got home from school. My first task was to light Pa's corncob pipe, even before I dumped the bag of stinking pee.

I didn't like blowing Pa's drool out of the stem, packing the loose tobacco in the bowl, or lighting the pipe. But I hated the first inhale. It was worse than the pee stench.

I knew that Pa looked forward to my stories, so I shared all the details, even when the teacher had put me in the cloak room all day because I refused to make my cursive letters march in the same direction. Pa laughed when I told him I had moved the lunch bags around. And mixed up the mittens and the scarves. What else could I do all day? Pa laughed. He was the one who signed my report cards. All A's, all the time.

I'd fetch whatever Nellie had left in the oven for our supper, usually soup or stew. Pa didn't have teeth, and his hands jiggled with tremors. I tied a dish towel around his neck and spooned soup to the side of his tongue. We ate supper around his bed. I came to understand that Pa had known he was sick long before we moved to 15 Vernon Street.

After I cleaned up our supper dishes and wiped his face, Pa regaled me with stories about his family. How the bias against the "Canucks," the French immigrants from Quebec, meant that the town clerk in Pittsford, Vermont, changed their name from Chevalier (a decorated knight on horseback) to Hostler (a caretaker of horses). Sometimes when Pa was feeling sad, he'd talk about his children—Pat, who was Hop's older brother and lived in South Carolina, and Hilda, but never Hop. Everyone in our town was White, but no one ever mentioned that. The teacher did point out the one Jewish girl, though.

At bedtime, Pa reminded me to shovel coal into the furnace, to bank the fire, and to turn the porch light on for Nellie. Pa understood I was afraid of the furnace, so he kept calling to me while I ran down and up the cellar stairs. Then I lit one last pipe for him.

Dr. Ryan came by every week or so to visit Pa. "It won't be long now," he said and squeezed Pa's hands in his. "I've always been grateful to you, Pa, for holding that school bell for me when I was late."

He pinched Pa's cheek, grinned at me, and picked up his doctor's bag. Pa and I listened to his footsteps on the stairs, the slam of the front door, and the sound of his car driving off. We were quiet, thinking about what Dr. Ryan had said. My life was focused on school and Pa. I didn't get to Susan's house much. We never saw Hop and only glimpsed Nellie coming or going to work.

One afternoon, I found only a few drops of pee in the bag when I got home. I knew that was not good. By then, Pa was struggling so hard to breathe that he could barely get a draw off the pipe.

Several weeks later, Pa refused his pipe. He took only a few sips of soup. It was long after dark when the death rattle started, Pa's breath gurgling through the junk in his lungs. Dr. Ryan had explained it was a little like Pa was drowning. I sat next to his bed and held his hand in the dark, but we were both scared.

That week, Nellie got home from work later and later. She'd made it clear what I was supposed to do. "Close his mouth. Straighten his legs.

Cross his right hand over the other," she said. She was matter-of-fact about it. "It'll be an open casket."

Pa died the week before Thanksgiving. It was around ten o'clock at night. I tried to do as Nellie said. I was nine.

The next morning, Nellie was focused on damning Hop Hostler at the top of her lungs. I worried that the whole neighborhood could hear her, but she didn't care. She scrubbed Pa's room and the downstairs on her hands and knees.

The undertakers brought Pa back home that afternoon for the wake. They set up the open casket in front of the double windows at the end of the living room where the couch belonged. Pa didn't look like himself, with rouge on his cheeks and his boney body in a shiny suit. I missed the old Pa. I wanted to talk with him about what was happening. Maybe he could have explained. But he was gone.

Women came with Boston baked beans, tuna casseroles, and yeast rolls. The kitchen reeked of powdered bodies, cigarette smoke, and beer. I wasn't included, but I got the gist. *Would Hop return? How would Nellie pay the mortgage without Pa's pension?*

The men hung around the dining room, keeping an eye on the casket and passing around pints of the hard stuff while the women scurried back and forth with food.

Nellie was three sheets to the wind when Hop appeared at the kitchen door. "Where the hell were you when your father was alive?"

Mourners came through the front door, handed me their heavy coats to take upstairs, and worked their way toward Pa. Some just crossed themselves, some kneeled before the open casket, some mouthed a prayer. The women fingered their beads and murmured when the parish priest from Mount Saint Joseph arrived to lead the Rosary. The men held back.

Pa had been a popular figure in Rutland. Teachers and students from over forty years remembered him. Every day, Pa showed up at Rutland High School with his huge ring of keys to ring the school bell for the start and the finish of classes. It seemed that Pa had held the bell at the high school for many town leaders like Dr. Ryan. Even the Benevolent and Protective Order of the Eagles, Pa's lodge, sent a wreath.

A neighbor whispered to me that Pa would sit upright when rigor mortis set in, so I stood on the landing watching for any movement of

Pa's body. He didn't. The men stood around the casket drinking and toasting Pa. They were singing when I fell asleep.

The day of Pa's funeral that November 1948 was cold, windy, and New England gray. I cried as the undertakers closed the coffin and rolled it out of the house into the hearse. It was a High Mass. The smell of burnt clove from the censers filled the church. When we came home from the cemetery, Mrs. Romano, our neighbor up the street, delivered a pot of steaming soup with tiny meatballs. "It's really Italian wedding soup, but it works for cold days, funerals, and sad stomachs," she said. "It's the bitter herbs."

Hop had come back to the house. He motioned me to follow him out on the back stoop. I wondered what he wanted.

"You're no athlete, kid, but Pa told me that you are pretty smart in school."

"Straight A's," I said without looking at him.

"If you keep that up, maybe you can go to the Normal School." He turned, sauntered down the driveway, and left without a goodbye. I had no idea what a "normal school" was.

The Christmas after Pa died, his Eagles lodge delivered a wicker basket tied with a red bow—a turkey and all the fixings. Nellie opened the front door just a crack, hollered, "We're not on the damn dole!" and slammed the door in their faces.

For Christmas dinner, the two of us had home-canned tomatoes over Nellie's homemade bread. She was a good baker. She'd learned how from the pastry cook at her restaurant. All that day, Nellie drank beer, cursed, and kept calling Hop at Rosalie's. I hated not having that turkey and trimmings, but not nearly as much as I hated Nellie's sniveling over the telephone that Christmas or describing the silver T-strapped heels she had worn for the Miss America Contest.

That winter, I started going to Susan's house every day after school. Her family had moved from the old downtown neighborhood into a modern house with lots of windows, flower beds, and landscaped lawns. A barn for Susan's horse, a potting shed, and a greenhouse for Mrs. Smith.

It was a different world at the Smiths. The living room was modern with low couches in gray leather, African violets, and white orchids in big baskets. Dr. Smith's library had floor-to-ceiling bookshelves, a human skull, and stacks of the *New England Journal of Medicine.* He had placed chess sets in various stages of engagement on every flat surface. Dr. Smith competed with opponents from around the world who sent their moves on postcards. And sometimes, after dinner, he sat in his leather chair and read medical journals.

During the day, Susan's mother wore overalls and a denim smock to work with her plants. By suppertime, she had changed into a silk blouse and pearls. "Ecru," Susan explained. "Ecru silk."

Susan explained that her mother had once been a show girl in New York City. Dr. Smith had courted her with bouquets and champagne. When he finally married her, he moved her to Vermont. At her garden club that Christmas, Mrs. Smith let us decorate evergreen trees with blue satin ribbon and sparkling green lights. When I told Nellie about my tree, she insisted that blue ribbon and green lights were absurd.

Sometimes Mrs. Smith allowed me to stay for supper, but not always. One night when Susan asked, Mrs. Smith snapped, "I have four pork chops. Four. If you want Sharon to stay, cut yours in half."

Every evening, the Smiths sat down for supper at a table set with china and silver, fresh flowers, and napkins. Dr. Smith asked us about school, what we were reading, and corrected our grammar. He expected Susan and her brother to recite sonnets. Not me.

By the spring of fourth grade, Mrs. Smith gave me a house key so that I could water the flowers, feed the horse, and check on things when they went out of town. I understood that I could use the key if I ever needed to even if they weren't away.

That summer after Pa's death, I had my first paying job. I didn't understand then why Dr. Smith hired me, but I worked there every morning.

His office was on Grove Street, the same street I'd explored as a four-year-old free of Nellie's harness. I was the only one in the office in the morning while Dr. Smith made house calls and rounds at the hospital. Sometimes a patient dropped off a crate of eggs or a sack of corn in barter. I knew to say, "thank you," make a note, and double-check the spelling of the name.

My duties included answering phone calls from Dr. Smith's patients and the local pharmacies, straightening up the waiting room, and removing the trash from the exam rooms. I had plenty of spare time, and I was an eager learner. After scanning the *Saturday Evening Post, Life,* and *Time* magazines, I searched the medical textbooks for anatomy diagrams, especially the sexual organs. When I ransacked through the top drawer of Dr. Smith's desk and found his personal checkbook, I discovered a balance of four thousand dollars. Astounding. Nellie made twenty dollars in tips on a good Saturday night. I was making five dollars a week.

The Friday before Labor Day, Dr. Smith shook my hand. "Good job, Sharon. Would you like to come back next summer?"

I grinned and nodded.

"Next summer, you'll have to say 'Dr. Smith's office' when you answer the phone. Okay?" I blushed with shame. *I was nine. How could I not have known the right way to answer the phone?*

Two years later, Hop finally showed up at 15 Vernon Street. I was in sixth grade. He was thirty-four years old and had been diagnosed with Hodgkin's disease. Dr. Ryan recommended experimental radiation therapy. Hop refused. He was as skinny as Pa had been at the end. Hop had been running a jackhammer for the city road works. Nellie insisted he sleep on the living room couch under the windows, where the casket for both Uncle Tom and Pa had stood.

I fixed soup for him, washed his laundry, and held his head when he retched in the middle of the night. He had navy-blue bruises all over his belly from the jackhammer. His bones protruded from his shoulders to his butt. Nellie continued to work the night shift, and sometimes she didn't come home at all.

Although I missed being at the Smiths' house, Hop and I eventually developed an after-school rhythm. He prepared pages and pages of math problems for me to solve, not difficult but tedious and repetitive. I preferred having him at home to an empty house. We listened to *The Shadow* on the radio and talked about the news and, sometimes, what was happening in school.

"Have you learned to dance?" he asked one day out of the blue.

I shook my head.

"You need some basic skills, sister. Dancing is one of them." He laughed, tuned the radio, and stood up, his arm outstretched. "Come on. Put one hand on my shoulder. Take my hand with the other one."

I got closer.

"Relax, don't hold your breath like that," he said. He started to sway, but I stayed put in place. "Sing along," he cajoled.

I giggled and hummed a bit. We managed to match a box step or two to the music. He laughed. "You got it, kid."

I had never been physically close to him. I couldn't remember him ever being kind or gentle in any way. My memories were of being five, trying to jump hurdles at the high school track and stumbling. Fumbling the basketball. Being hit in the face over and over by tennis balls I couldn't hit. I still remembered his disgust. The way he walked away.

I could remember snuggling with Nellie as a little kid, not often but once or twice when she had a night off and Hop hadn't come home. It was before the accident. She'd make white rice with butter, brown sugar, and milk for Sunday supper, read one of her women's magazines, and allow me to cozy up to her back. Once or twice, not since.

By the end of seventh grade, Hop was getting skinnier and skinnier. He even retched up the chicken broth I fixed. Nellie managed to ignore both of us.

One afternoon when I was walking home from school, I heard a car slow down behind me. It was Dr. Ryan. "I'm headed to see Hop, climb in."

"Can't you make him better?"

"He's getting worse every day. We talked about this before, Sharon." He turned in his seat to look right at me. "There is no treatment for what Hop has. It's Hodgkin's disease."

"But—"

"It's spread to his brain. That's why he's vomiting."

"You said it was blood cancer."

"It is, but it's gone to his brain, and the pressure is building. He'll start having fits like your Gram Hattie."

When we pulled up, Hop was on the porch reading the newspaper. He'd put on a clean undershirt and tucked it into baggy workpants, the rope belt clinched tight. He had on loafers but no socks.

Dr. Ryan took the steps two at a time, squinted at Hop, and leaned back against the porch railing. "Hop, how the hell are you?"

"Bitch of a headache." Hop held the newspaper in front of his face.

"What's in the *Herald* today, Hop?" Dr. Ryan made a point of staring at the newspaper until I looked. The paper was upside down.

"The usual. Royals lost again," Hop whispered and dropped the paper.

"How long? Hop, how long?"

"This morning."

Dr. Ryan bent down, put his arms around Hop, and swooped him out of the chair. Hop crumbled into Dr. Ryan's arms. Dr. Ryan patted Hop's butt, lifted him up, and carried him to the car.

"Not yet, Harry. Not the hospital. No insurance."

"It's time. Forget the money. Keep your head down and slide back. Relax your legs and let me tuck you in." He ruffled Hop's hair, grinned, and shut the car door.

"Sharon, let Nellie know. Remember what I said about Hop's brain."

I sat on the steps, watching as they drove off. The newspaper lay on the floor. The window boxes along our porch were empty, but a bank of blood-red peonies bloomed across the street.

Hop died that night at eight o'clock, before the priest arrived to administer his last rites. That meant Hop couldn't be buried in consecrated ground next to Pa, and we'd have to light lots of candles and say lots of Rosaries to get his soul even into purgatory. Hop was laid out in the living room, just like Uncle Tom and Pa, in front of the window.

The day after Hop died, Nellie's mother, Hattie, and her husband, George, moved into Pa's bedroom. They had their bags upstairs and unpacked even before Mrs. Romano brought over the soup with the bitter herbs.

After Nellie paid the undertakers, she used the rest of the burial money to buy a black-and-white television set. No one in our neighborhood had television. Nellie sat in front of the set, day after day. Fortified by a bottle of Ballantine Ale, a spare pack of Pall Malls, and her favorite ashtray. She watched the soaps, the *Ed Sullivan Show,* and even *Lawrence Welk* with his bubble machine.

Hop died in June 1952. I was twelve. I knew then that I wanted to be a doctor like Dr. Smith and Dr. Ryan. And when I did, I promised myself that no one would ever die of Hodgkin's disease again.

In eighth grade, the next year, the school principal wouldn't let me sign up for the precollege track in high school—who would pay for my college tuition? He said I had to be on the vocational track. I explained that if I was going to be a doctor, I had to go to college first to get into medical school.

Hattie told me I had to quit school. That I had to get a job to support Nellie. "No," I said. I was going to medical school.

Hattie and her husband, George, freeloaded until the insurance money ran out the next spring. Four people couldn't manage on $140 per month from Hop's Social Security benefits. The neighbors whispered about how Nellie couldn't pay the mortgage and took bets on how long before I'd have to quit school.

Every day, George had lurked in Pa's room with his fly open, waiting for me to get home from school. I went to Susan's most days.

As soon as they moved out, I mopped the floor, emptied out the chest of drawers, and took down Pa's crucifix from the wall. I pulled down the curtains, shoved the bed into a corner, and brought up an old table from the garage. I transformed the space into a laboratory.

I dissected a dead cat I'd ordered from one of Dr. Smith's medical catalogues. The cat was delivered through the mail, preserved in formaldehyde, and tightly sealed. I dissected the specimen without instructions, enjoying the cutting and the scraping, discovering what lay under each layer. Nellie complained about the stench, but she never budged from the television. Susan came over to keep me company. She poked at the cat corpse, asked a few questions, and then sat on Pa's old bed sketching.

One night the following January I woke up coughing from the smoke coming from Nellie's room. She'd fallen asleep smoking. I hollered at her to wake up, but she just cursed at me. I pulled off the smoldering covers and shoved them out of the window into the snow below.

Nellie waitressed at seedier and seedier joints. When she wasn't working, she sat in front of the television set. Nellie got drunk, lost jobs, and slid further down the ladder.

I couldn't count on Nellie. I would not grow up to be hungry and poor. I was thirteen, and I knew that I had to get the hell out of there. I knew then that I didn't want to grow up like Hop and Nellie, but I couldn't have begun to imagine a future with love that was open and kind. Unconditional.

· 2 ·

Finding My Way

1953–1965

When I started Rutland High School, I was not only placed on a pre-college track, but I became one of a cohort of high-functioning students assigned the best teachers and held to a higher academic standard. The new principal had created this exception when he recognized the group of twenty gifted students in the freshman class of 120. The cohort would compete against one another and remain together until graduation. I was relieved not to be in the vocational track.

But I still had to contribute to Nellie's and my living expenses, so I worked at a department store every afternoon, from 1:00 to 6:00 p.m. Most of the teachers at RHS had worked with Pa Hostler, and they understood my circumstances. They ignored my early departures.

Not the new principal.

He saw me leaving early in October. "You just can't walk out in the middle of the school day," he said. "What's your name?"

"Sharon Lee Hostler. I'm a freshman. And I've got to get to work."

"You can't."

"Check my grades, sir. All A's," I said and walked out the front door. He must have because he never stopped me again.

I always had jobs. All through high school, I babysat, I cleaned houses, I worked in Dr. Smith's office, I waitressed summers at nearby Lake Bomoseen, I worked as a chamber maid at a seedy motel, I tutored, I covered second-period geometry class for Mr. Floyd, the football coach; by senior year, I'd worked over twenty jobs and won many academic honors. I starred in the senior play, published a haiku, and had an affair with Tom the ski bum.

The Smith family provided a safe haven. The veterinarian next door, too young when he graduated to be licensed to practice, worked inoculating dairy cows against brucellosis for the Vermont Health Department. He edited my college applications, challenged my reasoning, and banged on the front door when I was home alone with the ski bum. The English teacher introduced me to the *Atlantic Monthly, Harper's,* and the Sunday edition of the *New York Times,* all free at the library. She wrote a note on my reading journal, "You can do this. You can get out."

Even the principal's secretary assembled the clothing required to attend Girls Nations in Washington, DC. It was a long, very specific list, and it included five pairs of white cotton gloves. Otherwise I could not have attended, but it was strange wearing clothes that smelled of girls I did not know. When the principal insisted that Susan and I had to attend the junior prom after we had single-handedly decorated the gym for the theme, Mood Indigo, I was again in the principal's office trying on someone else's hand-me-down gowns. During the country club cotillion, to which I had not been invited, I babysat for the family of a classmate. While the father drove me home, he said, "Give up the college nonsense. Learn to type. Get a job. No one is going to give you a scholarship."

On the other hand, the veterinarian next door drove me to college interviews. We never had a car, and Nellie couldn't drive. My teachers wrote letters of recommendation, and so did Dr. Smith. After all, he was not only Susan's father and my former employer, but chair of the Rutland School Board. I maintained a demanding schedule of classes, after-school work for pay, and extracurricular activities.

The old ladies of the family continued to berate me for staying in school. Nellie had a series of mostly derelict drinking buddies, but one was the photographer for the *Rutland Herald* and probably the reason I had my photograph in the local newspaper so often. I still remember the day I was on my knees scrubbing out a toilet bowl and the lady of the house checked in. "Aren't you the honor student I saw on the front page of the paper last week?"

Finally, on April 1, 1957, a large manilla envelope arrived from Middlebury College. Nellie was in front of the television puffing on her Pall

Malls and sipping beer when I ran in with the mail. Her eyes never left the screen as she held up her hand. "Wait for the goddamn commercial," she said.

I didn't wait. I ran up the hill to show the Smiths. The admission packet included a Jay Gould Foundation Fellowship—a full academic scholarship, including personal expenses and a requirement that I could not work during the school year. I was going to college. Over the years, I suspected that somehow the high school principal, an alumnus of Middlebury College, had conjured that magic, but he never acknowledged playing a part, not even when I was invited back to RHS in 1967 as a Distinguished Graduate to deliver the commencement address.

As the senior class recessed in academic attire, Nellie reached out for the sleeve of my robe. I kept marching. The Smiths had included me in their festive dinner celebration the night of graduation.

The dean of women gave a tea for the Middlebury College freshman girls before classes started. After she introduced me to President Stratton as the Gould Fellow, he shook my hand and referred to me as a calico girl. I must have looked offended because he added, "A calico girl is worth two velveteen girls any day."

On the first day of classes, the girls gathered around the breakfast table and discussed the height of the champagne fountains at their debutante parties. I called the veterinarian from the dorm pay phone. "I don't belong here," I said. "Come get me." He was headed to the Northeast Kingdom to give shots to a herd of cattle. He couldn't come until after work. I went to class.

That afternoon, bespectacled, straw-hatted sophomore Sumner Webber came calling. He showed me around in his VW bug. His cousin from Rutland had suggested he look me up. After an afternoon flying in an open-air crop duster over Lake Champlain, I called the vet back—I had decided to stay.

Middlebury College was magical. Classes were exciting. We had live theater on campus, string quartets, and Robert Frost reading poetry in the Old Chapel. All for free. Mandatory physical education meant golf, skiing, and dance. In the winter, a bus left every hour from the quad to the Snow Bowl, and there was no charge for the lift. Freshmen women had to sign out of the dormitory after dinner with a mandatory return by nine o'clock. My only restriction during high school was that Nellie insisted that I turn off the porch light if I wouldn't be home by dawn. "Because of the neighbors," not that she gave a damn.

Sumner, called Sam by his friends, was a history major, a miler on the track team, and spoke in rhymed, iambic pentameter when he had too many beers. Sam skied, sailed, and took me to meet his family in Hallowell, Maine.

Classes were fun. I wasn't allowed to work at school, a restriction of the Gould Fellowship. My challenges were extracurricular, in the realm of the social graces. Sam delivered the dinner tutorial. Hands in one's lap except when lifting a utensil from the table to one's mouth. Watch out for service to the left, clearing to the right. A long dress at dinner. My roommate, Mary, taught the thank-you note lesson. Heavy stationery, preferably personal, extravagant gratitude, and postmarked no later than the day of departure.

Knowing what I know now, I shouldn't have been surprised that Professor Hitchcock, chair of the Department of Biology, did not accept women as premedical students. I was no exception. The Gould Foundation would pay for fraternity party dresses, hairstyling, and graduate school anywhere to pursue fields such as French literature, religion, and philosophy, but not medical school. I majored in chemistry and English, took botany so I could help Sam pass his science requirement, and otherwise avoided the premeds, Professor Hitchcock, and the Biology Department.

Weeknights, I signed out to the Starr Library, where Sam had a study carrel with a window, wingback chairs, and a working fireplace. Weekends, I dressed up for football games, wore the mum corsage delivered by Sam, and dirty-boogied at Theta Chi.

In the winter, we stocked up on Ripple wine and powdered donuts at the general store in Ripton, Robert Frost's hometown, and skied at Middlebury's Snow Bowl. I was invited to the elegant homes of my friends, taught to fox-trot, and sip Dubonnet cocktails at lunch.

Summers, while my college friends sailed on Penobscot Sound, I rode my bike five miles to waitress at the Howard Johnson Restaurant. Nellie was the short-order cook. Lavonne, a crusty French-Canadian waitress in her late forties, took me under her wing. She assigned me to the booths with dressed-up customers, included me on her house-cleaning team, and sent me back to school with a case of her husband's home brew.

Pa's house on Vernon Street had gone back to the bank. That summer I shared a bedroom in Nellie's three-room apartment in the back of Dr. Leydon's old house where years before I had tossed the kid's shoe down the sewer. That was the last time I stayed with Nellie.

In Sam's senior year, my junior year, he took me to Burlington for a surprise jewelry store visit to look at silver and china patterns. Mary insisted that I would have more social status and influence as Sam's wife in Hallowell than as a struggling medical student. I disagreed. I was going to be a doctor.

Premed students usually sat for their Medical College Admission Test (MCAT) in the late spring of junior year so that their results could be submitted with the medical school applications in the early fall. The unspoken reason was to ensure a second chance to take the exam if the spring scores were insufficiently stellar. It was not a wise decision for me to blow my MCAT fees for lift tickets for one last weekend with Sam at Aunt Johnny's chalet at Stowe and great powder snow.

Professor Hitchcock gathered his premed boys around for tutoring for the MCAT, coaching for the application process, and practicing the medical school admission interviews. Although I partied excessively with my ski bum friend back from Colorado, my roommate Mary delivered me to the exams in Burlington after a hearty breakfast of oatmeal, bacon, and eggs at a diner on the way. One of the candidates complained to the proctor that I was intentionally distracting him when I rested my head on the desk between MCAT sections.

I applied to the University of Vermont's College of Medicine (UVM), as well as to Harvard and Columbia. When I was invited for an interview at UVM in early September, I had no idea what to expect. I walked into a room with five other applicants. We sat in a row in front of a conference table with six members of the Admissions Committee, some in white lab coats and some in suits and ties. I was the only woman in the room.

My position in the lineup was number two. One of the faculty asked a question, and then we answered in turn. The number-two position provided me time to think about the question while number one gave his response. Number six had a lot of time to listen to the five replies before him and to think what he was going to say but struggled to offer anything that hadn't been said. When they pointed out my C in physics, I replied that it was a "Dr. Wissler C," and I was damn proud of it. Some of them chuckled.

When asked about how each of us decided to study medicine, the others described the long history of medicine in their families starting with grandfathers and great-grandfathers, their summers working in science labs, and the practices they would join. I talked about Uncle Tom, Pa Hostler, and Hop. Dr. Ryan's house calls, working for Dr. Smith when I was nine. As I waited between the questions, I realized how different I was—obviously the only woman, but also, talking about the patients, how I wanted to be like Dr. Smith and Dr. Ryan. And to make house calls, to accept barter, to deliver babies in the middle of the night, to care about the patient and her/his family.

A week later, I was accepted. It was exceptional. It was unheard of. That year, I was the first person in the class of 1961 at Middlebury College to be admitted, and I was not even premed. It is still not clear to me why that happened, but I think my MCAT scores must have been high. Maybe the clinicians who interviewed me resonated with my dedication to patients, all patients, rich or poor. Maybe the personal letters from Dr. Smith and Dr. Ryan, both graduates of the UVM College of Medicine, made a difference. I don't believe that the UVM College of Medicine had any interest in recruiting women.

The structure of my senior year fell apart. Sam had graduated. I had been accepted early. My friends were getting married, going off to the Peace Corps, or—for my roommate Mary, sailing around the world with her family. I nearly self-destructed with partying, hitting the slopes every day, and being AWOL from the chemistry labs. After winter break, UVM sent a terse communication reminding me that my medical school acceptance was contingent upon graduation from Middlebury College.

I rallied, although the weeklong take-home exam from physical chemistry remains the cognitive challenge of my life. Mary's father picked up Nellie in Rutland and escorted her to our graduation from Middlebury College.

The Gould Foundation did not alter its policies about funding medical school. UVM College of Medicine offered me no scholarship assistance, and no loans were available because I was a woman. Mary's mother drove me to Woods Hole on Cape Cod for my summer job at the Landfall. I paid eight dollars for one of three beds in a shared room in a nearby boardinghouse. I bought a package of Ritz crackers, counted them, four stacks of thirty-two crackers each, and divided them up. The restaurant wouldn't feed the staff until the opening, nine meals and three days later.

I bartended at the Landfall that summer, while my medical school classmates concentrated on identifying the ideal cadaver mate. I learned too late that selection of the right cadaver mate was a critical determinant of first-year success. Instead, I selected Cove the wilderness guide for his good looks. We hauled Gray's 1,584-page *Textbook of Anatomy* for campfire review, but we fell behind in the cadaver dissection. Hopelessly behind. Cove was asked not to return for second semester—he failed anatomy, biochemistry, and physiology. I failed anatomy, but I had aced physiology, the cognitive Everest for first-year students.

I had a reprieve, but it was short-lived. Each morning, I found my cadaver not only unwrapped from the formaldehyde cloths but also sexually positioned with another student's cadaver. It was my responsibility to keep him wrapped and moist. My classmates were harassing me. In current times, we would label this as sexual harassment, but that was more than fifty years ago. The instructor had no sympathy. In fact, he assigned me to do the class dissection of the vessels to the penis, the only place besides the umbilical cord where there are two arteries per one vein. I showed up early every morning to rescue my cadaver. And I spent every evening in the library studying. I would, damn it all, not fail out of medical school.

In February, I ran out of money. I had enough to pay my fifty-dollar monthly rent for the cellar I shared with Paul, a curmudgeon of a chemistry PhD candidate. We each had a subterranean cubicle and shared the furnace room as our closet. I had already spent the tips from cocktail waitressing at the Lake Placid Club over the holidays. When my classmates took me out to Julie's for steak supper and dancing on the weekends, I emptied the breadbasket for breakfast.

The School of Medicine wouldn't give me a loan. The dean's secretary suggested I contact one of the local churches. I was getting skinnier by the day. I don't know how grumpy Paul and I negotiated an arrangement, but perhaps it was because I had taught him how to ski. I shopped and prepared supper every night for the two of us. Paul provided the cash for groceries out of his NSF fellowship.

The Fourth of July on Cape Cod was hopping as tourists, especially wealthy New Yorkers, celebrated summer by sucking lobster in melted butter and sipping a final cold beer at the Landfall before boarding the ferry to the Vineyard or Nantucket. When it stormed, the ferries were backed up, and the Landfall became standing-room-only, yielding exceptional one-hundred-dollar tip nights, which I needed for the next year. When, by the Fourth of July, I had received no word from UVM, I called the Dean's Office from the Landfall's pay phone. Hostler was listed on the second-year class roster.

Summer began in earnest. Skinny-dipping in the moonlight off Nauset. Sleeping all night on the beach. Late-night treks to Hyannis for Chinese food and Tiki cocktails. And late nights flirting with the red-bearded Viking who sometimes sipped cognac and read his paperback at the Landfall bar.

What did I really know about Alan Duane Dimock? That he was a handsome sailor scientist who hung out with the ebullient guys from Woods Hole Oceanographic Institute (WHOI), the regulars who requested my table at lunch even when it wasn't oceanfront. That he lived at Typhoon Tavern with the others when he was not out to sea on some oceanographic project. That he was eight years older, thirty-one to my twenty-three years, and had traveled a lot. That he was happiest on a boat. His eye colors didn't match. He called himself a warlock. He protested construction of the nuclear plants along the coast and came from a long line of peace-seeking Unitarians, but he had identified as a Druid. In the military. He was Welsh, not Scandinavian. All most intriguing. Seductive and thrilling, really, except for the detail that he had married at eighteen and was now separated.

There seemed no reason not to engage in a summer affair. After the competitive goody-two-shoes at medical school, Alan was brisk ocean air laced with humor, intelligence, and testosterone. You could assess the level of testosterone by his luxuriant, curly ear hairs. Labor Day would have me back at the academic grindstone: pathology, pharmacology, microbiology, immunology, and neuroscience.

Walking along the beach picking up turkey wings and quahog shells the morning after my first overnight at Typhoon Tavern, Alan told me about his childhood and his children, two girls and two boys. I didn't ask for ages or names. It seemed far too late for a midcourse correction. It was only a summer fling. Labor Day would be a hard stop. I was a medical student.

In September, I quickly settled back into the cellar routines with Paul and weekend dates. I was thrilled to be learning the pathophysiology of disease. It was one step closer to patient care, which was why I was in medical school. And I was invited into a study group. Best of all, the Nursing Office invited me to do "private-duty nursing" for post-op patients. Today, that role would be called a "sitter." I was paid forty-five dollars for each night shift, a fortune. I napped in the early evening, worked at the bedside from 11:00 p.m. to 7:00 a.m. I had a sponge bath in the public restrooms, picked up free coffee in the hospital cafeteria, and slipped into class by 8:00 a.m.

On the second Monday of September, red roses were delivered to me in the Pathology Lab. I placed them next to my microscope, continued the identifications, and ignored the quizzical expressions of the professor and my classmates. Deliveries appeared on the next Monday and the next. I ignored the raised eyebrows from the faculty and the questions from my classmates.

It was at the end of classes on the first Friday in October. I spotted my classmates milling around a sports car parked in front of the medical school. I was all the way down the stairs before I recognized Alan in the middle of the group, answering questions about the car, waiting for me. My class standing had risen with the red roses, but I attained star status when I opened the Ferrari's door and slipped onto the black leather passenger seat next to the red-bearded Viking.

On one level, I was delighted to see Alan, but, on all the other levels, his presence was a disaster. I had no time to squander. On my weekends, I needed every minute to study, do laundry, and to catch up on my sleep from doing two or three overnight nursing shifts during the week. I avoided thinking about his family status and focused on my survival. Second year for me had to be academically outstanding. Medical school was serious business.

I balanced study group, the demands of the overnight nursing shifts, and my enthusiasm for being at the bedside. It was helpful that Alan spent long periods at sea, six weeks and sometimes three months. My classmate George stayed the course, taking me dancing and skiing when Alan was not around. He knew he was going to be a pediatrician from the first day of school—his mother was a psychiatrist, and his father an obstetrician.

Gradually Alan became part of the cellar culture. Paul became a fan of Alan, noting how much less crazy I was than the first year. Alan climbed Camel's Hump on skis, snowshoed, and tobogganed with my study buddies for Washington's Birthday weekend. We celebrated the end of my second-year exams with Heineken beer, chips, and sour cream and onion dip. One weekend, Alan brought his son along. Timothy was around thirteen. We camped out in the woods. It rained, and he cried. Alan carried him down the mountain. I was not sympathetic to his whining.

The third year of medical school was a series of six-week rotations through surgery, internal medicine, obstetrics and gynecology, neurology, psychiatry, and pediatrics. As a student, I became a clinical clerk, the lowest rung on a vertical team headed by the faculty attending. In between, in ascending order, were the fourth-year elective students, the interns, the residents, the chief resident, the fellow, and the junior attending. Every patient was my personal mystery to solve. I loved presenting the patient, the history and physical exam, and my assessment and recommendation on morning rounds.

I thought about Uncle Tom, Pa, and Hop—how different it could have been. Back in Rutland, I talked with Dr. Ryan and Dr. Smith about articles in the *New England Journal of Medicine,* my patients, and the early discussions of national health insurance. They listened, laughed, and called me an idealist.

Sometimes the phone would ring in the middle of the night. Nellie would slur, "Slut!" and hang up. I cringed. Alan was separated but still married with four children. When Alan visited Burlington, we avoided talk about the future other than his trying to teach me how to make a rare rib roast and to drink tea from a china cup.

My last rotation of third year was pediatrics in the late spring of 1964. By then, I knew that I was not going to be a baby doctor. But I had not anticipated the unique learning experiences created by the UVM faculty. The chair, Dr. James McKay, was the editor of Nelson's *Textbook of Pediatrics,* the standard text used nationally and internationally. And Dr. Jerold Lucey, a neonatologist, edited the premium journal *Pediatrics,* known by all as the *green* journal. Dr. Lucey reminded me that we'd met before. We'd won the Twist contest at a local dive when I was a first-year student. And I had skied over the back of his skis one sunny afternoon at Stowe during second year when our class was being oriented to pediatrics.

It was the middle of the night. I was struggling to feed a bottle to a five-month-old huffing and puffing with pneumonia. It was a required assignment of my pediatric rotation to perform one week of 2:00 a.m. feeds. It made no sense to me. *Who didn't know how to feed a baby?*

That first night it took me an hour to cajole that five-month-old to take eight ounces. Sip by snort by sip. The second night was better. I settled the baby in my arms, leaned back, and rocked. A mother nearby whispered a lullaby. By the last night, I was looking forward to the intimacy of shadows and murmurs, the warmth of snuggled babies, and the nighttime network of mothers and nurses doing the 2:00 a.m. feed.

After my pediatric oral exam, Dr. Jerry Lucey invited George and me to attend a conference at Stowe. Dr. C. Henry Kempe from the University of Colorado presented the research behind his article describing the battered child syndrome—reporting his own case series, results of hospital surveys, and his court prosecutor interviews. After dinner, we twirled and hopped around the dance floor while the accordions and concertinas pumped out polka tunes. The next morning, Dr. Lucey and I walked around the grounds while Dr. Kempe met with George about internship possibilities in Denver.

"Sharon, where would you go if you could spend your fourth year in medical school away? Europe? Africa?"

"I can barely afford to live in Burlington, Dr. Lucey." I laughed. "No consideration of away rotations for me." I paused, "And I'm not so sure about pediatrics."

"I am sure about pediatrics. You're a natural. Now, listen to me. The department will sponsor an acting internship for you next year."

He waited for my surprise. "Dr. McKay and I have already asked the dean to substitute an acting internship in San Juan for your fourth-year classes."

I was stunned. Dr. Lucey added, "It's all set. What do you think?"

"Puerto Rico?"

I was twenty-four years old. The farthest I had been from Vermont was when I was sixteen and attended Girls Nation in Washington, DC. My only plane ride had been in the crop duster with Sam at Middlebury. But somehow, in September 1964, I arrived in San Juan with my suitcase, an early edition of the *Harriet Lane Handbook for Pediatrics,* and one hundred dollars in cash.

The chair of Pediatrics nodded a quick greeting, warned me about the dangers of traveling around the island alone, and forbade me to visit Old San Juan. Dr. Lucey had explained that the medical school was scheduled to be site-visited by an accrediting body requiring English, not Spanish, for the medical record. My chart notes in English would provide a teaching model. The chair's assistant assigned me a room in the nursing dorm, pointed out the hospital cafeteria where plantains were featured for every meal, and gave me directions to the hospital.

On the hospital wards, I was warmly welcomed by the Catholic nuns and the pediatric residents. My extra pair of hands were needed and appreciated, even if I didn't speak Spanish. They gave me a tour, oriented me to the hospital charts, and reviewed standard procedures like estimating the number of parasites passed in the first bowel movement after admission. Hundreds, it seemed.

The chief resident assigned me to start in the newborn nursery. My lack of Spanish would not be critical in that setting. He warned me against leaving the hospital grounds without an escort and reiterated the dangers of Old San Juan.

In the nursery, I was immediately recruited to three unexpected roles.

First, the Sisters insisted that every newborn be baptized in the delivery room, dead or alive. It was simple: *In the name of the Father, the Son, and the Holy Ghost, I baptize you.* Yes, I must baptize while I was doing the resuscitation. And no, it didn't matter that I was a long-lapsed Catholic. Sister made the sign of the cross over my head and swished off in her black habit.

Second, the grandmothers pressed tiny talismans into my palm and pointed out the intended baby. The *jigas* were gold, looped to either a tiny Black hand or foot. I was to attach the *jiga* to the newborn's wrist or ankle. The *jiga,* a practice of Santeria, served as an amulet to protect the infant against the evil eye. By some combination of Spanish and sign language, I understood I was also forbidden to cut the hair or the nails of the infants. The nuns paid no attention.

Lastly, I circumcised the boy babies. The father, uncles, and older brothers watched through the nursery window as I placed the bell on the baby penis and trimmed. Snip! Snip! My audience cheered, "*Brava, doctora! Brava!*" Sometimes I bowed to the gallery.

The nursery was Grand Central Station compared to my experience in Vermont. Bassinets held two babies, one up and one down. When too many babies streamed from the delivery room, we cantilevered bassinets to hold three and sometimes four babies. Babies stayed for twelve hours of observation and then were discharged. No teaching rounds in the nursery, just in and out.

The sick nursery was an intense experience in Puerto Rico. We took care of critically ill newborns with diarrhea and dehydration. Limited supplies and limited time meant that triage was quick, quiet, and nonnegotiable. We attended the alert, awake infant first—the child who had a chance of living if we could intervene with fluids. I understood why we couldn't start with the sickest, but I struggled with passing them by right from the start.

After my rotation in the nursery, I was assigned to the pediatric emergency room. It was a living hell. At all hours of the day, there were a hundred or more children and their families crowded into the waiting hall. It was a cacophony of sobbing, comforting, and praying. Families sat cross-legged on the floor, propped against the wall when the benches were full. The women fingered their rosaries and prayed. The patients, circled by family and neighbors, ranged in age from sick premature infants born at home to pregnant teenagers.

We had only six tiny exam rooms, two residents, and three nurses, but countless nuns and even the occasional priest. My assignment was to make the hourly triage—to identify the sickest patients to be seen first, to close the eyes of those who died waiting, and to guide families to the priest and then the morgue. No time for second-guessing. No time for consultation. No time for name-calling.

But I made some significant mistakes. I broke a platinum needle used to administer tuberculosis skin tests, snapped it right in two. We had hundreds of children lined up in the schoolyard waiting to have their arms pricked, but we had only one needle. Not just to use that day, but for the rest of the year. I started to understand about scarce resources. In the middle of the night on the ward, I commandeered a ventilator from the operating room for a twelve-year-old with breathing failure. In the morning, the anesthesiologist collected the machine for the scheduled surgeries, and I ended up manually breathing for my patient all day. Every few hours, one of the nuns relieved me long enough for a bathroom break. He lived, and I learned a valuable lesson about the role of rationing in medical care.

I was accustomed to presenting my patients in a combination of English and Spanish phrases, but one morning during rounds the chief resident became agitated with me as I discussed the patient I'd admitted from the emergency room the night before, a six-month-old infant with swollen, painful toes. I shared my working diagnosis of juvenile rheumatoid arthritis and my treatment with steroids. On rounds, the baby remained inconsolable, screaming in pain. The chief resident took me aside to point out that the baby was Négro, that the diagnosis was most likely sickle cell disease in crisis, and the appropriate treatment was morphine. He stood at my side as I changed the diagnosis in the chart and ordered a dose of IV morphine to be administered stat.

After rounds were finished, the chief and I went back to the infant, already in less agony. He took great pains to point out the differences between Négros (black-skinned people with ectomorph body build of African origin, a minority on the island) and Puertorriqueños (brown-skinned people with mesomorph body build of the Indigenous Taíno people, the island's majority)—differences not at all obvious to the White woman from Vermont. Sickle cell disease is a genetic hemoglobinopathy, a disorder in which the red blood cells sometimes contort into sickle shapes that block capillaries and cause severe pain. Juvenile rheumatoid arthritis is an immune disorder with episodes of swelling and pain in the joints. Treatment was very different: morphine and hydration for the child with sickle cell crisis and steroids for rheumatoid arthritis.

The nursing students showed me where to get flan near the hospital.

I'd learned my way around Old San Juan, how to nurse a cup of black bean soup for hours at La Mallorquina, and how to take the airport bus to pick up free copies of the Sunday *New York Times*. And the pediatric residents taught me the basic two-step of the merengue one night when the nuns were at prayer.

I was Doctora Americana from Hôpital des Niños by the time Alan arrived for Christmas. I showed him around Old San Juan with its El Morro and La Fortaleza, the elegant Condado barrio, and the rain forest at El Yunque. But Alan was distracted.

After Midnight Mass in Old San Juan in Spanish, not Latin, Alan delivered the news. He had left Cape Cod to take a position at Ocean Science and Engineering (OSE), a new company headed up by scientists from both WHOI and Scripps Institute. Alan had already moved to Washington, DC.

I'd planned to enter the national match for pediatric internships in February 1965, intending to list the Children's Hospital in Boston first and hoping that they would rank me. The match results would be announced in March, graduation from medical school with the recitation of the Hippocratic Oath would be in May, and internships started the first of July. Alan and I had never discussed the future beyond our next visit.

When Dr. Lucey visited the Hôpital de Niños in early February as part of their academic accreditation process, he took me out to dinner to celebrate. But I ended up crying. When I finally stopped sobbing, I told him I couldn't imagine life without Alan. Dr. Lucey leaned back in his chair and laughed out loud.

"Well, Sharon, is that all?" he said. "I'll take care of that. Now stop the crying. Everyone's looking at us."

I wiped my nose with my linen napkin and grinned. "Really, you'd do that?"

"Now, that's more like it. I'll give Bill Thurman a call when I get back home. Bill's a fine pediatric hematologist and the new chair at the University of Virginia. He'd be lucky to have you."

· 3 ·

Stranded in the South

July 1965–August 1965

It was July 1965. I had a secret.

I should have felt triumphant. I'd graduated from medical school. I'd matched with a university hospital within driving distance of Alan in Washington, DC. But Alan left to be an exchange oceanographer in Bergen, Norway, as soon as he moved me to Virginia. I felt abandoned. Yes, as my high school teacher predicted, I had escaped. But here I was, all alone. That was the secret I couldn't share. It was too risky to show any vulnerability.

I had no place to go. My friends were scattered. One was in Kuala Lumpur with the Peace Corps. Another was married with a kid in North Carolina. George was in Seattle starting his pediatric internship. I'd left New England to follow Alan.

I lived in a guest cottage at Beau Pré in Charlottesville, Virginia. The rent was $150 per month. My salary as an intern at the University of Virginia Hospital (UVAH) was $153.78 per month. I could eat in the cafeteria. The hospital provided uniforms. I had $50 left for emergencies from cocktailing on Cape Cod in June. No money to put gas in the red VW Alan left for me. No money to make a long-distance call. No one to accept a reverse-charge call.

On day #1 in the nursery, I was admonished by the head nurse about my shoes and the color of my stockings. In the emergency room, the surgical residents challenged my competency. The hospitalized patients were admitted to private rooms or wards by a formula that included: color (Negro or White), payment status (public or private), and medical service (pediatrics, medicine, or surgery). My landlady didn't believe me that I had night call when I declined her invitation to the Farmington Hunt Club to attend a horse-jumping competition.

I understood the messages, loud and clear. Skin color now made a difference for more than diagnostic reasons. This was not Vermont, and it was not Puerto Rico. New hospital expectations, new language, and new social rules. I did not belong here. Not at the hospital or the hunt club. Not as a single woman. Not as a Yankee woman. Certainly not as a working-class woman.

But I had no place else to go.

It was only 6:30 a.m., and my lipstick was already melting. It was day #12, and I was still struggling to find my way around the hospital. Alan was in Norway.

Predictably, the other interns in pediatrics were guys—two Southern gentlemen and an oddball who claimed he grew up in a bar. I'd met them for orientation the first day of July, but I hadn't seen them since. My only medical contacts were vertical. The resident, the chief resident, and the faculty ranked above me. The medical students below me.

As I wound my way to the nursery for morning rounds, I considered what was worse—being a Yankee, a girl doctor, or alone? That first month, I was assigned to the nursery during the day and the emergency room every other night, on call for very sick kids. A shift was thirty-four hours straight. I logged 127 hours my first week. And Alan was in Norway.

Dr. McLemore Birdsong was the faculty attending for the month of July in the nursery. "Dr. Mac," as he was called by everyone from the orderly on up, was a legend. The rumor was that Dr. Mac had grown up on a peanut farm in southwest Virginia, been a mandolin-playing, Stutz Bearcat–driving fraternity boy before going into medicine at UVA and training in Boston. Dr. Mac seemed to spend his day strolling around the hospital. He started the day early in the emergency room, then went ward to ward to check on new admissions, and by eight o'clock ended up in private clinic next to his office on Hospital Drive. He smiled and nodded to everyone, addressing them by name. In return, they smiled, nodded, and said, "Yes sir, Dr. Mac, it is indeed a great day."

My uniform was a starched white skirt and jacket over the scratchy, clerical collar of a Ben Casey shirt. It was soaked. The head nurse pointed out my flesh-colored hose and heels were not standard hospital gear. She suggested, instead, white hose and laced oxfords for safety purposes. I listened politely, smiled, and ignored her advice. Long ago, I'd made a firm decision against the pink ghetto of nursing, teaching, or secretarial work. I kept the heels.

First thing each morning, I examined the healthy new babies delivered during the night. I was responsible for the sick, small newborns, too. Each day, I graphed the morning weights on a chart.

When I finished examining all the babies, I visited the new mothers. Mothers who had Caesarean delivery or birthed twins stayed in the hospital for a full week. As did the "private ladies" who required a small respite, a toddy of sherry at teatime, and a baby nurse waiting at home. I didn't understand why sometimes—not always, but sometimes—the nurses on the obstetrics floor fussed at me. "No, not that corridor." "No, go back the other way!" "NO! You can't take that baby through here. Go back to the nursery." I turned red and retreated, not sure why I was being shamed.

Eventually, the nursery head nurse gave me explicit instructions for "walking with a Colored baby." She pointed out the somewhat circuitous path on the exterior corridors around the section for White mothers on the obstetrics ward. She explained, "Visit the White mothers first. Only if you have time should you bother with the Colored mothers. And never take a Colored baby on a corridor by the room of a White mother." It was the summer of 1965.

The chair of Pediatrics, Dr. Thurman, had explained to me that all US hospitals were required to desegregate by the Civil Rights Act of 1964. At UVAH, the nursery, labor, and delivery rooms appeared to be protesting silently, the last bastions of resistance. I didn't know that Virginia and Charlottesville had opted to close all public schools rather than desegregate as mandated by the *Brown v. Board of Education* decision of 1954. I didn't know that Vinegar Hill, the Black downtown of Charlottesville, had been razed in the past months and that families and businesses had been arbitrarily relocated in the name of urban renewal. And that the Black employees of the UVA Hospital had their own, separate cafeteria. So much I did not know.

Inpatient attending rounds were a ritual at teaching hospitals around the world. Dr. Mac preferred to make his rounds at 10:30 a.m. When he entered, we all stood up and remained at attention. Dr. Mac led the rounding procession, followed by the chief resident, the head nurse in her ruffled cap, the third-year medical student, and me.

Dr. Mac started rounds with the sick babies and finished with the puny ones, the ones failing to thrive. At each bassinet, the responsible nurse reported the day's weight—up or down, by how much—and commented on the feedings—robust suck, poor latch, or "inept mother." We looked for a pattern of good intake with weight gain before discharge, acknowledging that the weight gain of breastfeeding babies lagged behind that of the bottle-fed babies.

Rounding at UVA was like call-and-response in church, nothing like the crisis management of Puerto Rico. We'd crowd around each bassinet, and the head nurse would call out the name, "Baby Smith." The student or I presented the details in a formulaic response. "Baby Smith is a newborn White girl, now eight hours old, the 2,200-gram product of a full-term pregnancy, fifteen-hour labor and delivery complicated by breech presentation. Apgar in the delivery room was 6 at one minute (status in the womb) and 8 at five minutes (status in the world)." Newborn Apgar scores were like gymnastic scores at the Winter Olympics. Parents and even some obstetricians sought perfect scores. Newborn infants got scored on their appearance (color), pulse, grimace, activity, and respiration just like gymnasts were scored on form, originality, and technical skills.

Only interesting deviations from normal elicited comment from Dr. Mac; however, the chief resident might make a teaching point, "Those ears are low set. What's the head circumference?" I'd dutifully report the measurement, usually normal, and we'd move on to the next bassinet. When we were still rounding by noon, the head nurse made a grand gesture of looking at her watch, and Dr. Mac would hurry us along.

Finally, we'd finish at the back alcove where two or three Black women (neither nurses nor nursing aides, I was told) tended to the picky eaters. They cuddled these puny babies, repositioned them, and tried different nipples and different formulas—seeking the magic combination to get them to eat. They hummed and sang softly as they rocked. This was Dr. Mac's bailiwick, his favorite gig. We stood around him as he scooped up one baby after another, jouncing them, and making faces. By then, I was making a list in my head of what remained to be done. Eventually, he'd put them back in the bassinet, ask the ladies what they suggested, and nod in agreement. Rounds were then officially over until the next day.

In Virginia, the nursery staff preferred bottle-fed babies. They seemed to consider breastfeeding mothers to be hippies or, worse, feminists. In Puerto Rico, I'd learned to promote breastfeeding with a militant zeal. Mother's milk was associated not just with weight gain but with survival.

The newborn nursery at UVA was its own world—isolated from the rest of the hospital, orderly and quiet with abundant resources and attentive staff. Often I felt redundant, like I was just getting in the way. I attended the complicated deliveries, ready to resuscitate if the newborn was in distress. I rounded by myself morning and evening in the nursery, examined all the babies, entered handwritten notes in the chart, and visited with the mothers. I was competent. No one needed to contact the resident studying in the library or Dr. Mac outside of attending rounds.

By late afternoon, the Ben Casey collar scratched my neck, my pantyhose was bunched up at my ankles, and I was miserable from the heat and humidity. I dreaded every other night at five o'clock when I went for overnight call in the emergency room. By noon of those days, the tops of my feet itched in anxious anticipation.

The ER was a challenge for me as a pediatrician, a woman, and a Northerner. I was not welcome on all three counts, especially by the surgeons who dominated the ER hierarchy. They baited me. They called me Missy Doctor, Yankee Babe, and Baby Doctor. They touched me inappropriately and challenged my competence. They were disgruntled that the new chair of Pediatrics insisted his pediatric interns take care of the children who came to the ER. By early morning, even the lowly surgical intern was calling me the bitch baby doctor.

My first night on ER call was the Fourth of July. It was flat out with a steady stream of kids with impetigo, sore throats, and tummy aches arriving as rescue squads rolled in with knife wounds, heart attacks, or even a chain-saw injury. An ER nurse or orderly would put the patient in an exam room, record their vital signs, and hand the chart to me.

"Ten-year-old White girl in room #3." "Two-year-old *Colored* boy in room #12."

July was divided between the cozy cocoon of the nursery, the tensions in the ER, and the brief moments awake every other night at Beau Pré. No debates about sending troops to Vietnam. No concern about Medicare and Medicaid programs. No chitchat about the weather. I never saw the other interns, my senior resident, or Dr. Thurman, the chair. No newspapers. No mail. No phone calls. The highlights of my off nights were spooning vanilla ice cream straight from the container, a hot shower, and six hours of sleep, at best.

It was late afternoon midmonth when the ER nurse paged me before my shift began. "Come quickly. It's a four-year-old." I hung up and ran down the stairs.

Molly's father described how she'd been bitten by a snake in the woodpile. The mother tried to console the howling child as the nurse struggled to get a blood pressure. I was examining Molly's swollen, purple, and very tender ankle when the banging on the exam room door started.

"Hey, lady. We've got the snake," shouted the rescue squad guys. "You coming or not?"

"I'm busy," I said. The nurse shook her head at me, but I didn't read her warning. "I'm not interested in the snake. I'm taking care of the patient." I was terrified of snakes. Even earthworms. Why were they bothering me?

The nurse nudged me, "Go on, hurry up. I'll stay with Molly." The parents just stared.

The EMTs grinned. "You got to examine the snake, lady. It's part of the deal."

"They're right, Yankee Miss," the surgery chief resident said. "You've got to identify the snake and measure the distance between the fangs to determine the antitoxin dose."

I went out to the parking lot to the rear of the ambulance. The guys moved aside to provide me a full view of the snake. It was huge, lying in an ugly heap. Was it really dead? It looked ten feet long. Did I have to do this?

They closed a circle around the snake and me. I assumed what I considered a professional stance in my sweaty uniform, regarded the specimen, and took a deep breath. It seemed like an out-of-body experience. I paced back and forth, always maintaining a good distance from the specimen.

"Reddish in color, about three to four feet long," I reported out. "I don't notice a rattle."

An EMT stepped up to point out the "distinctive hourglass" pattern on the body of the snake and the "copper-colored" head. I noted the head's triangular shape. Another guy directed me to open the snake's eye to check the pupil. I struggled to remember why I would be examining the pupil of the snake's eye without surgical gloves.

I bent over the snake. I smelled its death and felt sick to my stomach. But, somehow, like I was some other, competent person, I continued to report out my observations—slowly and precisely. "The pupil is vertical, not round. This must be the heat-sensing pit."

One of the surgical residents demonstrated how to measure the distance between the fangs. "2.5 cm," I said.

From the parking lot tutorial, I learned Virginia has three poisonous snakes, all pit vipers—the copperhead, the timber rattler, and the cottonmouth. A copperhead bit Molly. I calculated the dose from the estimated volume of venom and Molly's weight, the nurse measured it into a syringe, and I injected the antitoxin into Molly's bottom. Her ankle continued to swell, becoming shades of purple and red, but her blood pressure eventually stabilized, and her EKG remained normal. Molly was admitted to the ward. The EMTs took the snake away.

As I wrote the chart note, the surgery chief resident leaned on the back of my chair and whispered, "We're the ones who know how to take care of snakebites. Why don't you get the hell out of here?" I shrugged and finished my note.

By two o'clock, the ER had slowed down. There had been no supper. No time to change my uniform. No time to shed my pantyhose. Since Molly, I'd seen three earaches, one bloody diarrhea, one broken arm, an acute appendicitis, and one status epilepticus. Last week, Dr. Mac had asked me if, *up North,* I'd been taught how to treat seizures.

It was time to check up on Molly on the ward. The monitors were steady, and Molly was curled up, fast asleep. I patted her bottom and peeked at her ankle. It was still magenta and still swollen, but there'd been no progression. Congratulations, antitoxin.

It was three o'clock when I walked out of the hospital into the steamy night air, stopped, and stretched. Ambulances were scattered over the parking lot, lights off, drivers dozing. I walked past the house-staff quarters where the other interns and residents had crashed—the males on call, that is. I slowly meandered by the hospital entrance and up through the arcade to McKim Hall, the locked dorm for undergraduate nursing students overseen by resident dorm mothers. Girl doctors were not permitted to sleep under the same roof as the boy doctors. Girl doctors slept with the nursing students.

I rang the doorbell to wake up the dorm mother to unlock the door for me. She shook her head and tsked-tsked at me, as though I were coming in from a late date instead of an ER call. I was due back in the nursery at seven for morning rounds. I thought about Alan in Norway as I fell asleep. I wanted to tell him about Molly and the snake.

The next day was Saturday. I had the afternoon and evening off. After ER changeover rounds and one more visit to Molly, I decided to poke around town—a grocery store suggested by my landlady called Foods of All Nations and a new shopping center. Meals in the hospital cafeteria were free. At Beau Pré, my supper was ice cream, but I was out of milk and cereal for breakfast. I had little money for food and certainly none for clothes. I should have known better than to go exploring.

The heat and humidity outdoors were relentless. I ventured into the air-conditioning of a froufrou dress shop and started fingering the fabrics, seduced by luxurious silks and crisp linens after my scratchy white uniform. Why couldn't I substitute a pale-blue, dotted Swiss shell for the hospital-issue Ben Casey? Really, it was baby's bottom soft. Dr. Mac hadn't commented on my heels and flesh-colored hose.

"Yes," I said when the owner invited me to open a store charge.

By then, the store owner, Robert Levy, knew that I didn't have the $16.95 to purchase the blouse, and I knew he had just moved his store from downtown to the new Barracks Road Shopping Center. When he discovered I was an intern at UVA, he shared that he was alone in the shop because his wife had uterine cancer. I was the only customer.

"Not a problem," he assured me. "You'll be a loyal customer and friend. Take the dusty rose one, you need two."

I hesitated. The pink seemed girlish. I was no longer concerned about charging *two* blouses. I'd dismissed the professional noncompliance of wearing a frilly shell as part of my hospital uniform. Why was I worried that pink might be too much? Was I already internalizing the implicit and explicit messages about being a girl doctor? I didn't have the vocabulary then to express such a thought.

"Thank you. I'll take both—the pale blue and the dusty rose." I was too pleased with my rebellion to consider the financial consequences. Mr. Levy offered the account voluntarily. I didn't solicit it. He didn't know how Hop bet on the horses or how Nellie wasn't allowed to charge milk or cigarettes at the corner store. He didn't know about my working nights as a private-duty nurse to pay my rent in medical school.

Once again I had passed, just like that morning at Foods of All Nations when the clerk assumed that I would charge the Cheerios, milk, and blueberries. I'd smiled and nodded yes. All they knew about me was the UVA nametag—Dr. Sharon L. Hostler, Pediatric Intern. Not even a billing address. I couldn't know then how very important Levy's Dress Shop and Foods of All Nations would become.

I traded the scratchy Ben Caseys for the soft, dotted Swiss shells. I smiled when Dr. Mac asked me on nursery rounds if I had run into Thomas Jefferson on the Lawn. I went bare-legged in the emergency room. I ignored the sexual innuendoes from the surgery residents except when it involved touching. I developed a sixth sense in the back corridor or when I was alone in the lab to avoid the slow graze of a hand across my rear. My first month of internship was almost over. I hadn't seen the other pediatric interns, my resident, or Dr. Thurman.

At the end of July, I turned over the pediatric service on a Sunday morning and walked out of the ER. I was exhausted. I had been up all night trying to care for a twelve-year-old Black girl who had been violated by her mother's boyfriend. She hadn't even had her first period and she had syphilis. We treated her with penicillin, but no one would help. Not the social worker. Not the nurse. I sent her home with her grandmother without follow-up. No referral for protective services in the community as Dr. Kempe had instructed. I didn't have the awareness to clarify if the hospital had protective services for White patients. The answer would have been "no." It was a miserable last night on call.

"Morning, Sharon. Congratulations," Dr. Thurman said. He was waiting in the parking lot. "The Dermatology chair called me early this morning about the young intern from Vermont who diagnosed primary syphilis."

I was beyond his kind words. "I don't understand," I said and backed away. "How could you and your damn hospital NOT have a way to protect a twelve-year-old girl from more sexual abuse? What the hell does it take?"

Dr. Thurman was quiet as we walked away from the emergency room entrance. When I started weeping, he passed me a neatly folded, white cotton handkerchief. We stood there in the parking lot until I stopped crying, then I drove Alan's red VW back to Beau Pré and put myself to bed.

It was July 31.

· 4 ·

Not My Kind of Medicine

August 1965

Each month of internship, I rotated to another clinical service as part of yet another team. Each month, I started all over—new geography, new nurses, and new protocols for getting the work done. Any moment I might have felt medically competent quickly faded. I had been naïve to think it would be any different. The medical degree was not an end point but, instead, the beginning of years of training, of proving oneself competent to move on. I'd long ago learned not to trust any suggestion of social competence.

I was assigned to the Children's Rehabilitation Center in August. The Center was about a mile from the University Hospital, west of town. It was located on acres of green lawn with gray stone walls and a funeral home next door. There was no indication that children lived there—no outside play equipment, no paintings in the windows.

Photographs of children with physical disabilities sitting in wheelbarrows on the grounds were posted in the Center lobby. Most rehabilitation centers in the United States emerged in response to epidemics of paralytic poliomyelitis to provide respiratory care to the sickest patients, the ones who required artificial ventilation. The so-called *iron lung wards.* The Center was different. Children with orthopedic disabilities were admitted there, ones who required long hospitalizations. The Center had historically been the sole domain of the nursing staff.

That changed abruptly in the summer of 1965. Dr. Thurman unilaterally introduced pediatric intern and resident rotations at the Center, predicting that the future of pediatric practice and medical education would focus on children with chronic illness and disabilities.

Head Nurse Tate met us the first day at the entrance to the inpatient ward. She had no smile. No greeting. No introductions. "Do not interfere with the children in their therapies, school, or the cafeteria," she said. "Adherence to the schedule is critical." I tried to pay attention, but the stink of disinfectant was distracting.

She waved toward a windowless cubby behind the nurse's station. "Sit in there."

The customary medical hierarchy was reversed at the Center. When the nurses ignored Dr. Thurman's arrival for attending rounds, he seemed unabashed. He outlined our month's work—to update the medical charts with an interim history, to perform thorough physical examinations, and to document a summary of medications and immunizations on each of the forty children.

Ms. Tate glared at Dr. Thurman, cleared her throat, and added, "Without disturbing our equilibrium."

"We'll round each day at four," he said to us and then smiled at Ms. Tate. "By the end of the month, I expect all forty children to have complete and accurate charts—consistent with the standards at the main hospital."

Dr. Thurman must have stood six feet four. His broad shoulders were stuffed into the long white lab coat. The sleeves, inches too short, ended way above his hairy wrists and huge hands. I'd heard that he'd played professional ice hockey in Montreal when he'd been a student at McGill. I was grateful he didn't mention my crying outside the ER, but I still held him personally accountable for the Commonwealth of Virginia not having child protection statutes. I was relieved that Dr. Thurman didn't bring up Alan. He'd met Alan that spring when we'd visited for an interview.

Even if we had had Nurse Tate's support, accessing the patients was difficult. The day shift at the Center started in chaos. The children woke up in cold, soggy diapers, cramping and hungry. They needed assistance with all aspects of their daily life—sitting up, eating, drinking, sometimes even breathing.

Many had spastic diplegia, a common form of cerebral palsy associated with premature birth. The goal of rehabilitation was to keep their legs in a functional alignment so they would eventually be able to sit and stand upright. In 1965, the staff accomplished that goal by positioning with pillows and bolsters, manual stretching, bracing, and surgical tendon-lengthening followed by more bracing and therapy. Very few of the children at the Center would ever walk independently.

Nurse Tate protested when we wrote orders for children to be weighed and measured, undressed and without their braces, but we persisted. We didn't understand at the beginning how helpless the children were without their postural devices—unable to sit up or move around in bed. And we had no idea what an ordeal it would be for both the children and the nurses to get those measurements.

I learned my patients' names, how long they had been at the Center, and whether their family visited. I identified inaccuracies of medication dosing, missing immunizations, and the overwhelming need for dental hygiene. There were loud protests from Nurse Tate when we wrote orders for toothbrushes and toothpaste, toothbrushing after meals. And then, hearing and vision referrals. That meant the nursing staff having to transport patients and their devices by bus to the main hospital.

Visitation was on Saturday afternoon. For two hours only, family and friends were allowed to visit the children—one visitor at a time. The nurses insisted on no holding, no picking up, no removing the children from their beds. Nurse Tate suggested that we not be present during the hours of visitation, but we had too much to accomplish not to.

There were murmurs of excitement as the parents congregated in the lobby, waiting for permission to come onto the inpatient ward to visit. I heard one little girl talking to herself, "Mommy's coming. Mommy's coming. Now, no crying and carrying on."

I don't think I recognized the impact of those Saturday visitations at the time, but I believe those early experiences informed my later focus on family-centered care for hospitalized children. Imagine children living for months in a hospital, enduring painful procedures, and not seeing family for weeks at a time. Not being held and rocked or read to.

I was taken aback on rounds when Dr. Thurman, the pediatric hematologist, discussed childhood development—about children taking turns, language development, socialization. I wasn't sure then that "play" was a legitimate realm of pediatrics. I shifted my feet, checked my watch, and wondered when he'd get to the medical stuff.

Finally, I was out of the Center without ER duty until Monday morning. No more talk of poop, too much or too little. I sang along with the radio as I drove home, winding along the back way by Farmington Country Club to Garth Road. "*It ain't me, babe. No. No. No. It ain't me you're looking for.*"

I was eager to shed my wrinkled uniform, finger-painted in drool. I turned into the dirt driveway at Beau Pré and checked the mailbox. No mail. Nothing.

I was stranded in Virginia, and people were asking questions. Dr. Mac was increasingly interested in what this Yankee young lady was doing "all by her lonesome in Mr. Jefferson's country."

I drove by the carriage house where the law professor lived, Roy something or other. He studied campaign law, whatever that was. I parked the VW behind the hedges and walked around front, following the flagstone walk to the main house and onto the grass. The bushes towered above me. I was afraid of those looming boxwoods after dark, but I had to pass them to reach the guest house attached by an arcade to the main house. I couldn't wait to get undressed and take a hot shower.

But as I rounded the boxwoods, I realized that my landlady, Berta Wood, was entertaining a gentleman. They lounged in wicker chairs with yellow-checkered napkins in their laps. The table was set with a pitcher of lemonade, frosted glasses, and a platter of cookies.

They were blocking my path. I had no choice but to greet them. I felt like a tired old servant in messy clothes interrupting her mistress at tea.

Berta was Swiss, a few years older than I but fifty years younger than her husband, R. Warner Wood. In her white peasant blouse, she was my childhood image of Heidi. Her speech was accented by the Swiss Deutsch of her childhood in Bern. When I'd moved in, Berta explained that Warner had discovered her teaching in kindergarten, wooed her, and brought her back to Virginia as his wife.

Her guest stood up as I approached, smiled, and put his bleached straw boater on the table. He was attractive, somewhere in his thirties. He wore a blue-and-white seersucker suit, a polo shirt open at the collar, and cream *cabretta* leather moccasins. I tried to pass by with a wave.

"Sharon, meet my friend, Bob Brown," Berta said. "He's a medical student." She giggled, "We're taking a child development class together."

When he pulled a chair out for me, I sat down and folded my hands over the drool stains. Mr. Brown explained he was a practicing psychologist who was then a third-year medical student. He planned on a psychiatry residency and was taking an elective in child development.

"Oh, Sharon," Berta said, "You'll be interested—we reviewed Piaget's experiments with young boys playing marbles. You know, the different rules for different cantons."

"I'm sure that Dr. Hostler is well-versed in Piaget," Mr. Brown interrupted. "Play is the work of childhood."

Who the hell was Piaget, and what did shooting marbles have to do with anything? Finally, I made the connection. Dr. Thurman had referenced Piaget with his talk on rounds about children taking turns in the sandbox.

It was September, and I still hadn't spent time with the other interns. I hadn't heard from Alan. But I had wasted a month learning about strange topics I didn't think represented pediatrics.

After a series of rebuffs, I'd accepted a social invitation to a Labor Day party. Roy from the carriage house and I were going out to cocktails and dinner at the home of one of his law school colleagues.

Roy looked me up and down, paused, and took my elbow. "Are you some kind of hippie?"

For sure, I thought, Roy was not. He managed to be scruffy around the edges but still quite buttoned up. He'd paired a burgundy shirt with a narrow, knitted tie. Chinos and a baggy, navy jacket. It did not meet blazer standards.

"I'm no flower child," I said with a broad smile, "but I am delighted to be headed somewhere besides the hospital."

Roy probably thought I lived in my wrinkled, never-quite-white doctor's uniform. I know Berta did.

That night, I was relieved to slip into my Marimekko green shift with huge black polka dots, pull on black fishnet hose, and don high heels. I pulled my dirty blonde hair up into a French twist, high and tight. Mascara, eyeliner, and eye shadow, not just lipstick. I held back on the red slip. Alan liked the lace edge peeking out from under the Marimekko, but where was he?

The house, a two-story brick with columns on the front, looked like the other houses on Rugby Road. Roy called it Greek Revival style. I wouldn't have known. We found the party in the backyard.

Women in linen dresses had fanned out around the potted red geraniums. Men gathered under the canopy of a massive magnolia tree. Everyone looked to be in their forties and fifties. Grown-ups, I thought to myself. At a bar midway between, a silver-haired Black bartender in a jacket and bow tie smiled broadly as he fixed my gin and tonic with extra lime and a Johnny Walker Red for Roy. I would have been a hell of lot more comfortable behind the bar.

I paid my respects to the well-coiffed hostess in pearls and followed Roy as he joined the men, dressed uniformly in navy-blue blazers except for one guy in pink madras. I listened to the introductions and the obligatory pedigree recitations—Princeton-Harvard, Harvard-Columbia, Yale-Harvard-Oxford. Their conversations, which ranged from the war in Vietnam to the unrest at the Farmington Country Club, were far better than exchanging recipes or fashion tips with the wives.

Roy told me that our host was highly respected, a chaired professor, whatever that meant. He seemed to be in his fifties, well-tanned and trim. As he listened to the others, he puffed on a fancy briarwood pipe which bore no resemblance to the corncob pipe I used to light for Pa.

The host comfortably assumed his role as moderator for the evening. The men vigorously expressed arguments around the burning of draft cards, the carryings-on in Haight-Ashbury, and UVA President Shannon's continued membership at the segregated Farmington Country Club. They disapproved of the troops and the protesters, for different reasons. Some wondered what should be done about the club. What they weren't talking about were riots in Watts or Bloody Sunday or the march on Selma. Or the past year's bulldozing of Vinegar Hill, the Black downtown of Charlottesville, in the express interest of urban renewal. I'd learned about Vinegar Hill from one of the ER aides, but I didn't realize the impact of that massive relocation until decades later.

Roy managed to interject one reference to his time clerking for Chief Justice William Brennan, but I guessed that clerking at the Supreme Court was a prerequisite for faculty appointment at the Law School. No one mentioned *Griswold v. Connecticut,* the decision finding oral contraception legal for married women, but that was understandable given the demographics of the group. I assessed these wives as solidly menopausal.

From Beau Pré conversations, I'd understood that Farmington was elegant and exclusive. No one had mentioned that Blacks and Jews and other ethnic minorities were not only not invited members but not allowed. I'd ask Roy about that later. Berta had mentioned more than once that Roy was Jewish.

The tall, thin guy in the washed-out madras plaid skillfully highjacked the conversation to a recent provost decision around faculty promotion and tenure. Roy whispered that the speaker was an endocrinologist from the School of Medicine. I was more interested in looking at the scarlet hollyhocks along the garage, which led me to daydreaming about my hundred-year-old great-grandmother and her hollyhocks, her dandelion wine, and the blackberry brandy in her bathtub. Dr. Thurman's name tuned me back into the conversation.

"The School of Medicine will never advance the research mission of the University by accepting federal money for community projects. Young faculty must excel at the bench doing basic science research if they are to advance academically. The last thing UVA needs are do-gooders like this Thurman, reaching beyond the walls, setting up neighborhood clinics."

Our host concluded, "Scholarship at the medical school has always been dicey, more like a vocational school."

I missed the end of the conversation. One of the wives whispered something about rescuing me and guided me to the wives' huddle. I thought better of protesting that I preferred being with the men. She was dolled up in a daffodil-yellow shirtwaist cinched tight at the waist. As we joined the others, I noted the group preference for poufy hair and perky headbands.

It wasn't long before the interrogation began. "How long have you known Roy?" "What do you do at the Medical School?" "What brings a Yankee to Charlottesville?" "Pediatrics? You must know McLemore and Charlotte Birdsong."

The women had assumed I was a nursing student when I told them I was training in pediatrics, but I corrected them, probably with more prickle and pride than required. Unseemly, I thought later, was the proper Southern expression to describe my behavior.

"Do I understand this correctly? You are studying pediatrics until you find a nice Southern doctor to marry? Isn't that right?"

"No," I said and clenched my fists at my side.

"But don't you see? You're taking the spot of a man," another wife interjected. "By adding another academic feather to your cap, you prevent one of our Southern gentlemen from earning his livelihood."

"I plan to do both," I said. "To practice medicine and to marry."

"Is the School of Medicine, I mean, is Dean Hunter aware?" The hostess paused for a beat, then said, "Does Dr. Mac know about this?"

The reference to Dr. Mac was troublesome. I was grateful when someone broke the tension. It was the only woman wearing pants. Capris, right out of *Roman Holiday.*

I was quiet the remainder of the evening. As we said our goodbyes, the hostess whispered to Roy, "What an interesting young woman your guest is."

And maintaining her saccharine smile, she said to me, "My dear, you know I haven't seen polka dots that size since the circus—or was it in kindergarten?"

Back at Beau Pré, Roy was ebullient, aglow from the evening's bonding with his new law colleagues. He escorted me to my cottage door, gave me a quick squeeze, and barely brushed his moist lips by my ear. Roy was neither flower child nor Romeo. I missed Alan.

"Thank you, Roy, for a most interesting evening," I said and shut the door.

Roy had no clue how interesting. It was naïve of me to think I was finished with judgments just because I'd marched to "Pomp and Circumstance" in academic regalia and recited the Hippocratic Oath. Did I have to worry about Dr. Mac? Was training in pediatrics the right choice of specialty? When would Alan return from Bergen?

The Marimekko put-down stung. It was my prize possession, my fabulous Finnish-block-print dress. The comments from my hostess took me back to Middlebury College President Stratton calling me a calico girl.

It's what I'd always be. Getting a medical degree didn't change that.

· 5 ·

Committing to It All

September 1965

Finally, I was assigned to the inpatient wards in September. I felt like I had been marking time in the nursery and out at the Center. The inpatient ward was the nexus of pediatrics with the sickest children and the wisest attendings. No more isolation on the margins for me. Though by then, I understood that I was not welcome in the Doctors' Lounge or the Nurses' Lounge.

I would interact with the senior residents, the pediatric faculty, and the referring physicians from downtown. I would work with all the specialties and subspecialties that made this place a university hospital: tertiary care, medical education, and research.

Children admitted to the hospital were assigned to the pediatric floor, but not all were admitted by pediatrician faculty. If orthopedics or neurosurgery admitted an infant, the pediatric team followed along to double-check drug dosages. I was assigned to pick up fifteen patients.

I was relieved the other intern was Dr. Peter Houck, a bow-tied Virginia gentleman with round glasses. His demeanor was gentle, almost courtly. I soon learned he was a double Hoo, meaning he was both a UVA undergraduate and medical student. I was writing on-service notes when Dr. Houck placed his hand on my arm. "Come to the morgue for Belinda's post," he said.

The morgue was on the hospital ground floor at the end of a long corridor that extended behind the emergency room and around several corners into what felt like a dungeon. The odors got stronger at the doors of the morgue. We were waved in by Turkey Bibb, a thin Black man of around fifty wearing a filthy rubber apron over his uniform and smoking a cigarette.

"You here for her?" he asked, gesturing to the body on the stone table. He was the morgue's diener, a word derived from the German *Leichendiener,* meaning the servant of the dead. The morgue was Turkey Bibb's domain—the only place in the hospital with a Black person clearly the authority, absolutely in charge.

I was overwhelmed by the smell of blood and disinfectant, the drainage noises, and the disarray of buckets and body parts on the counters. A heart rested on a scale, spongy lungs were plopped by the sink, and a nutmeg liver was in various stages of being sliced. Paraffin blocks and slides were being prepared for microscopic diagnosis. A peg board with dissection tools and a saw was mounted above a counter.

Turkey Bibb seemed to enjoy my distress as he flipped the sheet off Belinda's face. Dr. Houck started the presentation, "Belinda was an eight-year-old with cystic fibrosis diagnosed at six months of age when she presented with oily diarrhea and failure-to-thrive. She was initially treated with enzyme replacement and stabilized. But by four, she had repeated lung infections treated with antibiotics, physical therapy, and oxygen. Belinda struggled to breathe. She died last night after a prolonged hospitalization with acute respiratory failure."

"Cause of death?" Turkey Bibb asked.

"Terminal exhaustion." Dr. Houck sighed. "Belinda's heart and lungs finally gave out. She was simply too tired to take another breath."

I inspected her emaciated body, more the size of a five-year-old than an eight-year-old. Naked. No body fat, just skin and bones, a huge rib cage, and scaphoid belly. Her arms and legs were bony, the ends of her fingers and toes clubbed from chronic lack of oxygen like the old men I'd seen with COPD at the Veterans Administration Hospital. The nurses had closed her eyes and crossed her arms, but her mouth remained agape from the terrible air hunger she'd experienced at the end. Her light-brown hair was braided. I noticed that one was still tied with a red grosgrain ribbon.

"Ready?" Turkey Bibb asked.

Dr. Houck nodded. Bibb lifted his scalpel high above Belinda's sternum and quickly made a sweeping Y incision just as the pathologist arrived. He would complete the autopsy. Real medicine. The autopsy was the last examination of how and why someone died, a last opportunity to understand the pathophysiology of disease and to judge whether our treatment had helped or harmed our patient. It was the clinician's moment of truth.

The memory of Belinda lying in the morgue kept me grounded back on the ward. Dr. Houck and I remained respectful and gentle with each other from that first day. It was a relief to have no time to think about anything but the patients right in front of me. Every third night call should have seemed an improvement over every other night, but most nights I wasn't at Beau Pré until after eight o'clock and was back at the hospital by seven the next day. With only 168 hours in a week, there was no such thing as catching up on sleep.

My personal best on the ward was when I diagnosed a sickle cell crisis in Lamarr, a ten-month-old Black baby admitted from the ER. He was screaming bloody murder with swollen feet. I did not repeat the mistake I had made in Puerto Rico. I recognized sickle cell dactylitis this time around.

In Puerto Rico, my patient was still writhing in pain the next morning. But, after an IV drip with morphine overnight, Baby Lamarr was pulling on my stethoscope and playful.

At some point that month, Dr. Muller, the chair of Surgery, found me on the ward. I was puzzled about what he wanted, but Dr. Muller just wanted to fuss about my "nonstandard" attire. I smiled and nodded my head. I didn't seriously consider wearing white hose and nurse's oxfords.

By the time Dr. Thurman called me to his office, I didn't know whether to worry about fallout from the Labor Day garden party or to expect a dress code lecture. It was the end of my first month on the ward.

I sat quietly in the captain's chair while he folded his six-foot-four frame into an oversized leather chair behind his desk. I focused on not fidgeting. He complimented me on my care of baby Lamarr, and then, right out of the clear blue sky, he invited me to stay on as a resident in Pediatrics. I felt panic like a train speeding full throttle headed for a pitch-black tunnel in a solid-rock mountain.

He was asking for a commitment for another almost three years. He leaned forward with his elbows on the desk, scrunched up his bushy eyebrows, and grinned. "Sharon, you're a good doctor, and I hope that you'll stay," he said. "I will need your decision by the end of the month."

I gathered my wits, stood up, and shook his hand. "Thank you, sir," I said. "You've caught me by surprise. I've been totally focused on the ward, and I am on call tonight."

As I left, Dr. Thurman added, "By the way, don't let the fire-breathing chair of Surgery intimidate you. You're on my service, not his."

Later that night, I was paged. "An *overseas* call," whispered the hospital operator. Alan was at Heathrow and would arrive the following evening. Could I pick him up at 6:30 p.m.?

I had spent nearly three full months alone in Virginia. We had tolerated many separations during our three years together. Alan was at sea for six weeks or more at a time, off Bermuda recording whale songs. My time in Puerto Rico. This separation felt different. We were in different geographies and in different roles. This separation was open-ended and dangling.

I was in the Charlottesville terminal looking out at the tarmac when Piedmont Airline's fifty-seater landed. Alan was the second person down the steps, juggling a large cardboard box and his suitcase, grinning. Six feet tall, broad shoulders, open jacket and no tie. Alan's skin was deeply tanned, ruddy, his long hair flew in all directions, and his rusty red facial hair, scraggly as hell, needed a trim. From the persistent glare of the sun off the ocean, pterygia crept across the whites of Alan's eyes like a fine ink drawing. You couldn't tell from here that he was a warlock with different-colored eyes, but I knew. Alan readily stood out from the crowd of businessmen and academics. The hug that shepherded me out of the terminal and into the little red VW bug felt reassuringly the same.

"Lock the door," I instructed Alan at the cottage. He raised his eyebrows. We never locked our doors in New England.

"Berta," I said, "is never far away."

The evening was dark and quiet as we sprawled across the bed. I lay spent as Alan painstakingly drew arabesques from my hip bones to my belly button. Sheepishly he asked, "Is supper, perhaps, on the agenda? Or, at least, a beer?"

We sat at the table until midnight, stories stumbling over stories.

It was still pitch-black out when I smelled the coffee and heard the pings and clicks. Alan was playing his recording of humpback whales.

We scarfed down a quick breakfast. Alan skunked me at cribbage, but NOT a double skunk.

As we drove along Garth Road, Alan told me he had a flight early Sunday evening. That on Monday, he was headed to California. Long Beach. I didn't ask why, and I didn't mention Dr. Thurman's invitation. When Alan dropped me off at the hospital for overnight ward duty, I focused on smiling and waving to the audience of orderlies lounging by the emergency room. *California?*

On Sunday morning, when he picked me up, Alan was revved. "I have a surprise. I've been up all night too. You won't believe it."

In the middle of the nearly empty cottage, perched on a drop cloth and surrounded by wood shavings and odd tools, stood a six-foot-high, partially stripped wooden secretary. "I thought it might be pine, but I knew better as soon as I tried to carry it out of the shop. Way too heavy for pine. *Black walnut!* Look at that glorious grain! I scraped away all night. I need an hour or two more. You can read the Sunday *Times.*"

The secretary was the color of espresso. The top had two doors with four panes of glass each, and the hinged desktop dropped forward to reveal a series of cubby holes. The bottom had one large drawer across the width and two shorter ones below, a doored cupboard above. It was a combination of desk, dresser, and bookcase. It was, by far, the most imposing piece of furniture in the cottage.

We retired up the circular stairs for an athletic, almost frantic coupling and melancholic denouement. I leaned on my elbow, sighed, and shared the story of Thurman's invitation. Still naked, Alan jumped off the bed and bellowed out the window, "Ahoy! A landfall, and it's Beau Pré!"

"With you on the West Coast?" I asked.

"A lot closer than Norway!"

With that affirmation alone, I committed to three more years in Virginia. I waved as Alan's plane accelerated down the runway and took off into the night sky. I had no idea when he would be back.

Three more years in Virginia?

· 6 ·

Finding My Rhythm

October, November, December 1965

By October, I finally found my rhythm. The weather was what we called Indian summer in Vermont, a hint of crispness in the morning and no humidity. One Sunday I planted daffodil bulbs around the cottage. When Dr. Mac teased me about the man in my life, I smiled and changed the subject. I ignored the harassing surgeons in the ER, but I still resented the wives who delivered picnic suppers to their husbands on call, the same ones who'd delivered warm chocolate chip cookies to study group in medical school.

I'd finally made a friend in the cafeteria, Dr. Carolyn Brunner, a first-year resident in Internal Medicine. She still wore the Ben Caseys, the white hose, and the sturdy oxfords. She laughed when I told her about the chair of Surgery's complaints. "I follow the rules," she said. "I don't have the energy to protest." Carolyn reported that the hospital administration intended to seal off a section of the house-staff quarters to accommodate the women. We wouldn't have access to the pool table or the shared kitchen. She didn't care, but I did. I wanted to be one of the guys.

In November when I returned to the nursery, the nurses called me by name. *Good morning, Dr. Hostler.* The head nurse told me about an admission from West Virginia—a sick newborn with serious jaundice due to Rh incompatibility. We had no information except that the baby had been born in a jail. When Baby Turner finally arrived, his skin was orange, and his bilirubin was extremely elevated at 25. We stayed late to perform a double volume exchange transfusion through the baby's belly button to flush out the maternal antigens and the circulating bilirubin. Elevated bilirubin caused brain damage in newborns, but we didn't know how high was too high or how the baby's age impacted the process. The standard of care in 1965 was to perform an exchange transfusion when the neonatal blood bilirubin reached 20.

We had no idea then that Baby Turner would eventually require eight exchange transfusions. It wasn't customary to wear gloves to draw blood or to perform transfusions. We would learn weeks later that his mother had syphilis and had infected Baby Turner in utero.

As in July, I covered the ER on my nights on call in the nursery. It was unusual for the night nursery nurse to page me in the ER, but she needed me to evaluate a baby. I assumed it was Baby Turner, but it wasn't. It was a newly delivered baby girl. The delivery room sent her to the nursery as normal, but the experienced nurses recognized the stigmata of Down's syndrome and needed my confirmation. When the father came into the nursery the next morning, he shouted at the nurses and me, "That is no child of mine, and don't you dare take that 'mongoloid idiot' anywhere near my wife."

The nurses moved the baby to the back corner of the nursery so she couldn't be seen from the viewing window. She was left behind when the other babies were taken out to their mothers for feeding. She was not given a name, but the nurses held her and fed her. None of us knew what would become of her.

After a few days, Dr. Thurman stopped by the nursery to ask me to appear in court to represent the department. He explained that my role was to verify the diagnosis. The baby was to be made a ward of the state. She would be transferred to the Virginia State Training School in Lynchburg, where she would grow up. The Training School had initially opened in 1910 as the Virginia Colony for Epileptics and Feebleminded. The court date was set for Tuesday after Thanksgiving. The day to commit her to Lynchburg Training School.

To be honest, I was so caught up with the distinction of representing Dr. Thurman and the department that I didn't question the process. Only many years later did I learn that UVA and the School of Medicine had been the epicenter of the eugenics movement in the early twentieth century. In 1965, the Virginia Sterilization Act of 1924, which permitted legalized sterilization of the mentally ill and persons of low literacy, was still enforced.

I was on ER call the night before Thanksgiving, not preparing pumpkin pie or chopping onions and celery for the turkey stuffing. The hospital cafeteria put out such a sumptuous spread that even house staff not on call brought their families in for the feast. On Thanksgiving morning, I didn't linger after sign-out rounds. I went straight home and fell into the bed with my shoes still on. The cumulative sleep deprivation since July 1 was taking a toll. I intended to sleep until Friday morning.

I was deep asleep when the melee erupted. I transitioned from coma to consciousness and hit the floor still in my heels. I peered out my bedroom window. It looked like a medieval joust in the backyard—whinnying horses, blaring horns, and red-cheeked riders in velvet top hats and scarlet jackets. Men in polished boots carried whips. Women rode sidesaddle in long skirts. Children were on ponies, and hounds brayed all around. *The Thanksgiving Hunt.* I climbed back into bed, this time without my shoes.

Later, I would learn the correct terminology for the fox hunt—masters of the hunt, masters of the hounds, and the hilltoppers. The hounds had right-of-way once the horn was blown. Before the hunt, they gathered to bless the hounds and the animals of the field. Not the fox.

The following Tuesday was an adventure, starting with locating the courthouse in downtown Charlottesville. I didn't wait long before the judge directed me to approach the bench. "So, young lady," he said, "Dr. Mac says you're a doctor."

I stood in front of the judge's massive desk framed in flags. I was wearing my white coat with a stethoscope sticking out of the pocket. Couldn't he tell?

I nodded.

"I understand you know this baby has Down's syndrome. I'd hate to send a normal baby down 29 South, so tell me how you know this, Miss."

I assured him that the diagnosis was confirmed by the chromosomes and the physical findings. I reviewed the findings on physical exam as Dr. Thurman had instructed me.

"Tell me more about those special lines on the hands?" the judge asked.

I explained about the abnormal palmar creases. "Most normal people have two creases." I demonstrated the lines across the palms of my hand.

"I get it!" the judge said with a grin and extended his hands across that huge desk. He had single palmar creases on both hands. "Do you think I've got that Down's thing, too?"

I blushed and sputtered about the wide range of physical findings while he bellowed out a bunch of raucous belly laughs. He signed the decree, passed it to me, and looked up.

"Next?" he said to the bailiff.

I went back to hospital. Not to the nursery, but straight to Dr. Thurman's office. I had to give him the decree and tell him what had happened. He listened, nodded, and banged on the office wall. "Dr. Mac, you better get in here," he shouted.

The two of them lined up in front of me in their long white lab coats. They held their hands out, palms down. Then, in unison, they turned their palms up. I stared at them in disbelief. Dr. Thurman had a single palmar crease on his right hand. Dr. Mac had single creases on both hands. They started to giggle.

"We had to send you, Sharon. Judge doesn't believe us anymore." They chuckled away, two schoolboys tickled pink with their prank.

I blinked at my tears and fled.

That evening, as we cleaned up after Baby Turner's eighth transfusion, the head nurse said, "You know you've made it when the professors tease you."

I was confused for a beat or two, but then I registered her grin.

"You knew?"

Only then did I realize that for the entire month of November she had not commented on the absent Ben Caseys, my bare legs, or my high heels.

I was back on the wards in December.

Alan was coming for a long weekend, our first visit since September. He would stay through Monday so we could get a marriage license, receive the required counseling from the Unitarian minister, and get our blood drawn at the health department for the required Venereal

Disease Research Lab (VDRL) test. Once I learned that Baby Turner had congenital syphilis, I worried more about the results of my VDRL than the wedding.

By then, I was at one with the rhythms and the routines of the inpatient ward. I called the orderlies and the housekeepers by name when I walked through the hospital lobby. I greeted the other interns and residents by name when we got coffee at the cafeteria. I recognized parents in the hallways and asked about their kids.

I spent my call nights in the house-staff quarters, where three rooms for women had been walled off from the men's quarters. I didn't complain about the barricade, but I did complain, enthusiastically and endlessly, to Mr. Farish, the hospital's chief engineer. Mr. Farish, tall and slim with a well-trimmed, salt-and-pepper mustache, was the official Christmas tree commandant. He supervised the installations of holiday decorations from elegant wreaths and trees to tacky Santa Clauses and North Pole villages. There were crèches on the pediatric wards, but no Hanukkah candles.

Fire safety rules permitted live evergreens in the lobby and the parking lots, but only artificial trees on the inpatient wards. I was on call the week of Christmas, and I was lobbying Mr. Farish for a tree, a live Christmas tree, for my call room. At each encounter, he grinned and parried with another set of regulations—federal, state, galactic, or Farish forged. I countered with additional requests: bubbling lights—white, of course—and ornaments.

Christmas or not, babies born with bad hearts still came to UVAH from throughout the Commonwealth. Dr. Martha Carpenter, a no-nonsense pediatric cardiologist trained at Boston's Children's Hospital, had started a pediatric heart catheterization program which enabled detailed anatomic and physiologic diagnosis. Surgery, however, was mostly palliative, a mechanism to buy time until curative surgeries were developed.

Babies born in 1965 with a complicated set of heart defects known as the Tetralogy of Fallot could have a Blalock-Taussig shunt placed that would tide them over, ideally, until corrective surgery. It seemed miraculous to have these blue babies return from the operating room pink after the shunt was placed. But a definitive surgery had yet to be developed. When the shunts failed, as happened in adolescence, the children died. The wards were filled with survivors, no longer babies and not just blue, but deep purple and having Tet Spells. To relieve their excruciating chest pain, the teenagers squatted on the floor and squeezed their arms around their knees. The maneuver increased the blood flow to the heart which provided for momentary relief. Until it didn't.

David was a fourteen-year-old boy admitted with terrifying Tet Spells. Oxygen and morphine provided him some relief, but his nailbeds and lips remained intensely purple, the inside of his mouth the color of blackberries. David complained of relentless headaches and chest pain. His tissues were not getting enough oxygen. His mother was frantic. "Do something," she said to me.

It was scary to stand by and do nothing. When I paged Dr. Dammann, the cardiologist, for help, he reminded me that intravenous morphine was the only way to relax the spasms in David's coronary arteries.

"*Push the morphine?*" I repeated. "*Are you sure?*"

"Yes, do it now. Don't wait for me. I'm on my way."

David screamed and writhed in pain. He clutched his knees to his chest as I explained what I was going to do. When I slowly pushed the medication directly into the vein in his arm, David stopped writhing and became still. His mother cradled him, rocking and praying.

The cardiologist arrived and placed his stethoscope on David's chest. I leaned against the bedrails, not fully understanding what was happening. He listened for several minutes.

"It's over," he said to us. "I'm sorry."

"May God bless both of you," David's mother said. "May my son rest in peace at last. Let us pray."

The sounds of the ward careened around us. I pulled the curtains closed around David's bed for privacy. Dr. Dammann and I lowered our heads. David's mother prayed for David and for all the children born as blue babies. Then she laid her hands on the tops of our heads and blessed us once more.

The cardiologist pulled up a chair next to me in the nursing station. He reviewed the physiology and pharmacology of Tetralogy of Fallot as I entered David's death note in the medical chart. I'd had too little sleep and too much work. My only thought was that David had died because I injected the morphine.

In the corridor, carolers were singing "Silent Night," but the in-patients admitted around Christmas were too sick to notice. Families and doctors did everything in their power to keep children out of the hospital until after Santa arrived. The day after Christmas in the ER was a madhouse.

I missed the Pediatric Department's Christmas party at Dr. Thurman's house because of ward call. My colleagues in-house were distracted. They missed their families, especially those with little children at home. It was a dark stretch and getting darker by the day. I thought about the Druids and the fading light. Winter Solstice wasn't until tomorrow.

On Christmas Eve, I ate supper alone in the cafeteria and headed to the quarters for a shower and nap. It was my seventh straight night in the hospital, the last night of holiday call. Alan would be waiting when I finished rounds the next day, but that night I was in the dumps.

Once in the house-staff quarters, the spicy fragrance of evergreens floated into my gloomy reverie. I had to push hard to get my door open because a humongous Christmas tree filled my room. Its boughs scraped the ceiling and cascaded over the bedspread. I flicked on the light switch, and the tree lit up with white bubbly lights. Two boxes of ornaments lay open on the bed—gleaming reds, blues, and greens. What in the world? I started to cry, but it wasn't long before I began to chortle.

My very own Christmas tree! A gargantuan Norwegian spruce tree was stuffed into my call room. Bubbly lights, white lights, and elegant ornaments. A card was tucked in with the ornaments: *A Very Merry Christmas from Mr. Farish, Chief Clinical Engineer!*

It was almost dark on Christmas Day when I arrived home. It had been seven days in a half-staffed hospital with the sickest of the kids, despairing parents, and random snatches of sleep. All I really wanted was to climb the circular staircase for a hot shower, but there was Alan beaming with delight.

Santa Claus in his red Viyella shirt was delighted at my arrival. A bottle of Korbel Brut and two champagne glasses lay on a red linen napkin in front of the fireplace.

"Merry Christmas!" He gathered me up in a full-body, rock-and-roll hug.

"Alan, just a quick shower?"

"You'll collapse on the bed. You won't get close to the shower." He guided me to the black director's chair by the fire. A Christmas tree in the alcove was covered in tiny black and white packages, all alike, and tied with gold ribbon.

"My packages are still hidden in the closet," I said and sipped the bubbly. It seemed unreal, even surreal, to sit by the fire. Just half hour ago, I was admitting a toddler with meningitis.

"Open this," Alan said. "You're a beautiful woman. You deserve the elegance of Chanel!"

I sighed. It was one in a series of Pygmalion moments when Alan imposed the outside world on my monastic life in medicine. Just as he had presented me with Prince Albert bone china in my cellar apartment, discordant beside the collection of random crockery, now he was presenting me with beautiful *articles de toilette.*

I opened the perfume, Chanel. I was perseverating about my patients, the gift-giving opulence, and the messages of that Christmas afternoon. Why was Alan now referencing Coco Chanel? "*A woman who doesn't wear perfume has no future.*" What was he talking about?

Each package was another Chanel something or other, delicate scents, fragile soaps, soothing lotions, even a dark-red lipstick called something sultry and exotic. A silk nightgown.

"Periwinkle, not blue," Alan said.

Four days later, I awoke to the aroma of coffee and the shrill sounds from a bagpipe chanter. Not my pager. Not the alarm. After six months of night call, I had spent four nights in a row sleeping next to Alan in my periwinkle, not blue, nightgown. I stretched my arms above my head and poked my feet out from under the covers. Alan was practicing scales on the chanter. I was wide awake. It was Wednesday, December 29. Our wedding day.

The day whirled out of control. Alan embraced the chaos, but I was at sixes and sevens. Jerry let us know that he'd chartered a plane in Wilmington, Delaware, and would pick up the Typhoon Tavern guys in Woods Hole. We should expect them and a case of champagne to land in Charlottesville by midafternoon. The minister checked in for directions to Beau Pré. He'd arrive by five thirty.

Alan and I reviewed our vows, confirmed the omission of "obey," and marked the chosen lines from Gibran's *The Prophet*. The Unitarian minister insisted on a prayer or two, but there would be no reference to the Trinity or anything familiar to this lapsed Catholic/Episcopalian.

I had worried more about my VDRL test results than my wedding day. I called my friend Robert Levy at the store about a dress. Yes, he had a white, princess-line dress with long sleeves and a round neck.

I had no time to go shopping and cook. I did a quick check-in with Bill and Beverley Clover, the realtors who helped me find the cottage. We'd run into them at the courthouse.

"Don't worry," Bev said. "We'll bring supper."

Berta peeked in the alcove window and waved, excited about the festivities. Robert Levy delivered the dress and brought me a handful of tiny, white sweetheart roses. "For your hair," he said.

Alan and I whirled around the cottage until I was giddy. We had no thoughts beyond this day of champagne, good friends, and exuberant love.

The chaos continued below as I preened upstairs. Alan kept the fire roaring. Jerry, George, and Cookie arrived from Woods Hole with champagne, Veuve Clicquot, a few bottles of cognac, and a red cummerbund for Alan. Royal Stewart, his Welsh clan's assigned tartan. The toasts had begun.

I heard Bill and Bev Clover arrive, then the group's collective "ooh and aah" over the lobster Newburg and tiny wedding cupcakes. I cringed hearing Bev bang around in my little kitchen. The minister arrived, a resonant baritone, with his wife, an alto maybe. Finally came Warner's booming bass voice, Berta's sweet Swiss Deutsch accent, and their giggling girls.

Only then, showered and dressed, did I briefly consider the enormity of the day. We had had absolutely no discussion of the life ahead or how we intended to share it. Had there been a back exit, I might well have fled right then.

I took a deep breath and descended the circular stairs.

· 7 ·

Hostage in the South

1966

When Dr. Mac called me "young lady" that first Monday morning after the holidays, I knew I was in trouble.

I'd found that simple expressions in the South conveyed layers of meaning, sometimes signifying the exact opposite. Although it sounded respectful when Dr. Mac called me "young lady" on rounds, it was usually a scold. More like, "Listen here, young lady, how many times do I have to remind you about the way we do things at UVA?"

"Young lady," he said, "as you didn't afford me the respect of meeting your intended before the wedding, when shall I have the honor?"

"Alan's in California, sir."

"And you're here without him?" He took my arm, steered me into a corner, and lowered his voice. "Young lady, you do not belong here alone. Especially if you're in the family way." He shook his head. "I told Dr. Thurman it was a mistake—"

"I'm not pregnant, Dr. Mac," I said. "Alan will be back. You'll meet him."

I was grateful when Dr. Thurman interrupted. "Sorry, Dr. Mac. I need her before her clinic starts."

I had rotated in all inpatient settings until then. The outpatient clinic saw well children but also served as the daytime emergency room and the destination for diagnostic referrals. Last, but not least, it was the training site for medical students and house staff. The educational philosophy, now archaic, was articulated as, "See one. Do one. Teach one."

"Happy New Year! I hear you've been busy over the break," he grinned. "The Clovers were tickled to fill me in." At least he wasn't asking me about my last menstrual period.

"Now that you're married," he said and laughed, "you're eligible for some benefits."

I laughed. "The married house-staff stipend?"

"No, the hospital stipend is for the men to take care of their wives during training. But," he said, "you're eligible for a loan program from the American Academy of Pediatrics. Up to a thousand dollars a year. Here's an application. I hope it helps."

I laughed. "You have no idea. You know women are excluded from all the usual medical school scholarships and loans."

"I have some idea." He smiled. "It wasn't that long ago."

Maybe Foods of All Nations wouldn't be my full-service bank forever. Once I'd understood I was allowed to charge cash as well as groceries, the monthly bill had kept growing—no interest and no due date.

I turned off Hospital Drive and entered the public pediatric clinic tucked away under the staircase to the columned facade of the Old Medical School. Dr. Thurman kept walking to the Private Clinic Building where he and pediatric faculty had offices and adjoining exam rooms.

He hollered back, "I heard you were the belle of the ball on New Year's Eve!"

New Year's Eve seemed long ago, already a fantasy. Berta and Warner Wood had invited us to attend the New Year's Eve Ball at the Farmington Country Club. And Alan had accepted.

Such a roller coaster—from the despair of David's death to a Christmas wedding and a New Year's Eve Ball. And now I was assigned to the clinic, the public clinic, where the children of the country club servers received their care. Berta repeatedly commented that there were no poor people in Albemarle County. Only if you never looked beyond the boxwoods.

The Department of Pediatrics operated two outpatient clinics, one private and one public. Families of the children seen in the private clinic had health insurance or received professional courtesy from the faculty pediatricians because their parents were UVA faculty or schoolteachers or clergy. Sometimes neighbors or friends of the family. They were universally White.

Families of the children we cared for in the public clinic didn't have medical insurance, weren't members of a network of privilege, and couldn't pay cash. These patients were both White and "Colored," as Dr. Birdsong would say, or "Negro," as the chart read. I frequently heard the N-word or "Colored" used in the ER, rarely "Black," never "African American." I learned the derogatory terms for light-skinned Black kids who could pass as White: "You see the *high yella* in room four," "Take care of *Jefferson's redhead,*" and "The *Hemings girls* are in room three."

In Vermont in the early 1960s, the prevailing prejudice was directed at the French-Canadians from Quebec. They were called "Canucks." The shopkeepers posted signs warning that their Canadian money was not welcome. No one explained the source of the contempt—their Catholicism, their French language, the suspicion they'd bred with the Native Americans. When Pa had told me the story of our name change from Chevalier to Hostler, he'd made it sound like it was just the city clerk being mean.

I'd rarely seen a person of color before Puerto Rico. As an intern, we routinely used "Colored" to describe the Black babies and toddlers in clinic, probably the school-aged kids, too. Some staff used "poor White trash" and "piss poor protoplasm," even writing the latter term as the "Triple P Syndrome" in the medical chart.

One pediatrician in town used a covered back porch as a waiting room for his "Colored patients," examining them only after all the White children, rich and poor, had been seen. Another practice maintained separate waiting spaces indoors, but the "Colored children" still waited until all White kids had been seen. There were two Black physicians in Charlottesville that I knew about—one's office was on Ridge Street, and the other was on Main Street above the Greyhound Bus Station. Neither had admitting or referral privileges to UVAH or the community hospital, Martha Jefferson. Decades later, they were admitted posthumously to the Albemarle County Medical Society.

The first day of clinic was chaotic. The small waiting room teemed with harried mothers, kids horsing around, and screaming babies. In the mayhem, the head nurse maintained a stable state of disequilibrium. Nancy McCue was only in her late twenties, but she was a well-seasoned clinician with strong organizational skills and an informal network of connections throughout the hospital. She was married to Dr. Frank McCue, an orthopedist forging the new subspecialty of sports medicine and well-connected to local and state politicians. Most importantly for all of us, she recognized sick from not sick, sense from nonsense.

Ideally, the clinic was a place for monitoring child growth and development, as well as providing anticipatory guidance and preventive care like immunizations against tetanus, diphtheria, pertussis, and polio. Like most pediatricians, I believed in vaccines with a passion. I'd been in high school in the 1950s during the last polio epidemic in the United States. The Rutland city swimming pool had closed. A classmate ended up in an iron lung. But, in Virginia, a few families resisted the shots. Some remembered the contamination of polio vaccines in 1963.

The measles shot had just been introduced. Researchers were still working on a vaccine for German measles, or rubella. Complications of real measles in preschool children were serious—severe pneumonia and devastating encephalitis. But rubella was dangerous for pregnant women because of its potential to damage the developing fetus. Neighborhoods organized "rubella parties" to expose healthy children to kids infected with rubella so the girls would be immune when they grew up and became pregnant.

Nurse McCue and the senior resident controlled patient traffic, shepherded the sickest to the front of the line, and dependably emptied the clinic by five o'clock each day, Monday through Friday. By midmorning, the waiting room had a crowd of fourteen infants and toddlers scheduled for well-child visits, fifteen school physicals, seven follow-up visits, a twelve-year-old hit by a car while riding his bike, a seven-year-old with acute belly pain, a two-year-old with worms, and twenty Venable School third-graders to be checked for "cooties." Because it was January, we had a slew of preschoolers with earaches and sore throats. The inpatient wards looked orderly by contrast.

"How many silver trays?" Nurse McCue teased me as she passed me in the hallway, "You know, for your wedding?"

"None," I replied, shrugged, and entered an exam room. It was a six-month-old well-baby check. The mother jostled a gurgling baby boy on her knee as toddler twins, girls in matching pink dresses, tossed blocks helter-skelter around her chair.

"My name is Dr. Hostler and I—"

"Oh yes," she interrupted, "the lady doctor with the ruffles." She launched into the interrogation. "How many kids? Is your husband a doctor, too? How come you get to wear fancy blouses? Are you going to be our doctor from now on? We get shuffled around here a lot."

"We'd like a lady doctor. But no kids?" She paused for a moment and shook her head. "Bless the Lord, I'll pray for you."

I managed a few questions in between the barrage of her good-natured monologue. She listened as I explained the immunizations, but she started fidgeting when I launched into the child safety spiel—plastic plugs in floor-level electrical outlets, relocating pet food dishes, and cleaning out the poisons from under the kitchen sink.

"Okay, lady doctor with no children and none on the way! We'll see you next time!" She was done with me.

I left the room grinning and wondering about kids. Alan had four. We'd never talked about having kids.

The chief resident recruited me to the group of third-graders, teasing me, "You do recognize a louse when you see one?"

I nodded, remembering Hattie, Nellie's mother, checking me with her fine-tooth comb. Taking out my braids after school, brushing my hair hard, and then layer by layer, digging the teeth of her comb into my scalp, searching for nits in my fine blonde hair. No lice, but she enjoyed the hurting.

I lined the kids up in the hallway—lice positive on the right, lice negative on the left. I handed out the Kwell prescriptions to the kids on the right and the "no lice notes" on the left. I smiled, called each one by name, and kept my hands light and gentle as I combed.

A well-dressed White mother stormed into clinic, pulled her daughter out of the line, and announced, "My daughter does not belong here. We see Dr. McLemore Birdsong in the private clinic."

I handed a prescription to the girl, grinned, and whispered, "Give this to your mother." I nodded to the mother, "No need to bother Dr. Mac."

By midafternoon, I'd seen three toddlers with otitis media, one named Vagina Mae, most probably a delivery room prank by some obstetrics resident.

"NOW," Nurse McCue hollered, "Room four!"

A Black mother in a navy-blue suit and matching hat with both a veil and a feather struggled to get her uncooperative daughter, Eleanor, undressed and onto the exam table. She explained, "Eleanor is thirteen, a straight-A student in eighth grade. She called me at work saying she was sick. Only emergency calls are allowed." She shook her head. "You know the rules. I'm in Medical Records. By the time I got home, Eleanor was crying, hanging onto her head and confused."

Eleanor was clearly in distress, moaning and writhing on the exam table. She kept her eyes scrunched shut and resisted any attempt to touch her head. Her skin felt cold and clammy. Her pulse was too fast to count. When I tried to move her head, she screamed and collapsed, limp and whimpering.

Nurse McCue returned with supplies for blood drawing, a lumbar puncture kit, and IV fluids. She positioned Eleanor's arm while the mother held her shoulders against the table and hummed what sounded like hymns.

Why the hell are we in the clinic, way across the hospital from everything we need? Why aren't we in the ER? This child is in shock. She's going to die.

I couldn't see a vein in her ashy-charcoal arm, but I stroked her skin with my ungloved fingertips, felt a vessel, and slid the needle in. I squirted the blood into the culture bottles, then started the IV. That is when I saw the tiny violet spots, petechiae, bloom across the skin of her forearms. It was a telltale rash.

There was no time to do the lumbar puncture.

Nurse McCue loaded the syringe with penicillin. I pushed it into Eleanor's vein. Whatever the organism was, it was already in the blood and probably swimming around in the meninges of her brain. She was headed into septic shock. We couldn't wait for the transport team. We pushed the gurney upstairs to the inpatient unit.

It was past six o'clock when Nurse McCue locked the clinic door and we walked into the pitch-black in front of the Old Medical School. "What're her odds?" she asked.

"I don't know," I shrugged. "She's young and healthy, but she went downhill awfully fast."

"When I saw the petechiae start—" she sighed.

"Very scary. Thank you for being on top of everything."

When I called the ward before I went to bed, Eleanor was alive but unresponsive. Early next morning, I bumped into Nurse McCue outside Eleanor's hospital room. We both smiled as we spotted the bobbing feather in the shadows.

Midmorning, the lab called with a preliminary report, "Positive blood culture for meningococcus, sensitive to penicillin." Eleanor was awake by noon and asking for something to eat. Four years later, Eleanor would be the valedictorian of her high school class. Nurse McCue and I celebrated with her family and neighbors on Page Street.

I loved the clinic because of the pace, the variety of patients, and the chaos, but mostly, to be honest, it was because I had almost complete autonomy. The public clinic had no faculty, only a senior resident in charge and, of course, Nurse McCue.

That winter we had a real snowstorm in Charlottesville. Everything stopped, even the railroad trains. I skied into the hospital, stayed a week in the house-staff quarters, and filled in wherever I was needed. I was beginning to feel like a real doctor, like the times in Puerto Rico, Doctora Americana. When I ran into the mothers of my patients out in the community—at the bank, the grocery store, even the liquor store—they called me Dr. Hostler.

But I missed Alan. I was getting more and more sleep deprived with the every-other-night call schedule. Sometimes I became irritable with my colleagues. I made errors in judgment. Dr. Mac gave me an earnest tutorial about the importance of the opening of trout season, but I still chastised a third-year medical student when he missed rounds on April 1. Even the nurses were annoyed with me that day.

When I was invited to admire the azaleas in Dr. Mac's gardens, I didn't show up. It was on a Saturday afternoon. I wasn't even on call. I had no excuse.

On ER call, I complained of the stench in the ER. All hell broke loose when twenty-three adults and eight kids arrived at the same time—vomiting and groaning in pain after eating hot dogs at the greasy spoon across the street. Not enough mops, not enough towels, not enough staff. And I complained.

I was mad at the rescue squad. I was short with the ward clerk. I stomped around the ward. I was furious with the guy who shot his stepdaughter in the face with buckshot. She had tiny blobs and streaks of blood everywhere—splattered in her hair, dried on her arms, and puddled in her clothes. From the X-rays, we counted fifty-some pellets that had penetrated her skin—her face, forehead, nose, cheeks, lips, and chin. Even the edge of her left eye, the pinnae of both ears and her scalp. Four pellets had pierced her skull and were embedded in her brain.

I screamed at the psychiatric resident on call: "Tomorrow morning is not acceptable. Come see her immediately. Stat!"

Finally, I saw her off to surgery and hit the bed in the quarters around 3:30 a.m. It wasn't quite 5:00 a.m. when I was paged back to the ER. I had a full clinic starting at 8:00 a.m. I stormed across the parking lot and slammed the ER door.

The mother was a teenager in a ponytail, tie-dyed T-shirt, and rolled-up jeans. She bounced a chubby-cheeked baby on her knee. "I'm worried about my baby girl," she said. "Her little cheeks get bright red, really red, and she balls up her fists. She cries."

"And then?"

"She makes a great big, really smelly dump in her diapers." She giggled.

"Is there blood on her bottom or in her diaper? Mucous?"

"Oh, no. Never. I scrub up her little tush and she settles right down."

I leaned over the mother to examine the baby. I willed myself to be gentle. The belly was soft, no masses. It was a normal exam.

"Go sit on the commode, strain hard. Press down. Hold your breath." I gave the mother a small mirror. "Tell me what you look like."

She handed me back the mirror, scooped up her baby, and scurried out.

I hollered down the corridor after her, "No charge!" I ripped the visit form into shreds and tossed the confetti into the trash can.

For the rest of the day, all I could think about was the young mother and her baby, Priscilla Ann. It had just been a year since medical school graduation. I had recited the Hippocratic Oath. I vowed to keep my patients from harm and injustice. *First, do no harm.*

How had I become the kind of doctor who shamed a new mother for worrying about her baby?

How indeed?

The research about the effects of chronic sleep deprivation had been around even in 1965, but it was not until 1980 that the residency regulations would suggest to training programs that time should be allocated for education and personal pursuits. In 1981, psychologist Christine Maslach and her colleagues published the Maslach Burnout Inventory (MBI) for medical professionals. It measured increased emotional exhaustion, increased depersonalization, and decreased personal accomplishment as the components of professional burnout.

By 1988, the Board of Internal Medicine recommended an eighty-hour workweek for residents in training with one day in seven away from the hospital and overnight call only every third night. Finally, in 2003, the Accreditation Council for Graduate Medical Education (ACGME) mandated an eighty-hour workweek for all residents in training, and in 2004, the UVA School of Medicine initiated its first wellness program utilizing the MBI for residents in training and clinical faculty.

Throughout that internship year and my first year of residency, I insisted to Alan that I was fine. Just tired, sometimes cranky, and increasingly irrational. It wasn't until a bizarre experience in the nursery as the supervising resident in December 1966 that I would acknowledge how serious things had become.

It was the Saturday before Christmas, the day of the department party. My intern, Ben, and I were finishing nursery rounds with Dr. Thurman. Something went seriously awry as we approached the last crib. The baby inside was big and puffy but very still. He wasn't breathing. I opened the isolette. Ben listened for a heartbeat, then passed his stethoscope to me. There was no heartbeat.

And that's about when I left my body and floated away. Ben the intern started chest compressions. I heard myself shout to the nurse for an IV set-up and a butterfly needle. Dr. Thurman sat down in a rocking chair nearby and rocked.

From the ceiling where I was floating, it looked like a slow-motion ballet with Ben and the nurse doing some kind of pas de deux while I directed the choreography and Dr. Thurman rocked slowly back and forth, huge hands resting in his lap, quiet. Then Ben wafted upward toward the ceiling. We nodded as he floated by me.

Eventually, Ben stopped the resuscitation. I pronounced the baby dead. We'd lost a newborn baby, a full-term baby boy in the middle of rounds in front of our chair, Dr. Thurman.

At the end of the party that evening, Dr. Thurman asked Ben and me to stay behind. He explained the infant had Potter syndrome and was born without kidneys. Most such pregnancies resulted in stillbirth. If the babies did make it to term, they died within a day or two. He reviewed the pathophysiology, but mostly he tried to assure us that we had done nothing wrong.

But all I cared about was whether the chief knew I was floating around in the nursery with Ben. And did Ben know he was up there with me?

At home, Alan comforted me—rubbed my back, massaged my neck, and pulled out each toe on each foot, one by one.

"We might as well talk about it," he said.

It was months before Ben finally confided his experience to me. I think the psychiatrists call what we experienced dissociation, a folie à deux.

I worried for years and years about it happening again. It never did. It was eighteen months into residency training before I acknowledged to Alan—and to myself—the depth of my exhaustion, my stress, and the limits of my competency.

· 8 ·

Residency and Academic Rituals

1966–1968

That first year of residency was essentially a repeat of the internship year—the same clinical rotations, the same call schedule—except that I had a better fund of knowledge, I was more efficient, and I had moved up a rung. The interns were my responsibility, which is why I worried so about Ben in the nursery. We took care of our patients and made daily rounds as a vertical team, responsible to the next level up the ladder. It would be fifty years before academic medicine considered that the interdependence of a ward team composed of equals, a horizontal team, would produce better patient outcomes and better learning outcomes.

Even as a medical student, I had felt that I was the primary one responsible for the patient's care, and that didn't change as I moved up the hierarchy. I recorded every nuance of the medical history. I charted my physical examinations in precise detail. I composed thoughtful dispositions and thorough plans of care. I even included journal references in my patient notes. I relished the moments of mastery.

Alan remained in California. He had aways thrived on projects that involved wearing a wetsuit, collecting data, and solving complex dilemmas, but now he worried about the company's corporate aspirations and its evolving dependency on military contracts. I looked forward to Alan's return to Washington and spending weekends in Charlottesville. Alan was growing restless and increasingly ambivalent about his work as I was beginning to hit my stride in training. We had never talked about where and how we would live after my residency. We never discussed money, children, or shared values. Neither of us had considered that OSE might require Alan to shave his beard when Alan did return to Washington. I certainly had no idea that Alan dreamt of us sailing around the world.

I remained focused on the next clinical rotation, my night-call schedule, and Alan's next homecoming. Every two to three months, Alan would be at Beau Pré long enough to create a coffee table from cherry scraps and a slab of Vermont marble or to build a platform for the king-size mattress. In and around my call schedule, we managed to collect black walnuts, hike Humpback Rock, and entertain Peter Kaplan on Sunday afternoons. We'd met Peter through my friend Carolyn Brunner from Internal Medicine.

Peter had grown up in New Jersey where his father ran a haberdashery. I assumed that explained Peter's sartorial flare—the Harris Tweed jackets, the monogrammed shirts, the gray flannel trousers. He graduated Phi Beta Kappa from Princeton and Alpha Omega Alpha from the University of Pennsylvania Medical School. He matched at UVA, completed an internship in Internal Medicine, and was drafted into the Korean War. We met Peter when he returned to his residency and fellowship in cardiology. When I complained about the sexual harassment in the ER, he countered with his own tales of anti-Semitism at Penn. I am not sure exactly how it evolved, but Peter adopted us.

Sex had been the dominating focus of my reunions with Alan, but that was less freewheeling when we had to factor in Berta knocking on the door, Roy's dropping by, or Peter Kaplan's drop-ins. Especially on Sunday afternoons.

Peter would arrive in his tweeds and silk ascot, carrying cloth sacks of dry sherry or Spanish brandy delivered from his Princeton eating club—excited to share the uncorking and the tasting with us. Alan stoked the fire. I added more broth to the stew, knowing that Peter would still be there at suppertime. I felt our cottage in the middle of hunt country fueled Peter's fantasies of being to the manor born. Alan entertained us with news of the world outside medicine—the civil rights protests, the flower children and their shenanigans in Haight-Ashbury, the release of the Beatles' album *Sgt. Pepper's Lonely Hearts*

Club Band. Alan teased me that Peter was pursuing me, but decades later, I considered that Peter was probably more interested in Alan than me.

At the hospital, I was learning the rituals of academic medicine, the flavors of rounds from cursory turnover rounds at the end of the day to the weekly command performance called grand rounds. Every academic department conducted its own.

Pediatric grand rounds on Saturday morning at nine o'clock was the grand finale of the week. Dr. Thurman swept across the stage to his place behind the podium, an imposing figure in a long white lab coat and bow tie. His bushy eyebrows were scrunched into one as he made a quick eye-contact check-in with the audience—one by one—taking attendance. Dr. Thurman directed grand rounds with the finesse of a major symphony maestro.

The presentation centered on a child—Suzie or Ethan or Beulah—a child with a symptom and physical findings. The child with a parent or nurse would appear in the front of the lecture hall. Dr. Birdsong might ask about the pain or where the pain was located. Suzie might stick out her elbow to show us the redness and swelling. Then Dr. Thurman would smile at Suzie, bend down to shake her hand, and thank her for "teaching the young doctors."

After five minutes of the patient show-and-tell, a faculty member presented the scholarly portion of the conference, referencing Suzie's elbow pain to discuss the pathophysiology of the disease—the errant immune system in the case of juvenile rheumatoid arthritis and its myriad disguises. How to confirm the diagnosis? What were the treatment options? After the speaker responded to questions from the audience, he would step down and join his senior colleagues in the front row.

Dr. Thurman would reframe the patient, her family, and her disease in the context of home, school, and community—a reminder about school attendance or playing team sports. Or how the disease and its treatment affected normal growth and development. I'd remember then the Labor Day party when the law faculty called him a maverick for opening neighborhood clinics and focusing on social issues, meeting in Black churches. It wasn't just that Dr. Thurman was young; he had a very different vision of the role of academic medicine.

I looked forward to my rotation with Dr. Thurman in March 1967.

It would be my first time to work with him in the private clinic, to follow his hematology patients, and to interact with their families. He interfaced with the pediatric wards, the pharmacy, the subspecialty clinics from Surgery and Radiology, the blood bank, and referring physicians from throughout the Commonwealth. That month, we regularly visited the morgue for conversations with Turkey Bibb about postmortem damage from our chemotherapy agents. We attended funerals, graveyard services, and a family night or two. I learned to write sympathy notes.

My first hematology patient was Willie—a five-year-old kindergartener, referred by a pediatrician in Winchester, two hours away, because of a persistent anemia. Wille sat squeezed between his parents in the exam room—blue-green eyes staring straight at me, blond hair parted on the side, and cheeks translucent as china. Willie told me about school while I listened to his lungs, clear, and his heart with a too fast, staccato beat, consistent with anemia. I could feel the tip of his spleen, not normal. And I saw the petechiae on the tops of his feet under the crisscrossed shoelaces in his sneakers.

Willie was having an okay time, but his parents were not. They hadn't wanted to bring their child to the University of Virginia. They'd heard about experimentation on patients, "Colored people" mixed in with the White people, and the snooty people who lived in Charlottesville. Their pediatrician had insisted that Dr. Thurman would understand why the iron tonic wasn't working and that he had access to better treatments. No one had said aloud what they feared. It was serious enough for the father to take a day off from work to drive to Charlottesville.

I left Willie with crayons and a coloring book to go to Dr. Thurman's office to present our patient. The process was somehow different now. I recognized the most probable diagnosis, but I kept considering other possibilities—less fatal possibilities.

We returned to Willie and his parents. Dr. Thurman repeated my exam, but he reported out as he went along: "Your skin is really pale, young man. Willie's heart is beating a bit fast. These lymph nodes seem a bit large and tender. Oh Willie, your belly is soft as the egg custard my mother used to make me when I was sick. Yes, Dr. Hostler, I feel Willie's spleen down the width of your three fingers, my two." He chuckled and explained: "Willie, I played ice hockey once. Look at my paws. They're verrrry big!"

Dr. Thurman pointed out the petechiae on the top of Willie's feet and some I had missed on the big toes. He said to the parents, "Petechiae are little bleeding points under the skin. We can see these petechiae, but we can't see the other bleeding on Willie's insides, but they're there, too."

The parents fixated on each of Dr. Thurman's words, kind but foreshadowing what would come. Willie and I chatted about T-ball. He sputtered when I asked about jumping rope. Dr. Thurman introduced the necessity of a bone marrow aspiration to confirm the suspected diagnosis.

Willie and I went for a walk to the Corner, the historic district with restaurants and bookstores adjacent to UVA Grounds. We didn't get hot chocolate or a donut. The last thing we needed was Willie barfing during the bone marrow. I wondered if I would get to do the procedure or, because they were private patients from out of town, the chief would be the one to insert the trochar into Willie's hipbone. The goal was to aspirate bone marrow and study it under the microscope. Marrow contained the stem cells of the circulating blood—red cells to carry oxygen in its hemoglobin, white cells to fight infection, and platelets to clot the blood. Our working diagnosis was acute lymphocytic leukemia, and that is what Dr. Thurman was sharing with Willie's parents as we roamed around the Corner.

Willie had over 50,000 lymphocytes per cc of his peripheral blood. A count under 8,000 was normal for a kid his age. Dr. Thurman and I sat at the microscope to examine Willie's marrow. We counted stem cells, calculated ratios, examined the distorted morphology of the malignant lymphoblasts, and paid attention to the health of his red cell and platelet precursors. Once we started chemotherapy to knock out the lymphoblasts, Willie would need them. In those early days of clinical trials, children died from bleeding, sepsis, or other side effects of the chemotherapy.

At six o'clock, we gathered in Dr. Thurman's office with Willie's parents. The clinic nurse took Willie to the hospital cafeteria for ice cream, his treat for lying still during the bone marrow aspiration. I summarized the pertinent history, the physical findings on Willie's exam, and the results of the lab work, pointing out the crisis presented by the 50,000 number. Willie's lymphoblasts were increasing exponentially and could cause him other effects, even a stroke.

Willie's parents were barely able to sit up straight. They were beyond able to articulate their terror or to formulate questions. Dr. Thurman came from behind his desk, pulled a chair next to mine, and made a circle with the parents. We sat with knees touching knees. He put a box of tissues in the mother's lap. He explained that Willie's marrow was overgrown with primitive lymphoblasts, crowding out the other cells. Willie had acute lymphocytic leukemia (ALL).

Willie's mother's moan became a soft howl. Her husband steadied her. "Listen to the doctor. Willie might die. Do you understand?"

"What can we do?" He looked to Dr. Thurman, not me. "Willie's our only boy, the namesake, the heir. Our pediatrician tried to tell us, but we wouldn't listen." He held his wife and rocked her. Back and forth they rocked and sobbed.

Dr. Thurman stood up and said, "We'll be back in a bit. Would you like some coffee?" They shook their heads no. "When we return, you'll have to make some decisions. The first is whether you want Willie admitted here or in Winchester. Either way, Dr. Hostler will get him a bed." He sighed. "I'm sorry, but that's the easy part."

Usually, I was the resident receiving the newly diagnosed child, fuming because the admission hadn't been scheduled and the night team had no warning. But that night, I was trying not only to find a private room but to choose the best team, the one with the best hand skills for Willie and the best bedside manners for his parents.

I'd never been in a conversation like this. Dr. Thurman explained to the parents that Willie would not live six weeks without treatment, that he might have a cerebral event with the high number of malignant lymphoblasts crowding out all the other cells, or he might bleed to death. Palliative care meant giving him transfusions of platelets and packed red cells, but Willie would never leave the hospital, UVA or Winchester. The parents nodded when he asked them if they understood.

"Your pediatrician insisted that you come to UVA because he knew we're enrolling patients with ALL in clinical trials, national clinical trials. There are two major research groups, one out of Boston and one out of Texas Southwest. We're part of the latter. It's an experiment, not in a laboratory but in human beings, children." He paused and added, "Willie."

Willie's mother shook so much her teeth chattered. Willie's father sat up straight and stared at Dr. Thurman. "What're the odds of his coming home?"

"That's the right kind of question, sir. Willie is critically ill. First, we must get him through the crisis period." He paused. "Willie has a 50–50 chance of getting home from the hospital." We sat in silence for a few minutes.

"The question you are not asking is, Can we cure this disease? Will Willie live to go into first grade this fall? Will he get to grow up?"

I had never heard a conversation like this. I felt a little sick to my stomach. I was stunned by Dr. Thurman's direct, blunt, almost brutal stance. I concentrated on maintaining a neutral expression, avoiding eye contact with Willie's mother, wondering what flavor ice cream Willie had chosen.

The mother stopped crying and raised her head. "Will these drugs save our Willie?" she asked.

"This is a huge clinical experiment trying to find a cure for ALL. Everyone dies of ALL now, everyone," he paused. "Children are the subjects in this experiment. The questions we are asking are, Which of the potential chemotherapeutic agents, all of them dangerous and powerful, can kill off the lymphoblasts and not the child? What is the right dose? What are the side effects?"

The mother sobbed into her tissue. The father put his arms loosely around her shoulders, but he maintained eye contact with Dr. Thurman.

"The question we face today," Dr. Thurman continued, "is NOT whether we can cure ALL but whether we can achieve remission of the disease."

In desperation, I said to the parents, "A remission means that Willie would have time at home and at school without disease."

"Nationally, we've achieved remission in some children," Dr. Thurman continued, "Remission as long as nearly a year or eighteen months." He shook his head. "We have not cured a child of ALL. I believe we will, but the only way forward is to do these trials."

"Which of the agents is best, Dr. Thurman? That's what you'll give Willie, right?"

I shuddered. I couldn't imagine that we were debating the theoretical construct of drug trials while Willie was out and about with lymphoblasts raging through his body, ready to clog up one of his cerebral arteries at any minute.

Didn't they understand? There was NO *choice.*

"If you decide to participate in the trial," Dr. Thurman said, "Willie will be blindly assigned a protocol: drugs, dosage, and frequency." What Dr. Thurman didn't say was that Willie was unlikely to live more than a year or two.

The parents signed on. Willie was admitted. Dr. Thurman opened the sealed envelope. The pharmacy delivered the drug. The night team administered it by midnight.

Dr. Thurman and I filled out the patient's baseline data, the parental consents, and clinical research forms to fax to Dallas. He explained to me that major collaborative clinical research was the only way to answer questions about rare diseases. I was a bit overwhelmed by the fervor in his voice.

Dr. Thurman believed that ALL would be a curable disease—children would not only be disease-free but grow up to be parents and grandparents. Many children died in those early years of clinical experimentation before we learned how to induce remission, maintain remission, and eventually cure almost all the children with ALL. In the long run, Dr. Thurman had been correct.

The day I spent with Willie, his parents, and Dr. Thurman was life-changing. By the end of the month of the pediatric hematology rotation, I was a convert. I didn't ask Dr. Thurman any questions. I didn't discuss my decision with Alan. I don't think I even thought about Hop's diagnosis of Hodgkin's disease.

I signed up for a fellowship in pediatric hematology.

Ordinarily, I would have completed three years of general pediatric training (one year of internship and two years of residency) before beginning a two-year subspecialty fellowship such as pediatric hematology. But Dr. Thurman negotiated with the American Academy of Pediatrics that I would combine my last year of residency with the first year of fellowship. It saved me a year of training, but it required that from July 1967 to June 1968 I'd take double night call, hematology, and the other subspecialty rotations like pediatric cardiology and pediatric neurology.

My decision to complete subspecialty training meant committing to an academic medical center where the faculty shaped the future of medicine. And maybe, to be the doctor I vowed to be that day on the porch with Hop and Dr. Ryan. I loved working elbow to elbow with a giant like Dr. Thurman. I loved being a part of a national academic experiment. I loved being in control of the patient process from diagnosis to death. I developed intense, personal relationships with children and families that I never had with my own.

Under Dr. Thurman's leadership, the Division of Pediatric Hematology grew exponentially, both in numbers and in aspirations. It was no longer enough to focus on patient care, medical education, and clinical research.

By the late fall of 1967, after only months into fellowship, I was struggling. I had been the confident one, the competent fellow, Dr. Thurman's special resident and recruit. But now that the division was mandated to initiate basic science research projects, I struggled. I couldn't seem to articulate a research question and design an experiment to find an answer.

When Dr. Thurman reminded me that my clock was ticking, I resisted. I pointed out that I hadn't elected to do basic science, I didn't like being in the lab, and I was a superb clinician. He lowered the boom just before Thanksgiving, "You signed up for a fellowship in academic medicine," he said, "and you are running out of time."

I heard the frustration in his voice. I didn't like being cornered. I started to wing it. Perhaps, I proposed, I could learn the techniques for in utero red blood cell transfusions like they're doing in Europe, maybe work with the interventional radiologists.

Dr. Thurman asked about my experimental animal model, my study design, and the budget. But before I could answer, he suggested rabbits. "Size-wise, rabbits will work. I'll find a lab."

By the Christmas holidays, I was spending my evenings with the rabbits. *Sacrifice the pregnant doe*—that was the first line of my experimental protocol. It felt like murder to me, every time. I hated the way the doe stared up at me when I positioned her on the bench, put a towel over her head, and hit her over the head with a hammer. I hated the urgency to deliver the kit from the dead doe's uterus while the other rabbits thumped in their cages. I had to pierce the heart of the kit, withdraw a blood sample, and prepare slides. Only then could I clean up the gory remains.

I hated being in the lab alone in the evening after a busy clinic with patients. *How many more rabbits did I have to order to fill the empty cages? How many data points were required for statistical significance? Why was the animal incinerator so far from the lab?*

I had nightmares of the does and their kits, the thumping sisters, and the aunties, and the sicky, sweet smell of death mingled with feces. *Why didn't I have a research mentor?* I struggled to "array" the data for meaningful conclusions. For me, preparing an abstract for the Society for Pediatric Research was a task in creative writing. I obsessed over the library searches—I had to craft the perfect literature review. I found nothing of significant clinical relevance, but my research training requirement box had been checked for the fellowship.

On the other hand, I did master, with the assistance of the ultrasound imagers, the practice of slowly and delicately transfusing 100 ccs (about three ounces) of packed red blood cells through the abdominal wall of the pregnant human woman with Rh incompatibility, through her uterine wall, and finally through the abdominal wall of the fetus. Once deposited in the peritoneum, the red cells were quickly absorbed by the fetus and used for oxygen transport, modifying the often-fatal complications of the distressed infant at birth.

"Brava!" crowed Dr. Thurman after the first transfusion. I had guided the syringe.

I enjoyed the precision. I loved the immediacy of the solution. The results were evident right away on the ultrasound. The cells were delivered precisely into the belly of the fetus. The baby was healthy at delivery. It was a happy outcome. The procedure required a team—the obstetrician, the neonatologist, the interventional radiologist, the wide-awake mother, and me. A few years later, researchers at Columbia developed Rhogam, a drug that prevented the hemolysis in the infant from occurring. Immediately, fetal transfusion became obsolete.

I was at my best working with patients—children with cancer as well as children with routine pediatric diseases, but I loved the intense focus of the inpatient wards. Sometimes parents rebelled against the hospital rules, especially rules developed by the nurses to maintain order and control. Especially those parents whose children were regularly admitted, the children with cancer.

One morning on rounds, the intern and I waited outside a hospital room as a mother harangued the nurses. I explained to my intern, "Father's faculty, mother's not easy, and Dr. Thurman's the attending physician. VIP status."

He nodded and buttoned up his white jacket.

"Tommy is an exceptional five-year-old," I said, "diagnosed with retinoblasma as a newborn, had enucleation of his eye, and been in endless chemo trials. I've followed him for the past year."

The door opened. "We're ready now."

The mother was not much older than we were. She was crisp and chic in a navy linen shift with a lime monogram and matching espadrilles, but she had dark circles under her eyes. It had been a long night. I secretly cheered her efforts to decorate the hospital room with Cat in the Hat linens and drapes—against all the nursing rules. A tape recorder played music at low volume.

Tommy looked like a battered Buddha propped up on the *Green Eggs and Ham* pillows, but I knew him to be formidable. Sweat dripped off his nose. His blue and white porcelain tummy protruded over his pj's. No matter how much he struggled to breathe, he couldn't get enough oxygen.

A pirate's patch covered the empty left socket, and the oxygen mask dangled around his neck. He hated it over his face. I twisted the knob on the green tank to up the oxygen flow to 100 percent. Tommy had fought mightily, but he was battered and bruised.

"Sorry, Tommy," I said, "I know you didn't want to come back in, but packed red cells may help your breathing."

His mother sighed, "We couldn't do it at home." She gripped the bed board with both hands.

"Not another stick," he groaned.

"The cells are here." I nodded to the mother, "Please wait outside."

The intern concentrated on the top of his swollen right foot. "Maybe this one." He collected tiny scalp-vein needles, alcohol swabs, and gauzes. I retrieved the packed red cells and an IV pole. The vein rolled when he pricked the surface.

"You can do it," Tommy urged.

"Bingo!" Red cells flowed smoothly in the tubing. Mama Cass was singing "California Dreaming." I opened the door for his mother to come back in.

"Excuse me," Tommy said to the two of us. "I need to say goodbye to Mommy."

We closed the door quietly. Our team seemed far away, laughing and shouting orders at the nurses' station.

"Did I understand Tommy correctly?"

"Yes." I nodded. "You sure did."

The charge nurse made questioning eye contact. "A little longer. Let her have a little longer with him," I said.

Not five minutes later, Dr. Thurman barreled down the corridor. By this time in my training, I no longer questioned how he knew. He just did.

"Thank you, both," he said to us and knocked on the door. "May I come in?"

I wrote Tommy's death note and called the morgue. I was relieved to be covering the public clinic for the afternoon.

As I got off the elevator, I could hear the din from the clinic waiting room. The easygoing chaos of well-baby clinic was a relief. The intern would go to the morgue with Tommy.

"Orange juice, bacon and eggs, toast, milk." That's what the public clinic mothers reported their preschoolers ate for breakfast. I didn't realize at first that they were making fun of me. They described images from popular women's magazines—children with well-scrubbed faces sitting around a breakfast table with a cheerful father at the head of the table and the aproned mother serving with a smile. I entered their dietary histories word by word in the medical chart. They snickered behind my back, nudged each other, and rolled their eyes. I didn't have a clue what families ate for breakfast in the public housing of Westhaven or the country club neighborhoods around Farmington. And they knew it.

I was jealous of the clinic mothers with their bravado, their know-it-all grins, their joking comradery. The way they greeted each other with laughter and teasing. How they knew the names of each other's kids, corrected them, and comforted them as their own.

They teased me. The lady doctor with a husband but no babies. I was aware of their giggles and eye-rolling but not of my own gullibility.

After the requisite "shots" in well-baby clinic, the nurses made a show with stickers, but it was the big sisters and the aunties and the grannies who gathered around with hugs and granted the real hero status—lollipops, the promises of an ice cream cone, maybe even a visit from Daddy before nap. In the emergency room after the broken bone was set, the waiting room cheered. Even the security guards would clap. They had community.

I was jealous. I wanted to be one of them, the laughing, full-of-themselves clinic mothers. I wanted to go to the playground, to have picnics.

I wanted to be more than a stepmother, was not really connected to Alan's kids on Cape Cod. Being a stepparent—or a stepchild—wasn't easy. Timothy called me a witch for making him collect kindling for the campfire. Gioia, even after I bailed her out of the Woods Hole jail, referred to me as the blonde floozy. And Dorothy insisted I was giving her mother headaches. I hadn't yet met Adam.

I was jealous of the clinic mothers. I wanted a family. My own family. I wanted a community. I wanted to belong.

I wanted a baby.

· 9 ·

Medicine and Motherhood

Fall 1968

After two years of marriage, Alan and I finally lived within driving distance of one another. We had phone contact and spent most weekends together at Beau Pré. But Alan was challenged by his company's focus on becoming a publicly traded company. He was required to shave his beard, wear a jacket and tie, and, every now and then, attend company socials with his wife.

For me, that meant finishing clinic early, driving two hours to DC, and changing into a cocktail dress at a gas station somewhere along the Beltway. I soon learned that there was nothing social about these affairs—OSE was being scrutinized by larger companies seeking acquisition or diversification. My role was simple—to stand by Alan, look pretty, and smile. No conversation about medicine, UVA, or the two of us living apart. I had no concept of the depth of Alan's distress.

With regular weekends at Beau Pré, we developed ways of being together—out of bed. We played cribbage and drank Heineken at the laundromat. We argued about how important it was that I learn to make pie crust. It wasn't. Alan knew how. Or scrub the bathroom floor. Again, I refused. I had done that in high school.

We never talked about money, but I worried about it all the time. Alan still didn't know about the Foods of All Nations charge account. We eventually did talk about babies. Rather, I did. At some level I understood that Alan hadn't intended to have more children—he had failed the brood on Cape Cod. I talked more and more about the clinic mothers, how I wanted a baby of our own, a baby with DNA from the both of us. Alan laughed, hugged me, and changed the subject. And I kept taking my birth control pills.

The decision about becoming pregnant had implications beyond Alan and me. I was still in training with long hours and night call. No health insurance. No leave policies. Women were an exception in medical school, training, and practice. We were "other"—tolerated, not welcome.

While I was in training, a woman physician in Boston was fired from her internship when she became pregnant. I loved that later the same woman became editor of the prestigious *New England Journal of Medicine.*

The UVA labs started providing rubella antibody tests to women of childbearing age on the staff, a public health campaign to bring awareness to the risks of congenital rubella. Dr. Thurman handed me my positive test result, grinned, and said, "You're good to go." At some irrational level, I believed that he was giving me permission, maybe even inviting me, to get pregnant.

I didn't think about Alan's wishes, the responsibilities remaining in fellowship, or my fitness as a mother. Magically, I extrapolated not being at risk for transmitting rubella to Dr. Thurman suggesting I should become pregnant. It was a complicated, inappropriate, and probably illegal message even in 1968. After an excited conversation with Alan, I stopped the pills.

The very next month, I fell asleep reading bone marrows at the dual-headed microscope, Alan applauded my breasts, and I gagged frying bacon. The baby was due early in September 1968.

Dr. Mac did not smile. "It's not seemly," he said and explained about confinement. Pregnancy was not a public process for White ladies in the South. He espoused that I should remain at home once my pregnancy was visible. My resident colleagues groused that they would have extra work, but I easily covered my clinical responsibilities. I ignored the whispers that I would not return after the baby's birth. I was healthy and carried my clinical load plus some.

Alan was exuberant. I thought it was totally due to my pregnancy, but it might have been the United Nations project that took him away from the politics of the DC office. Alan was supervising the building of an aluminum scallop boat at a shipyard in North Carolina. He was delighted that the yard was still building wooden boats, a rarity along the East Coast.

By June, my pregnancy bump was prominent, and we were excited to feel fetal movement. Alan rubbed my tummy and named the baby Dinky. On Sunday afternoons at Beau Pré, he carved and bent aged cherry into a cradle for Dinky. It looked like a cross between a rocking horse and Noah's ark.

That September I went into labor. I fussed that Alan wasn't allowed in the labor room. I fumed about being referred to as an "elderly primip" in the chart. Labor lasted fifteen hours. The pediatric anesthesiologist placed an epidural and sat with me through the second stage of labor.

Our girl baby was born face-first at 7:32 p.m. on Sunday, September 8. She was squalling, squirming, and red-faced. Alan named her Kathleen Ann because she was such a lusty little Celt. I counted fingers and toes, felt her fontanelles, and checked out her spleen to rule out congenital leukemia. Under my breath, so that Alan the Unitarian wouldn't notice, I did as the nuns had trained me and baptized her.

The next morning, Alan snuggled the two of us in his arms. I'd showered, dressed in a new peignoir, and was ready to receive the rounding teams of obstetricians and pediatricians. I brought the baby to my breast. Alan soothed me. "You're a natural, Sharon, take a deep breath." Alan knew what to do. I did not.

Dr. Thurman was our designated pediatrician, but it was Dr. Mac who walked in with outstretched hands. "Congratulations, young lady," he said. "Let's see if your milk is in." He palmed one tender breast, then the other, and chuckled. "This baby's not going to starve—well-done for a Yankee first-timer."

The following Monday was our first day alone at Beau Pré. Alan had gone back to North Carolina. The early-morning sunlight created patterns on the oak floorboards and across the cherry cradle. My plan was shaping up. We were going to get know one another. I was done with Berta's lectures about night nurses. I was tired of the resident wives and their eye-rolling comments about my not returning to work before Dinky was in kindergarten. I especially resented the queries about the whereabouts of my mother. I wouldn't let Nellie anywhere near my baby.

Friday evening, Alan was all smiles. "I hardly recognize either of you! How could you change so much in five days?"

For the first time ever, Alan and I behaved like normal people who lived together. I saw him off early Monday morning and welcomed him home on Friday. I talked about Dinky, and he talked about the aluminum boat. During the weekdays, I caught up on sleep and reading. At one month, I invited the lab team out for lunch at Beau Pré. I yearned for news of the patients, the hospital gossip, and adult conversation. They seemed surprised that I would be returning.

Dinky was six weeks old. Monday was my first day back at work. Alan was already on the road. What had I been thinking?

I looked at the stuff spread out on the cottage floor—Alan's battered leather bag full of clean cloth diapers, extra onesies, and blankets piled on top of Similac cans. My purse stuffed with patient files and a bag lunch. The bursting-at-the-seams laundry bag.

Dinky watched wide-eyed as I twitched around. At six weeks, she was cooing, smiling, and mimicking my facial moves. She was a perfect baby in all ways, but I was itching for adult contact, grown-up conversation. And feeling guilty about it.

The cocooning time was over. My first day back at work and I had made a major tactical error. I hadn't calculated the number of trips it would take to load up the VW bug to take Dinky to Mrs. Chase's home day care.

Do I leave you here in the cottage, *alone?*

Or under the boxwoods at the parking lot, *alone?*

On the first run, I was surprised to find the new neighbor Beverley running on the same schedule. When Roy left the UVA Law School for his sabbatical in July, Beverley had rented his carriage house. I'd waddled over with a loaf of warm banana bread when she arrived, but I hadn't seen her since.

I would gladly have avoided anyone bearing witness to my flustered first day back, especially Beverley, who was looking cool and professional in an aqua Lacoste dress, pumps, and shoulder bag. Her hands were entirely free—as opposed to mine, now the bag lady pediatrician. We nodded hello before she revved up her red Alpha Romeo and drove off. I returned to the cottage for the next run.

I drove away from Mrs. Chase's day care that first day with vivid images of her as a serial killer, infanticide her specialty. I forced myself not to turn around for a Dinky rescue.

Even before I got to the hospital, I was sweating. I ignored the stack of mail on my desk and focused on the list of hematology consults. So far so good, until I felt the warm wetness spread across the bodice of my Paisley shirtwaist. Not as dramatic as the night I flooded our bed and Alan had to wake me up, but not under control. I made a detour into the ladies' room to stuff Kleenex into my nursing bra, pat my dress dry, and check for stains on my lab coat. The breast pump was tucked in my bag back at the office, but there was no time. I'd have to detour around the nursery. The cries of the newborns were guaranteed to cause me to leak.

How could I pump every hour and get my work done?

Dinky must have somehow understood, at some basic physiological level of newborns, the change in our routine that first day. Even though she was only six weeks old, she slept straight through the night. I awoke in the same, curled-up, almost fetal position I had fallen asleep in. I was surprised but hopeful that that pattern would continue. Pediatricians *know* that babies usually don't sleep through the night until they weigh ten pounds. Dinky weighed only eight pounds, four ounces. I knew that because Frank Daniels, in his white apron, the butcher at Foods of All Nations, weighed her on his meat scale every week.

My account at Foods continued to grow slowly. Foods became my official bank when I learned I could charge cash as well as groceries. I worried about the growing balance, but Foods never added interest or included past-due comments. I hid the monthly bill in the drawer of the walnut secretary. But I hadn't needed to worry; Alan paid no attention to money. The small increase in my fellowship stipend covered the cost of Dinky's day care.

The second morning, I decided to schlep Dinky on the first trip and leave her in the carrier on the grass. Beverley appeared after my second load. I smiled and asked her if she would keep an eye on Dinky while I made one more quick run to the cottage. She paused, crossed her arms, and thought for a minute.

"That's absolutely all I will do. Keep an eye on her." She leaned back against the Alfa. "I don't do babies."

In the middle of that morning, I made an unannounced visit to Mrs. Chase's day care. Dinky was lying wide awake and playing with her fingers in a big baby crib. All she had on was a diaper. The room was warm, but there were no mobiles. No rattles. No toys. Mrs. Chase said she was saving Dinky's onesie from getting stained with spit-up. I assured her the bag had enough for lots of changes.

By noontimes, the bodice of my second dress was usually wet. I asked Mrs. Chase not to give Dinky formula after the two o'clock feed so she'd be ready to breastfeed as soon as we got home. My breasts were painfully engorged by midafternoon, even if I did sit on the toilet to pump whenever I had a break. There was no acceptable place other than the women's restroom to pump. No matter how efficient I was, it took me five minutes to express an ounce with the handheld suction pump. Then I had to empty it out, rinse it, and start over. Everyone at work ignored my leaking breasts. Everyone, that is, but Dr. Mac. When he'd pass me in the hall, he'd grin, mimic cow-milking, and give me a thumbs-up.

It was Wednesday morning, the third day, when Beverley, in another tidy little Lacoste dress, grabbed the laundry bag. "Where does it go?" she asked. "And when will it be ready to pick up?"

By Thursday night, I had consult reports to write after I nursed Dinky and had my own supper. Honestly, that night it was French vanilla ice cream straight out of the container, flashing back to my internship year, but then I had topped it off with Vermont maple syrup. Alan had brought me a gift last weekend, a record with *How to Belly-dance* on one side and *How to Strip* on the other. I didn't need reminders that my belly was no longer taut and flat. No maple syrup on my ice cream that night.

By the time we climbed the circular staircase, it was eleven, and I hadn't bathed Dinky. Who had ever told me a daily baby bath was required? I sudsed Dinky up, supported her head, and washed behind her ears and her neck—as though she could possibly have gotten dirty at day care.

As I picked her out of the basin to dry her, Dinky slid through my hands. I was frantic as I reached for her slippery little body. I had terrifying images of her hitting the floor. But, at the very last second, I secured a firm grip on her ankle. Dinky was dangling upside down. She let loose a bloody howl. I wrapped her in a towel, rubbed her dry, and snuggled her close My adrenaline surged. I had almost dropped her on her head. When I tucked her in, I thanked the powers that protect little babies, and I vowed to screw daily bathing. I would never, ever tell anyone, not even Alan. Especially not Dr. Thurman.

By Friday of the first week back, I was relieved to sit quietly at the microscope, reading and reporting out the slides from the bone marrows done that week. I was grateful to be alone in the lab when, once again, I fell sound asleep at the scope. At supper, Alan kidded me about the red indentations around my eyes, just before he checked in on my progress with the striptease moves. Every aspect of my pregnant and postpartum body seemed to remain a powerful aphrodisiac for him.

Alan was in constant motion all weekend. He had to introduce Dinky to the trees and the falling leaves in the yard. He guided her tiny palms across the rough furrows of American black walnut bark, tossed walnuts up in the air as she shrieked in delight, and then identified the patterns of the leaf veins. Alan modified her cherry cradle to carve out handles midway on each side so that I could move it from by the fire to by the window. We went to the laundromat in the afternoon. Dinky napped in her carrier while we played cribbage. I marveled that I, Sharon Lee Hostler, the barmaid and the party girl, now yearned for a washing machine and an early bedtime on a Saturday night.

The next Monday morning I spotted Beverley waiting by the Alfa. Thank God.

"The laundry?" she said. I thought I detected the trace of a smile.

"I'll get it." I set the carrier down in the grass. "Keep an eye on her?"

She laughed. "I guess I've signed on for the duration."

"I'll be right back."

And so the routine was established. No discussion. No fanfare. Beverley assumed responsibility for the daily laundry run: drop off in the morning, pickup and delivery after work. She didn't talk to Dinky. She didn't look at Dinky. She managed Dinky's laundry.

Initially, she dropped the laundry package by the cottage door for me to find. But, after a few weeks, Beverley would call the cottage and ask, "Are you done?" By "done," she meant had I finished breastfeeding. Berta disapproved of my return to work even more than my not having a night nurse. She was clearly miffed when Beverley started dropping off the laundry. I didn't realize how isolated Berta was.

After a few weeks of this routine, I shared my chili or beef stew with Beverley. She'd arrive with her Scotch on the rocks in hand. Dr. Thurman had recruited her from Miami, where she'd worked with families of children with disabilities at the Mailman Child Development Clinic.

Beverley moved to Virginia to work with Dr. Miriam Birdwhistle, the chief of social work from the University of Pennsylvania. Dr. Birdwhistle was a tiny woman physically, but she had an outsized intellect and was an unapologetic feminist. She challenged the pediatric faculty in the middle of rounds and advocated for immunizing teenage girls against pregnancy. I would never have admitted it at the time, but I was intimidated by Dr. Thurman's new recruits—nurses, social workers, psychologists, and social science researchers. They operated as independent professionals, very different from the hospital nurses. But I learned a lot from these recruits, especially Beverley.

Beverley would ask me a few questions, then settle back by the fire to listen. I talked about my sick patients, the different kinds of leukemia, and the big clinical trials, the Group B and the Southwest groups. I couldn't wait to tell her when I was the one from UVA to call Paris to register the one-hundredth child in the world to live five years with ALL. Beverley listened, nodded, and sipped her Scotch. I explained it was not a cure, but it was progress.

We shared stories about work and then, gradually, where we'd come from. Beverley was the oldest of four children, two girls and two boys, all of whom water-skied on the bayou behind their home in Bradenton, Florida, sometimes right over the backs of sleeping alligators. Her mother, Alice, had her own tree house where she regularly retreated. Harry, her father, owned a shoe store where all the kids worked. It was a lot different from growing up with Hop and Nellie.

On Thanksgiving, Alan told me about the official launch of the aluminum scallop boat. My presence was required by Alcoa and OSE.

"Dinky's only three months old," I said. "You want me to drive with Dinky all the way to New Bern?"

"It's only four hours."

At work, I made excuses when Dr. Thurman wanted to review my experimental rabbit data. No way that data was going to be helpful clinically. The National Cancer Institute (NCI) in DC had an opening for an inpatient clinician for pediatric cancer trials, and Dr. Thurman thought I should interview. I was set to complete my fellowship in June 1969.

So many questions. What was I going to do with Dinky when I had to go into the hospital at night? Would Alan and I live together in DC next year? Should I restart my birth control pills? How long was I going to nurse Dinky? What was I going to wear to the christening in North Carolina?

It would be windy and bone-deep chilly on the pier in New Bern in December. When I complained to Beverley about my wardrobe dilemma, she offered me her new leather coat. She was only five foot four, and I was five foot seven, almost eight, but I fit into her full-length, coffee-colored leather coat. On me, it was closer to knee-length, but it was still elegant and toasty warm. I'd wear leather gloves and an orange silk scarf.

Dinky and I started our adventure in the dark and drizzle. She babbled for a while, even laughed aloud some, and then slept the rest of the way. My overnight things were stuffed in her diaper bag. The sun peeked out of the clouds by the time we reached New Bern. The decorated bottle cracked smartly on the first swing. Champagne flutes were passed. Sips were taken and photographs snapped. News summaries released to members of the press. The self-satisfied men shook hands, nodded a lot, and patted each other's backs. Alan was pleased.

I smiled and jounced Dinky around the pier. She gurgled and giggled until she burped. She burped up what we knew in the family as a wet blouie—a blouie all over the shoulder of Beverley's leather coat.

That next Monday morning in the parking lot at Beau Pré was awkward. I handed Beverley the laundry bag, but I kept the suede coat. "I'm taking it to the dry cleaners."

"It's only the second time it's been worn."

"There's been a blouie."

"A Dinky blouie?" Beverley laughed and slammed the door to the Alfa. "It's just a coat."

The stain never came out. Beverley and I got to be best friends anyway.

· 10 ·

Juggling in a Long White Coat

Christmas 1968–July 1970

That Christmas, I decorated the cottage with shiny magnolia leaves I'd soaked in pails of acetone when I was home with Dinky. There was no dancing on New Year's Eve, but Peter brought champagne and black-eyed peas for New Year's Day. Dinky entertained us with blowing bubbles and belly laughs. I was wound up about my interview at the National Cancer Institute in Bethesda for an inpatient attending position. Alan had his nose in books and atlases preparing for an international project—the collaborative measurements of the depths, temperatures, and currents of the Indian Ocean with a team of Russian oceanographers. Beverley was in Florida with her family. I was back on hematology night call after my laboratory stretch. There was no such thing as family leave in 1968—the Family and Medical Leave Policy wasn't enacted until 1993.

The UVAH maintained a small day care for nurses working the night shift—11:00 p.m. to 7:00 a.m. I assumed that if I had to go into the hospital in the middle of the night, I would be permitted to plop Dinky down there in her carrier. I wouldn't be gone for long, less than an hour. My strategy worked the first time and the second, but not the third. The head nurse read me the riot act—the very special day care, nighttime-only service was for the infants of nurses, not doctors. Even Dr. Thurman's intervention failed. Dr. Mac refused to try. He didn't believe I should be at work, certainly not taking night call or bringing my baby along.

I carried Dinky to bedside when the ward team needed assistance with one of our hematology patients. I had no other choice. It was January 1969, the last six months of my fellowship. During the day, I saw patients referred to Dr. Thurman in private clinics.

"How many times have you been pregnant? Miscarriages? Births?" Standard questions from the medical history I asked the mother, Lillie, who had brought four-year-old Sammy from Kentucky for consultation with Dr. Thurman. She was my age, poised, and well put together in a cashmere sweater dress with a matching teal scarf. Her son had a rare tumor of the smooth muscle in his middle ear, a rhabdomyosarcoma, an almost always fatal cancer. It was a strange tumor in a strange place. Sammy challenged us. He was, as we'd whispered before they arrived, an interesting case.

"Two pregnancies, no miscarriages, two children. Sam's little sister will be two next week. My health is great now," she paused, took a deep breath, and continued. "I had a double mastectomy and chemotherapy between their births. I was godawful sick and very nearly got divorced in the process. Now this."

My eyes must have widened, for she added, "It just gets better and better. He's still mourning the loss of *his breasts*—his words, I swear to God. You can guess how he's handling this development with Sammy. He refused to come here with us."

I passed her the box of Kleenex from the bedside table.

"No question in his mind—it's all my fault. He can't get it up in bed, either. My fault again, he misses my tits!" She sobbed quietly. Sammy abandoned playing with his truck. He sat cross-legged on the floor, leaning against his mother's knees.

Even after three years of training, sitting quietly with someone in distress was an acquired skill for me. Abiding did not come naturally to me. I had to remind myself to keep quiet, to focus on her, to follow her cues. Beverley coached me. Social workers were good at nodding, not interrupting, and listening.

Lillie wiped her eyes, ruffled Sammy's hair, and lifted the corners of her lips into a smile. "Now, where were we?"

I learned that her mother, two maternal aunts, her mother's mother, and maybe a great-aunt had all died of breast cancer. It was unusual enough that Sammy had a rare rhabdomyosarcoma, but now to learn that his mother's family had such a strong history of breast cancer was puzzling. As I put the pieces together in my own mind, I wondered if she had considered Sammy's little sister and her future health.

After clinic, I headed to the library, conducted a literature search, and found a few case reports of rhabdomyosarcoma in the offspring of mothers with breast cancer. It was eponymously called Li's syndrome after the physician who first reported the association.

In the late 1960s, scientists recognized that some cancers were associated with and probably caused by chemicals like coal tar, radiation, and viruses—Epstein-Barr virus in lymphoma or hepatitis B in liver cancer. Risk for some cancers like breast, thyroid, and ovarian seemed to be inherited, but the genetic mechanisms were not yet understood. Since 1953, when Watson and Crick had demonstrated the double-helix structure of DNA, scientists had hypothesized that alterations to DNA by agents and viruses induced cancer. My patient Sammy and his mother presented ideal subjects for such an exploration.

"An intriguing clinical study, Sharon, has fallen into your lap," Dr. Thurman beamed. "The National Cancer Institute (NCI) is right up the road, and you're headed there in July." I grimaced as he continued, "So many laboratory tools to explore their cells. We've no idea of the genetic and metabolic paths to carcinogenesis. Plus, you've established great rapport with this patient's mother. And you're good at skin biopsies!"

I was reluctant to consider Lillie and Sammy research subjects. Lillie had ended up sleeping on the couch at Beau Pré when Sammy came back to the hospital for experimental chemotherapy.

I recognized the signs of pregnancy in April 1969, even though I had restarted the pill and just stopped breastfeeding. Alan wrote on the chalkboard in the OSE conference room, "ATTENTION: *I've knocked up Sharon a second time! Hurray.*"

It was Lillie who brought the champagne the night when Alan arrived home with two dozen red roses. Lillie easily joined Beverley, Peter, and Alan as they toasted me. Later, I traveled twice to Kentucky—to gather more family samples and to attend Sammy's funeral.

In Minneapolis that May, I gave my first national presentation, a classic ten-minute talk at the annual meeting of the American Public Health Association (APHA). It was a very short story about Sammy's, Lillie's, and Lillie's family's cells. No feelings. No adjectives. Not even proper names.

I found myself, unexpectedly, in a press room surrounded by science writers from the leading science journals and the major newspapers in North America. I was stunned as they asked sophisticated questions about carcinogenesis, fluidly comparing my work with recently released abstracts from around the world. They shouted questions, interrupted me, and elbowed one another for the microphone. I focused on the exit door, but the exit door was behind the mob of reporters. Their haranguing was at a theoretical level beyond my basic fund of knowledge.

I smiled confidently and gave very short answers. I repeated the points of my talk exactly as Dr. Thurman had drilled me to do. Finally, the cadre of very smart reporters let me go. I worried that, somehow, I had failed Lillie and Sammy. I felt like a scientific poseur, an imposter.

Dr. Thurman shook my hand with great formality. Lillie sent yellow sweetheart roses. I received congratulatory calls, long-distance even, from friends. There were my photo and an article about the APHA presentation on page three of the *Washington Post.*

I still remember the terror of being cornered in the press room in Minneapolis, my brain going blank, and yearning for an escape route. I belonged at the bedside with patients and their families. I never told Dr. Thurman how frightened I was.

Dr. Thurman interceded with the NCI to delay my official start for a year. My due date was early November 1969. Officially, I'd complete my fellowship in July, but I would continue working in hematology, attend in the Children and Youth (C&Y) clinics, and postpone the start of my position at the NCI until July 1970.

I had another conference to attend in May, the Society for Pediatric Research in San Francisco. I had no research abstracts to present. Alan was back from the Indian Ocean project and stayed with Dinky. It seemed very strange to be the one flying off.

At the conclusion of the first day's program, someone touched my elbow and whispered, "The weather tomorrow is going to be sunny. I'd be honored if you'd join me."

I was startled, but unwilling to ignore the handsome man, so formal in his posture, accent, and mustache. "Skip the meeting?"

"Yes, let's explore the Napa Valley, pack a picnic, and sip pinot noir." Zsolt Koppanyi was a pediatrician from Johns Hopkins University.

"Sounds like a plan," I replied.

The next morning, we headed out of the city, north and a little east to Napa Valley. I read the map. Both of us wore gold wedding bands.

We sat on the ground by bushes loaded with ripe blackberries for our picnic. We laughed and told stories. His wife was the first violinist of the symphony. They had a son. My husband, an oceanographer usually traveling hither and yon, was caring for our ten-month-old daughter. No names were shared.

It had been a long time since I'd had this kind of adventure. I was past the fatigue of first trimester. I enjoyed how my breasts had popped the top button on my dress.

Zsolt grinned and helped me up from the ground. I felt the briefest touch on my waist. It was delicious. We strolled around the vineyard, my pregnant hand within his protective hand as we inspected the lushness of the spring growth. Back at the hotel, Zsolt gave me a grown-up hug at the elevator.

"What time shall I collect you? I'll find a Hungarian restaurant with goulash with just the right amount of paprika, a little gypsy music for dancing."

"I'm not sure," I said, blushing. I got on the elevator. "No, I can't," I said and pushed the button for my floor.

I called the airline to change my return flight. Alan sounded puzzled, but he agreed to meet the red-eye at Dulles in the morning, two full days earlier than scheduled.

The summer of 1969 brought many changes. Dinky was crawling and managed to start up the circular staircase in the cottage. Alan was back wearing a coat and tie as OSE prepared to go public. I completed residency in pediatrics and fellowship in pediatric hematology without ceremony or celebration, but my lab coat was long, with *Dr. Hostler* embroidered in red thread over the left pocket—the symbol for faculty status in the hospital.

At the beginning of July, I learned about the C&Y clinics from Dr. Thurman and Beverley. The C&Y Project was part of President Johnson's War on Poverty program. Dr. Thurman had lobbied for the funding for Charlottesville and Albemarle County—the system of neighborhood clinics scoffed at by the faculty from the Law School and even some at the School of Medicine.

My real mentors were Clariece Harris, the Black nurse in the city clinic, and Helen Wright, the Black nurse in Esmont. It was an ongoing competition. Helen was the country sage to Clariece's city diva. I was often caught between their conflicting philosophies of healthcare and life. In the city clinic, we had a bathroom right off the waiting room with a tub. Clariece required that our patients be scrubbed with soap and hot water before they were put in an exam room. "How else are they going to learn?"

Helen fussed at me from day one. "How many times do I have to remind you that this family has no running water? Stop telling folks to soak in hot water and scrub with soap. Not going to happen. If you want the sores to heal, prescribe the topical antibiotic. Why are you so darned stingy?"

The city clinic operated daily. It was located on the UVA Corner tucked between the pediatric public clinic and the railroad tracks. Families either walked or took a city bus to reach the clinic. I examined fifty children a day in the city clinic, most of them initial well-child checks, but each day a few children were acutely ill. Clariece was skilled at triage. She kept all parts moving, including me. Each day at five o'clock, the clinic was empty. This pregnancy, it was Clariece, not Dr. Birdsong, who fussed about my swollen ankles.

The county clinics met weekly in four locations. Each clinic had a primary nurse and what Dr. Thurman called an indigenous outreach worker, someone who was raised in that community. The Earlysville patients seen in the firehouse north of town and the Crozet patients seen in the Women's Center west of town were predominantly White. Patients at the Keswick clinic in the railroad station to the east and the Esmont clinic to the south were mostly Black. Transportation was a major problem in the rural area. Many children in the county had never seen a physician or gotten any of their shots. In 1967, immunizations were not required to attend school. Many had been born at home.

When I arrived at C&Y, Helen protested the weekly meeting I instituted for staff. Medical rounds was my soap box to advocate for immunizations and preventive care. I shared the data about tetanus—50 percent survival even in an intensive care unit; the sequelae of measles—blindness, deafness, even encephalitis; and polio with paralysis. My goal was 100 percent immunization. Helen spoke for the others when she noted that there were things that I still needed to learn about healing. Once a month, the staff were the teachers—the medicinal use of herbs, the right season, and the best places to collect them, how to dry and store them. As they started to trust me, they took on language—high blood versus bad blood, meaning hypertension and syphilis. Finally, they addressed the proper etiquette of the home visit. I should take off the white lab coat, wear flats, and accept the food offered me. Decades later, after many seminars on organizational behavior, I would recognize that Dr. Thurman, Beverley, Clariece, and Helen had been my first and finest mentors.

The clinic core teams included not only the medical team but also social workers and nutritionists. Each morning, the county teams packed up exam tables, trunks of medical equipment, and clinic charts in an old VW bus. Their last stop before driving out to the county clinic was to pick up hot vegetable soup, cheese, and the PB&J sandwiches prepared from USDA excess. All families received a morning snack and lunch. I had the luxury of arriving after the clinic was set up and the families registered, with the kids waiting to be seen. Initially, I worried that I didn't have easy access to the hospital lab and X-ray, but I learned to trust my clinical acumen. I learned to love clinic.

One evening early that November, Alan and Beverley watched me sewing lace on a borrowed bassinet. Dinky was asleep in her big-girl crib, unaware of how her world was about to change. The baby was past due. I was scheduled to be induced the following morning.

Alan had oiled the cradle. I'd wrapped wooden building blocks for Dinky to open when she visited me in my hospital room. I still had a pile of medical charts to finish from clinic. Both pregnancies had been easy for me, but I dreaded another long labor. I remembered Dinky's face-first presentation and that prolonged second stage. So much for the myth about the amnesia of childbirth.

I failed the Pitocin drip, not even a tiny cramp. I was dismissed at the end of the day, instructed to return for another trial in the morning. I went into labor while I was getting dressed and delivered a boy in thirty minutes. It was my turn to do the naming. It would be Dylan, the Welsh word for ocean, with Alan as the middle name.

When Dinky visited, she unwrapped the wooden blocks and, one by one, threw them at me in the hospital bed. She ignored the baby. I realized later that she could have thrown the blocks at Dylan.

A week later, I flew with baby Dee to Shreveport, Louisiana, to check out the mobile clinic under construction for C&Y. Breastfeeding was a piece of cake this time. At home, Beverley not only picked up Dinky from day care but shared sleepovers. Alan was in DC, being corporate.

All hell broke loose two weeks later. Alan called to announce that OSE had gone public and his shares were worth fifty thousand dollars. He was on his way home. I had brief thoughts about the Foods of All Nations bill, a washer-dryer, and, fleetingly a diamond ring, but I was busy with Dinky and Dee.

Alan arrived two hours later. He was grinning from ear to ear. When Dinky grabbed his pant leg, he swung her up on his shoulder. I kept nursing Dee. What was happening?

"We're going sailing," he said. "We're going to sail around the world. It's a great way to raise the kids." He danced with Dinky, laughed, and popped the champagne cork.

"I've found a solid fifty-foot sailboat in Annapolis, beamy and comfortable, easy to sail. Don't worry," he said to me. "You'll be able to handle the helm."

I wondered if Alan had lost his mind—*sail around the world?* In medical school, we'd talked about immigrating to the north end of New Zealand's South Island. The application process was long and tedious, but we completed it. The government welcomed Alan's oceanographic engineering skills, but they had no use for a pediatrician. No chance for a license to practice. No room on the faculty. Maybe I could tutor the medical students.

In the spirit of adventure, I had applied and interviewed for the position of maternal and child health director for the Virgin Islands—St. Thomas, St. Johns, and St. Croix. The salary wouldn't cover our cost of living. Fresh produce, dairy products, and fresh water had to be imported. Then there was the question of the schools. Besides, I had had a position waiting for me at the National Cancer Institute in Washington, DC.

I watched as Alan spun around with Dinky, spouting about the adventures that lay ahead. It wasn't until he asked me if I wanted to drive to Annapolis the next day to check out the boat that I lost it—totally lost it.

What the hell will I do with Dee's diapers? Rinse his bottom with sea water?

And Dinky? Put her in a harness like Nellie did me?

And what about me? I finished sixteen years of school, four years of medical school, and four years of postgraduate training. You think I can pick up a few locum tenens positions in port, bartending a shift or two while you teach the kids to fish or go find shells on the beach? Let's look at the listings for an academic pediatrician in the Virgin Islands. What about the requirements for medical licensing and malpractice insurance in Jamaica?

Dee was three weeks old. Dinky was fourteen months old. Yes, I had just gone on a business trip, breastfed Dee, and everyone survived. But sailing around the world? No damn way.

Disappointed, Alan drove back to DC the next morning. By afternoon, he'd bought a shipyard in North Carolina that built wooden boats. His business partner was Peter Johnson, another disillusioned scientist at OSE. That weekend, they located a houseboat to share as living quarters.

Alan and I didn't discuss sailing around the world again.

My return to work after delivering two children to day care was a challenge even with Beverley's assistance. I was grateful that my days at C&Y clinic had a later start than the days on inpatient service. I needed a different day-care set-up. And a larger place to live.

When I was late picking up the kids, Mrs. Chase was not interested in my excuse. She had the kids dressed in snowsuits, strapped into their carriers, and the dirty laundry packaged—all lined up at her front door.

In desperation, I convinced one of the taxi drivers who parked on the Corner, Mr. Brown, to be on call late afternoons. If I were in the ER performing a spinal tap on my C&Y patient, I'd call him. He'd pick up Dinky and Dee and drive them around town until I was done. The kids loved the excitement. The handover to me was never more than an hour. But Mrs. Chase wasn't happy handing over the kids. She was White. Mr. Brown was Black. I didn't have time for better problem-solving. My working strategy was to hope that we would make it until we moved to DC in June.

On Christmas morning, Alan put out a doll with blonde braids and red bows under our tree. I dressed Dinky in a red velvet jumper and white tights. She took one look at the lights and spewed her orange juice. I have a photograph of Alan in a red Viyella shirt and red socks. He's sitting in an armchair feeding a bottle to Dee. Dinky stands at his arm and watches, dangling the baby doll. All I remember from that Christmas is that Beverley gave us a set of Georg Jensen stainless flatware with a check tucked inside the chest for three thousand dollars, the balance of my Foods of All Nations account. It was a lot of money. She couldn't stand my anxiety and had accessed her life insurance policy for the cash.

Alan had never known about the Foods bill and still didn't.

Mr. Brown's being on call at the end of the day reduced my stress, but I still had night call. Inpatient call for Dr. Thurman's patients in February 1970 was an unexpected challenge. I was called to the hospital for a dying three-year-old with leukemia around ten o'clock. I had no choice but to bring the kids, both asleep. I tucked Dinky into the second bed in the hospital room on South Two and put Dylan in the corner on the floor in his infant carrier. I sat with the parents at bedside as their three-year-old struggled to breathe.

She died around midnight. My kids didn't wake up.

It was two when I crawled into my own bed after consoling the family, obtaining the autopsy permit, and writing the attending death note. Dinky never stirred, even when I tucked her into her own bed.

I was deep asleep when my phone rang. It was the nurse asking about the kids.

"What are you talking about? It's five o'clock in the morning," I said. "My kids are sound asleep." The ward nurse wouldn't hang up. She kept haranguing me.

"Okay, okay. I'll check, but this is crazy." I turned on the light. "I just got to bed! Alright then, okay, I'm awake. I'm out of bed." I put down the phone. "I am going to check."

Moments later, I grabbed the phone. "I'll be right there."

I pulled my trench coat on over my nightgown, slipped into my sneakers, and left Dinky asleep in her bed as I went to retrieve Dee. I'd left him sound asleep in his infant seat in the corner of the hospital room.

I parked illegally in front of the hospital and raced up the stairs. The bright lights were disorienting, but there was four-month-old Dee in his infant seat on the counter of the nurses' station. He was blowing bubbles. Relieved, I snuggled my flushed face in his baby belly. He pulled at my hair and giggled.

"This is Dee, formally Dylan Alan Dimock," I announced to the nurses standing nearby. "And I bet he needs a diaper change."

"Dr. Hostler," the head nurse said, smiling at me, "we were pretty sure he belonged to you, but you came on the floor before our change of shift at eleven."

"Did you call Social Service?" I said and remembered that Kaki was asleep at home. Alone.

"No way, Dr. Hostler. But the day shift might have."

I picked up Dylan and fled. I worried that my car had been towed. What if Dinky woke up all alone—like that Christmas when I was six?

What was I doing? My routine was as crazy as sailing around the world.

Dr. Thurman and I usually met at his office for our weekly check-ins, a process that was part and parcel of my junior faculty status. He expected updates on C&Y, the hematology consult service, and the status of my scholarly writing. It was a sunny day, even though it was late February. We walked on a path up from Hospital Drive to the Lawn.

When it was my turn to speak, I said, "Dr. Thurman, I'm having second thoughts about the NCI position. Maybe I should get a degree in public health—do something without emergencies and night call." It was a relief not to be sitting across the desk from him—without eye contact or my shame.

"Well, now," he said with a chuckle. "I hear that Dee was the center of attention the other morning."

Of course, it had been naïve to think that Dr. Thurman would miss anything that happened in the hospital. Of course, he knew. The nurses probably called Dr. Thurman before they called me. And told Dr. Mac when he strolled in for early-morning rounds.

I clenched my jaw to control the tear ducts. My breasts were leaking, too, but I had my lab coat for cover.

"Let's think about it. July is five months off."

Then we discussed the fifteen-year-old girl who had died from sepsis. Three days ago, she'd come to the C&Y clinic in rural Esmont. We admitted her. Her grandmother had botched the abortion. She had used a hanger. *Did it matter whether it was rusty? Why was abortion only available for the rich and famous? And when would there be access to oral birth control?*

What about the protest at the University of Michigan demanding admission of Black students? Could we imagine the coat-and-tie undergraduates at Mr. Jefferson's University inviting President Shannon for dinner and staging a massive sit-in? Unlikely.

The local division of the American Dental Association had hired someone to tail the C&Y van as the driver picked up children for dental appointments, protesting government interference with local competition. Kids living in poverty—and, what was unspoken, Black children—didn't deserve clean teeth and braces.

The very next week, Dr. Thurman was in high dudgeon. I was barely settled in the chair when he announced that Dr. Dimitri, the C&Y medical director, had had a heart attack and died last night. Dr. Thurman had recruited Dr. Dimitri from Chicago to be the C&Y medical director. I only knew him by sight. He was a behind-the-desk kind of doctor—writing memos, developing protocols, preparing reports for Congress. I'd never seen him with a patient.

"You'll make a strong medical director," Dr. Thurman said to me. "What do you think? You're a competent clinician, and the C&Y staff work well with you. You're still too demanding as a teacher, and that needs to change, but you understand the goals of the C&Y Project."

"Not go to the NCI in July?" I asked. "Stay here? Seriously, I could stay at UVA?"

"Absolutely!" He laughed, "I heard you've made some home visits out in the hollers."

I nodded and grinned.

"You didn't really wear your lab coat? Did you?"

Yes. I'd worn the lab coat, but I didn't take a folded newspaper to sit on like the public health nurse instructed me to do. I'd accepted and eaten the cake offered. The C&Y team had mentored me well. I gave up my heels, but I refused to give up the lab coat.

"I'd like to send out a memo to the staff and faculty. What do you think? No night call. No need for an MPH."

"I feel bad about the NCI, especially after they held the position for me."

"I'll call them, if you'd like. We're colleagues, blood club buddies from training years and the Southwest Collaborative."

I nodded yes. I was already thinking about finding a larger place to live and a better day-care arrangement. I was relieved not to be moving to DC, especially when Alan might end up at the shipyard in North Carolina. Peter would miss Beau Pré the most.

I drove home to call Alan.

"Hurray!" he said. "What's the salary? What kind of office? I'll get the Dom Perignon and see you by six."

The pressure was off. I weaned Dylan from the breast. I didn't tell Alan about leaving Dylan in the hospital.

It never occurred to me to ask about salary or an office. I still shared an office space with the fellows by the lab and in the city clinic with Clariece.

I never knew what kind of annual raise I would receive until I opened my August paycheck. My intern's salary in 1965 had been $2,100. Each year of training, it went up a little. I eked out living expenses with my residency loans from the AAP and the float from my account at Foods. Money wasn't something we talked about at work.

And certainly not at home.

It was a privilege for me to be a doctor and to be at UVA and, secretly, to be one of the boys. Dr. Thurman was not only my department chair but my academic mentor and the pediatrician for our kids.

Perhaps that explains why I trusted him.

Completely.

· 11 ·

A Safe Landing

July 1970–July 1971

Dr. Thurman sent out the memo. Alan and I toasted my faculty appointment with Peter and Beverley over the weekend of the Fourth of July 1970. Right away, Alan started talking about a farm in the country. Beverley lobbied for a place big enough for Great Danes. I hoped my faculty salary would cover in-home childcare. I wondered about the meeting scheduled with Dr. Merrill on Monday. I didn't know what it was about.

Professor Robert E. Merrill had been recruited from Vanderbilt University by Dr. Thurman to direct our residency program. He was known for his sense of humor and his bedside teaching. Our only interactions had been at the bedside and had been professional. I had no idea why he had asked to meet with me, but I soon found out.

"You're staying on faculty?"

"Yes, sir." I smiled. I was pleased to have a three-year faculty appointment as both assistant professor of pediatrics at the University of Virginia and attending pediatrician at the UVAH. I had never considered the possibility of academic pediatrics.

Women were rare in academic medicine, but a little more frequent in pediatrics, psychiatry, and public health. In 1970, women constituted 1.2 percent of US medical school faculty (AAMC data).

"It's a damned mistake!" He slammed his fist against the desk.

I wasn't sure I'd heard him correctly. I squeezed my hands together in my lap, took a deep breath, and tried to sit quietly.

"Sir?" I felt the flush begin. "I don't understand."

"We trained you to be one of us. Trained you to be one of the boys."

"Yes, sir." I couldn't imagine what could be wrong with that.

"We trained you to be an alley fighter. That's not going to work."

I felt the tears forming. I squinted my eyes to keep them at bay.

"You're a woman in a man's world." He took a deep breath. "In the South." He scowled, stood up behind his desk and shouted, "*You're an alley-fighting woman in the South.*"

"Dr. Merrill?"

"Instead of the rusty pipe we hoodlums use in the alley, I guess we could get you a ladylike pipe, sterling or something."

He sat back down, lowered his head into his hands, and muttered, "You don't have a snowball's chance in hell!"

I let myself out. I didn't sob until I got in the car.

Five years earlier, Dr. Thurman had defended me when the chair of Surgery wanted me to wear a starched shirt with the Ben Casey clerical collar, sturdy oxford shoes, and white hose like the nurses wore. I wasn't a nurse. I was a doctor.

Three years after that, Dr. Mac called me unseemly when I was eight months pregnant on the inpatient ward. "In the South, we believe in confinement for our women."

Dr. Aldrich, the pediatric surgeon, regularly expressed to me and anyone else listening that he preferred his *Southern ladies on pedestals. Not on call. Not at the podium.*

One month ago, UVA had a week of coat-and-tie protests on Grounds that ended May Day. Admission of women to the University was one of five demands on the petition presented by students to UVA President Shannon. In objection, the *Cavalier Daily* printed a column projecting the end of the Honor System should women be admitted. "Women Have No Honor" was their headline.

I didn't get it at the time. Dr. Merrill wasn't being deliberately mean. I would learn in time that he had been correct.

I had worked hard at being one of the boys since before medical school. As a resident, I'd worked at being smarter, earlier to morning rounds, and later for evening sign-out. And at being a bully just like them. Dr. Merrill understood the consequences of those behaviors. I did not.

Being one of the boys had become a negative for me, an obstacle in my professional life. Being a bully was unseemly for a woman in medicine, especially in the South. If I could have really heard him, maybe I might have asked him for help. Maybe he would have agreed to mentor me or to identify a wise role model—man or woman—to take me on. But I didn't understand.

Dr. Merrill predicted I would fail as a faculty member. I didn't.

But, if I had understood what Dr. Merrill was trying to say, I could have smoothed out my many rough edges, acquired some new skills, and succeeded sooner. I was twenty-nine-years old, married to Alan, mother of two toddlers, and newly appointed to the School of Medicine faculty. It would have been a perfect time to change. Maybe even flourish.

I didn't.

The position of medical director turned out to be more complicated than I had anticipated—far more than scheduling coverage for the city clinic and the outlying clinics. In my first week, I had meetings at the health departments and the public schools, a cameo appearance at an anthropology class at the University, and a sex education course for a private school in town, St. Anne's–Belfield School. I worked on C&Y reports on the weekends.

Dr. Thurman received a US Public Health Service (USPHS) training grant for ten dental school graduates to spend six weeks at UVA that summer. They were to learn rural public health practices by rotations through the C&Y clinics, home visits with the family health workers, and a curriculum on childhood diseases. It was my responsibility to create the schedules, design the curriculum, and deliver the daily lectures or recruit other faculty to do them. And Dr. Thurman asked me to host the graduation party at the end of the summer.

The numbers of newly registered families, clinic visits, and interim status reports were shared freely with me, but not the details of the C&Y budget.

"Don't worry," Dr. Thurman said. "Peggy will take care of everything." Peggy was Peggy Denby, an attractive, well-dressed young woman whose political and social status seemed equal to or greater than that of most faculty.

I could handle fifty patients a day in the city clinic with the support of Clariece. She managed the medical supplies, the clinic schedule, and the clinic flow. She knew the families and their histories. She recognized sick from skipping school. She established the priorities. Clariece was a licensed practical nurse (LPN), educated at the Jackson P. Burley High School in a segregated program created by the UVA Hospital in 1951 to address the nursing shortage. Black students were not permitted to study at the School of Nursing on Grounds. It was these nurses who desegregated the UVA Hospital in the early 1960s.

The C&Y research coordinator, Patty Cormier, prepared reports to the federal funding agency, the Office for Maternal Child Health (MCH). Patty was from Boston, accountable and precise. She hounded me for the numbers of new patients registered, annual health screenings, return visits, subspecialty referrals, hospitalizations, and immunizations. I wasn't interested in the data-crunching, but I was always enthusiastic when Dr. Thurman suggested new electives for medical students or a rotation for second-year pediatric residents. Of course, I'd develop an outreach strategy for Head Start programs.

We needed physicians to work in all the C&Y clinics. I needed help as I took on what seemed to be burgeoning responsibilities. Dr. Thurman concurred.

"See Peggy." he said. "She'll know."

I found Peggy's office in the private clinics, next door to the offices for Drs. Mac and Thurman. The nameplate on her desk read "Department Administrator." She directed me to the Human Resources Department, where I was handed additional paperwork to justify new positions. I was still working in city clinic and with the teams out in the county.

The C&Y Project had social workers trained in community organization with whom I had little contact. It seemed they hung around the general stores out in the county, talking up the locals and learning about the local political dynamics. Beverley explained their intent was to achieve more low-income housing, coaching our families through the red-tape barriers to sign up for Food Stamps or Aid to Dependent Children (ADC) benefits, and the creation of entry-level jobs. I was surprised when the community organization guys invited me, as the new medical director, to listen to a Dick Gregory tape with them. *They had some suggestions for me.*

I accepted the invitation.

I'd never heard of Dick Gregory. He was a Black stand-up comedian who had, on live television, insisted on sitting *on the couch* with Jack Paar. It seemed the couch had been reserved for White guests. When Gregory was jailed and beaten for protesting in Birmingham, Alabama, he told reporters, "It was just body pain, though. The Negro has a callus growing on his soul, and it's getting harder and harder to hurt him there."

As the Gregory tape opened, we heard a few jokes. Then, very gradually, Gregory became more and more intense about the use of the "N-word and Colored," as in the "NO Coloreds Here" signs by water fountains and rest areas throughout the South. He scoffed at the terms "Negro" and "Negress." He described Stokley Carmichael's writing about Black nationalism and Black Power. He concluded with an endorsement of the word "Black." *No more N-words, not even Negro. No more use of Colored!* BLACK *and* BLACK *only! In language, formal and informal, oral and written. Black was beautiful. Black was power.*

By the end of the tape, I felt uncomfortable. I was unclear what the message had to do with me, but the group was quick to clarify my role.

Which was why, after clinic on the following Monday, Clariece listened as I summarized the tape. She shook her head a couple of times but did not interrupt me.

"Clariece," I said, "I recommend that we start referring to the C&Y patients and their families as Black. I'll see about getting Medical Records to print us sheets that say 'Black' and 'White,' instead of 'Colored' or 'Negro' and 'White'—"

"Absolutely not, Doctor Hostler," Clariece interrupted in her church voice. "Not another word. You'd insult our families—take away the little dignity we all have."

She paused, shook her head at me, and continued in her usual clinic voice, "I agree that using the N-word is a disgrace. 'Colored' is wrong, but some country folk still prefer that. But you listen to me. The words 'Negro' and 'Negress' show respect, standing, and history. This is the South, Dr. Hostler! We are a million years from Black Power."

I pleaded my case, or rather the social workers' case. Sometimes Clariece had modified my wording, but she had never said no before.

"This is the University of Virginia, Dr. Hostler. This is my community. Are you listening, Dr. Hostler? We are in the South. You will not disrespect our families and our friends. Do you understand?"

"Yes, Ma'am," I said. "I understand."

When I bumped into controversy with Clariece or Helen, they did not hesitate to share their truth and set me straight. The staff in the Department of Pediatrics were less clear.

I needed to recruit doctors for the clinic. That summer of 1970, I was committed to the goals and activities of outreach to the rural poor families. I knew Albemarle County had 726 square miles and twenty-seven schools who reported no children with mental retardation and no children with handicaps. I knew endless details about the county, but I didn't know what resources I had to hire doctors. Or how to find out.

Peggy Denby understood that I needed to see the budget, but she didn't make it available. I was ready to hire Dr. Margaret McChesney, a pediatrician who was moving to Charlottesville from California.

When I finally did get a copy of the budget, the numbers were clear. The medical director before me had a salary of $28,000. The pediatric dentists were allocated at $20,000. My salary as medical director was $15,000.

I'd never reviewed a budget spread sheet like this before. What was I missing?

It couldn't be true.

I felt ashamed and embarrassed. I remembered how thrilled I'd felt when Dr. Thurman offered me the medical director position. How relieved that I wouldn't have to move to DC for the NCI position. Why had I been embarrassed to ask about my salary?

I started to cry. Alan put his arms around me. "Steady girl, steady. Ignore the gusts. You'll be all right." I couldn't tell Alan why I was crying.

Be all right? I doubted that. Dr. Thurman was my trusted mentor, but Dr. Thurman had betrayed me. I hadn't felt so ashamed since I wet the bed in the upper bunk at sleepover camp when I was six.

The following Thursday, I juggled Dee in the crook of one elbow, shrugged the diaper bag and saddlebag purse over my shoulder, and clutched Kaki by the hand. How had I, the barmaid, the one who scoffed at becoming a baby doctor, the one who never dreamed of having babies—how had I become this early-morning juggler of baby stuff?

Dr. Thurman balanced Dinky on his knee and fed her breakfast on his side of the desk. Not at the very end of my list of agenda items, but more than halfway, was the C&Y budget. It was 7:35 a.m. I could hear the office coming to life. It was my turn.

"Why do the dentists make more than I do?"

"I'm not sure that's accurate."

"It is accurate. I saw the budget. They make $20,000 a year. I make $15,000."

"Fiscal year 1971?"

"Whatever the year Denby provided—they make $5,000 more than I do."

"Well, they're subspecialty dentists with pediatric residencies."

"I have done an internship, residency, and fellowship after my MD." I reminded myself that there would be no whining and no crying. "Sir, the numbers are in the budget. It is not a debate."

"Dr. Deputy has an MPH."

"I'm the medical director!"

"They're in a very competitive market. They make far less in academic practice than they would in private practice."

Market? Pork bellies? What market?

My cheeks were hot. Kaki stared up at Dr. Thurman. Dee grabbed my dress bodice and whimpered. There was no easy egress. No dramatic storming out. I had the kids and all their paraphernalia.

As I closed the office door, Dr. Thurman said, "I'll look into the salaries."

The next week, Dinky smeared her blueberry muffin across her cheeks, and Dee protested his sippy cup. They sensed the tension. Dr. Thurman and I ran the agenda, but we didn't talk about the C&Y budget again.

I had failed salary negotiation, but I had learned several important lessons.

The easy ones were: *Negotiate from strength. Never negotiate salary while breastfeeding. Never negotiate salary with your children in the room.* The harder ones served me well in academic medicine: *Be the one to develop the budget. Never delegate titles. Always maintain control of the budget.*

On September 1, I saw the increase in my monthly paycheck. My salary had been corrected to $20,000 per year. No one discussed it—neither Dr. Thurman nor Peggy Denby. As the C&Y medical director, I earned as much as the dentists. Finally, I had access to the C&Y budget, but not yet the department budget.

It was a long spell of barely getting by—the balance of children and patients, usually sick and sometimes dying. The expectations of family at home and the even larger family at work. Alan dreamed about leaving OSE and running the shipyard in North Carolina full-time. Alan's daughter Gioia was pregnant and refused to marry the father. When I shared my frustrations, Alan suggested inviting Amy, his first wife living on Cape Cod, to move to Virginia to help with childcare.

Hell, no. I was not that desperate.

It would be Yvonne who joined Beverley and Mr. Brown to keep me afloat that fall. Yvonne had cleaned for us once a week. She always had been happy not to have me around. I understood.

I'd cleaned houses in my day. I hated it when the lady of the house followed me around, watching, and waiting for me to make a mistake.

I was a little afraid of Yvonne, but the run of barely getting by couldn't go on. With what I paid Mrs. Chase for day care and with the C&Y salary increase, I could pay Yvonne for five days at her established cleaning rate. Yvonne signed on without negotiation. Little did I know then that Yvonne would remain part of our family until the children went off to college and got married. I didn't ask who took care of her little girl.

Alan announced it was time for Dinky to be called by her given name—the name he had given her in the delivery room—Kathleen Ann. But, at two, she struggled saying Kathleen and soon became Kaki. And Dee became Dylan.

Yvonne was beyond description. She explained that she was "mahogany, not Black" and that her husband, Spencer, wanted no "Black mamas in his bed." When I called out, Yvonne would answer in a little-girl voice, "Here's me." Most days I'd come home from work to find all three of them in the bathroom. Yvonne on her knees by the tub lathering them up, washing their straight pale hair, and ceremonially dumping a pail of water over their heads while they squealed.

Yvonne would put the children into her old sedan without seat belts and go pick up groceries at Foods of All Nations. She competed with freckle-faced Lucille in the bakery for Dylan's affections, but she understood not to take on the butcher. Frank still weighed the kids and provided the weekly "baby pack" containing a filet mignon, a boneless lamb chop, and a ham slice. It cost one dollar. Hand in hand with the tow-headed toddlers, Yvonne cruised through the checkout, scribbled the house charge, and allowed the bag boy to carry the groceries.

I left daily notes and lists. Yvonne ignored them. It seemed that everyone was happier when I trusted the three of them to structure the day as they saw fit.

Yvonne and I never discussed behavioral limits or consequences. I was easygoing, but I could escalate quickly to become a top-of-my-lungs screamer and a wave-the-meat-tenderizer-mallet-around kind of parent. Yvonne acted rather than threatened. One time, I found her washing laundry. She had Dylan pinned under her arm, indifferent to his hollering. Another time, Yvonne was ironing table napkins with Kaki glommed between her knees. Naptime was never a problem—the three of them napped together.

Mister Dimock, as Yvonne addressed Alan, approved the arrangement. They seldom interacted, but Alan was relieved the household chaos had quieted.

Both Alan and I had a touch of obsessive-compulsive behavior, but my crazy didn't manifest in the household as much as it did on the wards. Alan believed that the house should be ordered like a sailboat. Yvonne and Alan's tug-of-war escalated from a chance skirmish to bordering on war. A war limited to kitchen utensils, but still a war. The kids and I were happy. And the house was tidy.

Yvonne and I walked around each other respectfully. We learned how to maintain the peace, identify the critical compromises, and settle on safe topics.

Yvonne was the "housekeeper" now, her chosen title—not the maid. Not a nurse, not a nanny, not a cook. We all called her Yvonne, including the kids. She called me Doc. We argued about the importance of the kids learning to use "Yes, Ma'am" and "Yes, Sir" when they spoke to adults. Yvonne prevailed. Yvonne organized lunch for the kids from the obvious contenders in the refrigerator, but she refused, even when asked, to start supper preparations. I assumed she didn't know how to cook.

Yvonne's behavior changed when people came by the house. I heard the tone of Berta's voice as she told Yvonne to bring her a cold drink. Yvonne ignored her. I laughed out loud when Berta chastised me for not having Yvonne in uniform. I started to pay closer attention to the words, the tone of voice, and the expectations of friends who dropped in while Yvonne was around. Yvonne seemed comfortable with the ever-present Doc Kaplan and Miz Butler, but I learned not to take that ease for granted.

After several months, we couldn't imagine life without Yvonne. The kids ran the hose in the backyard, got bloodied, and were frequently bandaged. Yvonne would bring the kids to the C&Y clinic when I was running late with a sick patient. Eventually, Yvonne started to fix supper when I was late. We loved her fried chicken and biscuits.

One night I had to drive to Lynchburg, about sixty miles south of Charlottesville, for a dinner at someone's home related to work. It was unusual, it was during the week, and I didn't know the host and hostess. Yvonne would stay with Kaki and Dee.

"Be careful, Doc," Yvonne said as she followed me out to the car. "Lynchburg is the beginning of the Deep South. It's dangerous."

"Don't be silly."

"Doc, listen—*they lynch people down there.*"

I thought about what Yvonne said as I drove away, but my mind quickly wandered to what this dinner was about and why Dr. Thurman had asked me to go.

The designated address was a neighborhood of modest homes with white picket fences. A card table was set up in the side yard as a bar, and a uniformed Black man served drinks to the guests and the host couple. It seemed a strange setup, but not dangerous.

Later, I reported out to Yvonne. "Two people worked this dinner for six people. They were in uniform—with white gloves! It was like something straight out of *Gone with the Wind.*"

"I knew it," Yvonne shook her head. "I shouldn't have let you go there, Doc!"

It was decades before I started to understand what Yvonne was telling me. I still remember how worried Yvonne was for me as I headed down to the Deep South and how completely safe I felt in my Northern White skin.

Yvonne took the kids on adventures to Louisa County, where she lived. I only knew because Kaki reported on Yvonne's mother's beautiful rose garden. It would be years before I learned that Yvonne lived in a gray shingled house smack dab in the middle of forty acres with vegetable and flower gardens, and a family cemetery. And that Spencer, her husband, was not only not working then but an insulin-dependent diabetic and a raging alcoholic.

It was the end of spring semester in 1971. By then, Alan and Yvonne got along better, maybe because of their shared taste for Glenlivet, a single malt Scotch he'd bring home for her from DC.

And, amazingly, the statue of Thomas Jefferson remained upright in front of the Rotunda even though 350 first-year women had enrolled, matriculated, and successfully completed first-year exams.

In a similar spirit of optimism, we were moving to the country.

· 12 ·

Daylilies for the Mill

Fall 1971

We were buying an old mill on a creek in North Garden, about ten miles south of Charlottesville. The Mill, built in 1841, cost twenty-eight thousand dollars. It was a stretch. I'd had two raises, the first after I read the C&Y budget, and the second, a "midyear correction" communicated a week before UVA faculty salaries were disclosed in the local newspaper. I learned that junior faculty could borrow 10 percent of their first home cost from a special UVA fund toward a down payment. However, not female faculty members, it appeared. Dr. Mac made a few phone calls. "My colleague insists it was his secretary who refused your request, not him." Dr. Mac laughed. "Apparently, she wasn't aware that UVA allowed women on the faculty."

Alan was scheduled to make a major presentation in Washington during the time scheduled for our closing. He insisted that I could sign the mortgage without him. It was just routine paperwork. On the morning of the closing, I received a call from Dr. Mac's friend and real estate lawyer, Mr. George Gilmore, letting me know the exact amount of cash I needed for the closing. I was five thousand dollars short due to the delay in the funds transfer from the University.

When I couldn't reach Alan on the phone, I blurted out the story of my shortfall to Dr. Thurman. I hoped that he could pressure the University to expedite the cash transfer. I remembered how Nellie lost the house at 15 Vernon Street to the bank. What was I thinking? Me, buy a house? How could I be so stupid?

Dr. Thurman pulled out his checkbook. "Five thousand? Correct?"

I nodded. "Allison won't need her college fund for another fifteen years. Here you go."

"Are you sure?"

"Absolutely, but you may regret buying a ramshackle place out in the boondocks. I hope Alan knows his way around house repair."

I took the check and nodded yes. I didn't move. Instead, I blushed and teared up. I didn't know what to say, how to express my gratitude.

The Mill was built to grind wheat into flour. It was sited at a curve in the creek. Water from the creek turned the millstone. The ground level of the Mill was filled with mud and leftover furniture from Camille, the Category 5 hurricane that devastated southern Albemarle and Nelson Counties in 1969. It had been two years since anyone had lived in the Mill.

Originally, the external walls had been clapboard, but over the years they'd been encased in gray stucco with cement overlaying wire for insulation. Working farms and modest houses surrounded the Mill.

The next weekend Alan and Beverley went off to explore kennels. They returned with two Great Dane puppies, a blue and a black. The Danes were clumsy, falling over their big feet, but soft and cuddly. Max, the blue one, was Alan's. Mattie belonged to Beverley, but she lived with us. Yvonne and I fed the mother tiger cat and her kittens we found under the porch, and they soon moved into the kitchen.

The Mill had three levels but no inside connection between the main floor and the ground level. You had to go outdoors, walk down and around the house to enter through the ground-level door. On the main floor of the Mill, there were two front doors. One door led into the kitchen and one into the foyer.

Our official front door was the foyer one. Along the right wall of the foyer was a mahogany table with carved legs we'd purchased for ten dollars at a yard sale. We couldn't afford the second ten dollars for its matching mirror. Instead, Alan massed prints of vintage sailboats on the wall above the table. A closet was tucked under the staircase to the left. From the foyer, you walked through a dining room into a living room with high ceilings and open beams. The stairs from the foyer led to the second floor with four bedrooms and two baths. Each child had a bedroom. The guest bedroom would be shared over time by Beverley, Yvonne, Patty, and Gioia.

The front doors faced west to a long, narrow plot, stretching between the road and the creek. The second door led into the kitchen. Alan immediately sledge-hammered an existing wall to expand the kitchen. We called it the common room. It was large enough for the kids and the puppies to run around and build forts. The only furnishings were two round oak tables we'd bought when the Library Restaurant went out of business. Sunlight poured into the common room from windows along the south side overlooking the creek.

Soon after we moved in, Alan built floor-to-ceiling bookshelves in the southeast corner room. Closest to the creek. We put down a braided rug from Vermont, and that became the library. No furniture, just lots of books, newspapers, and magazines. It wasn't long before Alan decided we needed a circular staircase in the library going down to the ground level. Weekends back home from DC always meant the next project for Alan.

Our friends the Hagens—Jim, Erla, and their three children—were renovating and living in Neve Hall, an old stone-walled Episcopal monastery off Route 29 South. Jim was a sculptor in the Fine Arts Department. He had immediately converted the chapel into his studio. Alan and Jim traded tools, architectural ideas, and the occasional salvage expedition. Erla and I traded casseroles, childcare, and consultations, most recently about marriage.

On Halloween, the Hagens hosted a costume party at Neve Hall. Patty Cormier from C&Y was nine months pregnant and showed up in a nun's habit. It was perfect, from the starched white guimpe to the wimple. Her husband, Ray, was a junior faculty member in the French Department who researched courtly love and published poems written in Latin and Greek. He arrived in an abbot's robe and wooden crucifix. During the party, Ray crowed about their open marriage.

We were cleaning up after the party when Erla and I overheard Jim and Alan talking about Ray's comments. Erla shut them up: "Don't even think about it!" I concurred, but then I remembered that Alan had suggested his ex-wife might be willing to move in and assist with Kaki and Dee. *Had Alan been suggesting an open marriage?*

I found this new socializing of couples confusing. How could Patty be so rigid in her research expectations at C&Y and be flexible with either of them taking lovers as long as they weren't students, and the trysts didn't take place at home? Beverley laughed it off, but Erla and I worried. The most I ever saw my husband was on weekends and not even every weekend. It was the first time I even considered all the weeks and months of separation when Alan was away—Norway, California, India—and I was on call.

A few days before the first frost of 1971, Mr. Gilmore, my realtor, delivered a sack of daylily bulbs with a handwritten note. He cautioned me to be patient—"with enough time, I'm sure you'll get the hang of living in the South."

But it wasn't just getting the hang of living in the South anymore—it was the constant shape-shifting of roles—wife, mother, doctor, gardener, community leader. And now, worrying about living separately from my husband.

One weekend, Jim and Alan went off on a salvage expedition and returned with an eight-foot bow window. Alan imagined the window would open-up the kitchen to more light. That Monday, he stayed home to install it. That afternoon, he called and interrupted a team meeting.

We were discussing a fourth-grader with Fanconi anemia and his pending removal from his family. We had found the child asleep on a pile of dirty laundry when we made a home visit. A front window had been shot out. His mother was passed out on the floor.

The team scowled when I took the call. "Jim can't get here," Alan said. "You've got to come home, sorry!"

I fumed all the way down 29 South. When I pulled in, I saw a huge hole gaping in the side of the Mill. It was an emergency. Alan hugged me and said, "I couldn't let Yvonne and the kids see this."

I steadied the bow window, all eight by three feet, as it twisted in gusts of wind and rain. I wore heels and hose, my lab coat over a sweater and skirt. No raincoat. The window frame was heavy, awkward, and splintery. I pushed it against the house and juggled one knee up to support the bottom edge. I got soaked. Fortunately, Alan was fast with the nail gun. The window was installed fifteen minutes later. I went back to work. By supper, Alan had installed a six-foot-long plank door in the kitchen beneath the bow window and painted it fire-engine red. It was our kitchen table.

The circular staircase was another adventure.

Which was why, the next Saturday morning, we were in earnest pursuit of a forty-foot or taller southern yellow pine or western red cedar, essentially a used telephone pole. Virginia Department of Transportation (VDOT) not only had a used pole, but they agreed to deliver it on a Saturday—for free. So much for finishing up my clinic notes.

"The VDOT guy was intrigued with the idea of a circular staircase." Alan grinned like a mischievous kid. At two, Dylan already had a reasonable imitation.

After we installed the telephone pole, Alan spent the next day with pencil and protractor, drawing shapes and angles of rise for the staircase. Jim dropped by in the early afternoon to check out the pole and the calculations. It wasn't long before he had a pencil and protractor, too. We let them be.

No time for clinic charts. Instead, it was my time for weekend laundry, figuring out the supper menus for the week, and laying out Alan's shirts and ties for his Washington workweek. We dreaded Sunday nights. Alan resented returning to the buttoned-down expectations of OSE's culture instead of the boatyard or, better, being at sea. I was relieved by a schedule and the structure of my workweek, but Alan resisted. I pushed aside my growing worry that Alan was beginning, ever so gradually, to resent my commitment to medicine.

Of course, Alan invited Jim to stay for supper. Erla and the kids would bring a salad and brownies. I started spaghetti sauce for supper and a batch of minestrone for weeknight suppers. I tuned out the children. I tuned out Alan and Jim and the dogs. My thoughts were focused on the meeting with Dr. McChesney about Frankie, my C&Y patient who was in foster care.

The foster father was a Baptist minister, and the family had become focused on praying out Frankie's badness. I wasn't clear if they believed prayer would correct his genetic disorder or save his soul. Frankie was only ten years old. His disease was terminal.

Dr. McChesney and I were slowly crossing lines: clinic lines, medical lines, ethical lines. Each week after school, she transfused Frankie with packed red blood cells in the C&Y treatment room. We didn't say it out loud, but we both understood we were only prolonging the inevitable end. We both agreed Frankie deserved a few more normal days and weeks of living, whatever that might require.

Alan came up behind me at the stove and whispered in my ear, "Where have you gone?" He hugged me. "Sharon, come back—it's Sunday night. Stay with us, babe." Jim laughed and opened more beers.

At the clinic the next day, Clariece met me and nodded toward the treatment room. Dr. McChesney was listening as Frankie complained.

"I've been to church five times this week. Sunday services, Sunday school, and Bible study in the afternoon, and then evening prayer on Wednesday and Fridays. What's enough?" Frankie glanced at me standing at the door and kept going. "Mommy may 'whore around' like the pastor says, but she's still my Mommy. I miss her."

Clariece motioned me into the office. "Dr. Thurman asked me today if we really were doing transfusions in the clinic?"

"Well, yes, but only for Frankie."

I knew better. We were crossing lots of lines for Frankie. The C&Y Project was funded for primary care and community outreach, not subspecialty care. I was fellowship trained in pediatric hematology. I knew Frankie would die of his Fanconi anemia—these transfusions were simply prolonging the inevitable. But these days, he went to school in clean clothes, slept in a warm bed, and had a stable, if *judgmental,* foster family.

We knew that keeping Frankie alive with transfusions was a double-edged sword. The iron from the transfusions would eventually become toxic to his liver—but maybe we could get him to fifth grade. I'd discuss Frankie's care with Dr. Thurman, but not tonight.

"Who's taking Frankie home?" Clariece asked. "He's missed the bus."

"I'll drop him on my way home," Dr. McChesney said.

Right, I thought, on her way to take care of her own family. I secretly wished I could go home with Dr. McChesney and let her take care of me, too.

· 13 ·

Weaving the Bridge

Spring and Summer 1972

The chaos at the Mill continued. Alan had more projects than money or time. He was reclaiming the furniture left over from Camille in the Mill basement and setting out asparagus crowns for the next season. Even though I no longer had regular night call, I rotated on the inpatient ward with the attending call and daily rounds. I even agreed to attend a home delivery at a nearby hippie commune, and that was very poor judgment.

I tried to meet all the expectations—back-to-the-earth hippie housewife, gracious Southern lady and hostess, academic peer at the University, sexy partner to the red-bearded Alan, and the neighborhood mother who makes popcorn balls for Halloween trick-or-treaters. I had trouble sorting out my roles as wife, mother, doctor, and friend.

The kids hid from Yvonne in the attic, climbed trees, and escaped to the creek. The Danes grew more rambunctious the bigger they got. Now, when strangers came knocking on the door, the Danes herded the kids under the red kitchen table or into the pantry. Max developed arthritis in both of his shoulders. Too big to be held, he put his huge head in my lap for soothing.

Beverley had been working with a fellow social worker to develop yet one more of her business schemes—setting up a handyman company for small house repairs. We socialized with Erla and Jim and their three kids, usually around a project needing both men in one place. Yvonne was unflappable. She became our anchor in the growing chaos.

After the first summer, our pantry was lined with my homemade tomato sauce, pickles, and preserves. I had one crock of sauerkraut brining, and Peter dumped fruit into another crock to make brandy. Under the bed, I had Mason jars of peaches soaking in brandy for holiday presents. An exhausted eighteen-year-old Gioia visited for a few weeks with newborn baby Stevie for respite before she joined Big Steve on the Air Force Base in Utah. I thought she looked depressed. I should have urged them to stay longer, but I didn't.

At work, the C&Y Project was thriving. Dr. McChesney was a strong clinician, unflappable and wise. She managed the C&Y city clinic. I staffed the rural clinics. Medical students, pediatric residents, and nurse-practitioner students now competed for rotations. At home, Beverley and Yvonne remained the safety net for Kaki and Dylan. The daycare center had put me on warning about pickup time.

I was accustomed to standing in for Dr. Thurman in the classroom, on call, around the hospital, and in the community. Both Dr. Thurman and Dr. Mac regularly asked me to cover their patients—I examined one of the five daughters of President and Mrs. Edgar Shannon on the Lawn. The C&Y clinic had so many truancy cases that Judge Zehler in Juvenile and Domestic Court greeted me by name. Substituting for Dr. Thurman, I flew on the University plane to Roanoke for a working session to design a sex education curriculum for the public schools.

Those assignments paled when compared with representing Dr. Thurman and the Department of Pediatrics at Alumni Hall at a small-group discussion about abortion. The evening session was to be chaired by Dr. Joseph Fletcher, a former Episcopal priest in Boston and a distinguished ethicist. Dr. Fletcher had published the controversial *Situational Ethics* in 1968 and postulated circumstances in which, morally, the end justifies the means. Love and justice were the same. Love was the only intrinsic good. Fletcher concluded that love's decisions were made situationally.

In preparation, I'd gone to the library and reviewed the history of abortion. Colorado had been the first state, in 1967, to legalize abortion for rape, incest, or permanent disability to the mother, as determined by the woman and her physician. Alaska, Hawaii, New York, and Washington state had enacted similar laws, but abortion remained a criminal act, a felony in the rest of the United States.

Dr. Thurman's request hadn't seemed out of the ordinary at the time, but before that evening, I'd not interacted with faculty from the other schools within the University. I hoped that I'd be able to speak about my patient, the fifteen-year-old Black girl who died from gram-negative sepsis secondary to a backroom abortion. When she died, only the police had been interested in talking about it.

When I arrived at Alumni Hall, I was greeted by a stranger. "Dr. Hostler," he said, "it's wonderful to see you." He continued with a familiar Boston accent. "We were both at Middlebury, Sharon." He laughed, squinted his eyes, and tilted his head upward in kind of a tic. "Of course, I was years ahead of you."

I liked his confidence and his lively eyes, but still, I was uncomfortable. I didn't know what was going on. Why did we have to do this damnable social stuff?

"Professor Alec Horniman from Darden," he said. "I saw your name on the list. Be my supper companion." He took my arm. "Have you met Professor Fletcher?"

"No, but I've read his book." I knew by then that the Darden Business School faculty thought they hung the moon, but Horniman seemed pleasant enough.

We entered a huge hall. People milled around an elaborately set buffet table and chatted in small clutches. Chairs were arranged in a huge oval. I tried to count, maybe twenty. I'm a counter—telephone poles, cracks in the sidewalk, or redheads in an audience. That night, it was chairs.

As we passed the chair of Obstetrics and Gynecology, he glanced at me and said, "Dean Hunter mandated this event for Thurman and me, but I see Thurman sent his lackey." I nodded and kept moving.

Horniman and I found a corner, balanced buffet plates in our laps, and observed the crowd. One by one, they sought out the evening's host. Fletcher was dressed in a black suit, not religious robes. He had white hair, shiny pink cheeks, and a benevolent smile.

I told Alec Horniman the story of the fifteen-year-old, pregnant by a cousin, who died after her grandmother attempted an abortion. I complained that all anyone at UVA wanted to talk about were the student protests, not abortion in back alleys. Finally, I would tell this group what it meant for teenage girls around here. No legal birth control pills.

No family planning. No antibiotics for gonorrhea. Illegal abortions in filthy backrooms.

Horniman listened as I ranted on. After I was finished, he spoke—slowly, deliberately, and quietly. His tone, the timing, and the intensity of his soft voice warned me against interruption.

He pointed out that the session was an academic gathering of scholars representing the entire gamut of interests around the concept of abortion. The idea of abortion. The possibility of legalized abortion. They represented the various schools at UVA—Law and Business and Nursing and Medicine for sure, but also departments like Psychology, Sociology, and Religious Studies. And the community—the Catholic monsignor, the superintendent of schools, even a judge or two. Professor Fletcher was seeking a theoretical discussion of ethical, moral, religious, and legal perspectives.

Fletcher's imperative was to build a community of trust.

"They don't know what it's like on the front lines," I said, about to cry.

Horniman placed my hands in his and looked me in the eye. "Your time will come," he said. "Tonight, play by the rules. Listen."

I shook my head no, but I said that I would try.

"If you blow it tonight, you won't get another chance to make a difference. Not just about abortion."

We joined the larger oval of twenty-two chairs. Horniman pulled ours together and stretched his arm across the back of my chair. There was one other woman in the room, the dean of Nursing. Once again, a group of men would discuss the rules and regulations about women's bodies.

Professor Fletcher established the ground rules, then invited us to introduce ourselves and to share what brought us to the circle. After the first round, Fletcher discussed the four principles of situational ethics: pragmatism, relativism, positivism, and personalism.

After several rounds of orchestrated comments, the Catholic monsignor requested that we consider the perspective and rights of the fetus. Then, one of the local judges asked what the impact of legalized abortion would be on the University of Virginia and the community.

That is when the chair of Obstetrics and Gynecology stood up.

Horniman put his hand on my forearm, tightening his grip as I shifted forward in my seat.

"Legalized abortion means the total and absolute destruction of our training programs. It would make my residents into garbage collectors. Why should my residents be the ones designated to extract the bloody garbage of society's loins?"

He paused and rubbed his hands together as if he were scrubbing for surgery. "We will never be clean again." He looked around the circle. "And we become the souls damned."

Professor Fletcher walked across the floor until he stood in front of him. Fletcher slowly reached over, touched him, and spoke quietly. The room was still. The chair sat down and Horniman released his grip.

Fletcher gracefully assumed control of the conversation and guided us to a theoretical, philosophical, maybe even an ethical conclusion to the evening.

Suddenly, it was over.

I said a proper thank-you to Horniman. It would be years before I grasped the importance of that evening—not only the requirement and power of self-restraint, but the privilege it was to be a member of the academic community of a major research university.

Driving home, I thought back to Woods Hole, when I was a medical student. The first summer, I roomed in a boardinghouse for eight dollars a week and shared a room with two graduate students, both Catholic and both from Boston. One was working toward a MSW and the other, a PhD in psychology. During that summer, they both shared stories of unwanted pregnancies.

Both had relied on the infamous rhythm method of birth control. One was sent to a Catholic home in Alaska, where she spent a semester living with punishing and unforgiving nuns. She labored alone without anesthesia for twenty hours and was not allowed to hold her baby girl. The other one had an abortion in a dingy backroom and remained worried that she was sterile after a lingering infection. Neither shared her story with the other. I was a trustworthy confidant solely because I was in medicine, I guessed.

The next morning in clinic, I received a page. Professor Fletcher invited me to join a group meeting at his cottage on Spruce Lane. "I've heard you're passionate about this topic. You'll keep us oriented to the issues on the front line."

It never dawned on me that I should have sought Dr. Thurman's approval to participate, but I did tell him about the work group at our regular Thursday meeting. Later, I realized that Dr. Thurman was already viewed with some skepticism among the academic hierarchy because his social activism extended beyond Grounds. Abortion might have been one challenge too many for him.

Joseph Fletcher was named the first professor of medical ethics with his academic home in the School of Medicine. His domain included students and faculty throughout the University and beyond. He was instrumental in creating an Ethics Consult Service for the inpatient services, unique because any member of the team or the family could initiate or request a consult. In 1972, the US Supreme Court established the right for unmarried people to possess contraceptives on the same basis as married couples, a right established by *Griswold v. Connecticut* in 1965. The landmark decision known as *Roe v. Wade* ruled that the Constitution of the United States protected a pregnant woman's liberty to choose an abortion without *excessive* government restriction. We would never have believed then that that landmark decision would be overturned by the Supreme Court in 2021.

Was I present in Alumni Hall that fall evening of 1971 for Joe Fletcher's discussion about abortion as Thurman's lackey or Thurman's mentee? I never knew. I did recognize that the freedom to be both in and outside of the University was a gift for me as a young doctor, wife, and mother. At the time, I was unaware that Dr. Thurman had appointed me on a tenure track or what that meant about eventual academic review. I'd had no academic projects since my fellowship.

I never thought of myself as Thurman's lackey, but I wasn't one of the boys. I wasn't invited to the weekly poker night. I didn't play squash or gossip in the men's locker room. We weren't members of a church or a country club or any social groups. It would be years before the Faculty Wives considered inviting me to tea. And, of course, I refused. At the same time, Dr. Mac did volunteer advice on my retirement benefits—avoid the stock market and stick with the traditional stuff.

Advice even extended to our marital life. Dr. Merrill suggested that

Alan and I should regularly get away for weekends. Sometimes on Fridays, Beverley or Yvonne fed Kaki and Dylan so that I could meet Alan at the Mousetrap for a beer and a burger. In a frenzied, five-minute free-for-all, we'd decide which one of us got to talk first—who really had a legitimate crisis, who had the worst or the best week. Whoever listened on Friday got first dibs on Saturday. It worked for us.

None of them had any idea what my life was like, but that didn't restrict the fatherly commentary.

I was growing in the role as medical director, proud and protective of our programs and our people. We registered over a thousand patients in those early days of C&Y. It was relatively easy for the families in public housing to walk or take a city bus to get to our city clinic at the Corner, although perhaps "easy" might not have been the word used by the mother hauling a febrile toddler with three little ones hanging onto the hem of her skirt.

I wrote grants for state and federal funding as principal investigator (PI). I lobbied for a process for state licensing of in-home day-care facilities and was awarded a grant to train providers in health concerns and child development—like the appropriate age for toilet training. When the Maternal and Child Health team from DC made C&Y site visits, Dr. McChesney suggested we entertain them at the Mill. I would not have had the confidence, but the site visit was a great success.

I could still be bossy in the clinics. I could become stubborn and self-righteous without much provocation. A call from UVA Human Resources turned out to be that kind of provocation. The call was alerting me that the candidate for an open C&Y nutritionist position was the wife of the vice president of development. She would be *a perfect fit.*

I set up the interview at the clinic in Esmont, a poor, farming community of predominantly Black families about twenty miles south of Charlottesville. Helen shrugged and shook her head when she interrupted a patient examination to introduce Mrs. Ann Vernon Sullivan.

I took an instant dislike to Ann Vernon Sullivan. Was it the preppy linen dress with the monogram and piping on the cap sleeves—hot pink on navy—or the matching espadrilles?

There she was, completely at ease, introducing herself to Beverley and some of the mothers, smiling and nodding. She seemed to know one of the mothers by name. My interview wouldn't take long.

"Call me AV," she said. I nodded and asked about her work history. She grew up in the Valley, majored in home economics, married Gilly, who played football at UVA, and had four kids. The youngest was starting first grade. "It's time for paid work," she said with a laugh.

I dismissed her at the home economics, but she wasn't finished. "Home economics and life experience trump biochemistry any day." I ignored her.

I was oblivious to how inappropriate our questioning was—I asked her how she'd manage work and four children. Helen emphasized the dangers of home visiting in the hollers—the men with shotguns and hunting dogs.

The other candidate was single, well-schooled in nutrition, but none of us thought she could work independently. There were no other candidates.

So, AV returned to the Keswick Clinic for a second round. She arrived in sneakers, put on an apron, pulled out index cards with recipes featuring USDA surplus known as welfare cheese, and worked the room. It was unanimous—we hired AV.

Helen and I were both embarrassed and delighted when AV folded right into the team. I'd learn that AV could talk to a rock, a great job skill for someone in development and, it turned out, making home visits. Soon, I was seeing her children as patients in my private clinic—first six-year-old Susan, then Sara, VG, and Mike. It wasn't long before I was fully absorbed into her family.

Even with the network of C&Y vans, transportation in the rural areas was a major challenge. The dentists called Dr. Thurman and the C&Y staff "communists." I thought about third grade. I had been a charity patient treated for trench mouth. Each week for months, I took the city bus to the dentist for him to scrape my swollen gums. Toothbrushing hadn't been on Nellie's list. That dentist withheld pain medicine, lectured me about being poor, and shamed me for having a mouth full of pus. I didn't cry then. I wouldn't give him the satisfaction. Years later, when I read *A Tree Grows in Brooklyn,* I couldn't stop crying.

Beverley was the one who hired Bonny Wilson, a fresh graduate from Smith College, to run the C&Y bus system. Bonny's major credential was that she'd run the basement sale at Filene's, a department store in Boston with a notable free-for-all summer sale with customers changing clothes in the aisles. Bonny mastered the county roads, the directions to hard-to-find hollers, and remembered which families would be ready for early-morning pickups. It was Bonny's controlled confrontation at the dental society meeting, not Dr. Thurman's protests, that ended their harassment.

It was a heady time to be on the front lines of the War on Poverty—very distant from reading bone marrow slides under the microscope or sacrificing pregnant does. I loved being called "Doc" when I ran into my families in the grocery store. I wondered how the C&Y team would have described a home visit at 15 Vernon Street with Nellie. The team was always surprised when I asked patients difficult questions about sexuality and abuse. Not my patients. They were relieved when I used language they understood. I didn't fidget when I asked them questions. I didn't interrupt their answers.

I made a lot of mistakes, egregious ones I still recall with shame. The worst was when I asked Clariece who in *her* community had stolen the laundry out of my unlocked car the evening I'd attended her choral performance at the Baptist Church. In those days, I understood the classism in Charlottesville far better than I recognized my own internalized sexism and learned racism.

I was learning lessons in medicine and in leadership. I was teaching others and making a difference. I connected with my patients, their families, the C&Y teams, their families, faculty, and staff. I had family and friends who were not doctors. But I worried endlessly about my competency as a mother. Dee was now two and mispronouncing the word "truck." He pointed at the eighteen-wheelers and hollered, "TWUCK, TWUCK!"

My concerns led me to the new speech therapist in the clinic. I overheard her counseling a new mother. "She'll learn to talk from listening to you. When you feed her, describe the applesauce. When you change her diaper, talk about her knees and her hips and her belly button. Make it fun." The mother laughed, that was different.

The therapist was striking—tall and dressed in a tailored pants suit and a cream-colored silk blouse. She had huge brown eyes, rosy cheeks, and a lively mouth. She didn't mind the rural clinic or the audiology booth in the mobile van parked next to the railroad station. Jan

Allaire had spent the last two years in Newfoundland. She was happy to be in the lower forty-eight. Helen interrupted Jan to tell me that Frankie had been admitted to the hospital.

Clariece greeted me at the clinic door. "Frankie is dying. Beverley's out looking for his natural mother. No one is with him. Dr. McChesney went home to get her things. She'll stay bedside tonight."

Clariece, the backbone of the city clinic in her spotless uniform and starched nurse's cap, started to cry.

"We did our best. Frankie made it to fifth grade." I reached over and hugged her.

"Dr. Thurman came by clinic to thank us. He was looking for you." She shook her head. "He even thanked me."

The next evening, Yvonne stayed at the Mill while I sat with Frankie. Beverley was still trying to find his mother.

Frankie's body was blown up from the steroids. I rubbed Vaseline on his cracked lips, brushed his hair, and puffed up the pillows. Frankie needed a pile of pillows behind him to breathe. It was after midnight, but he wasn't asleep.

"Doc, am I going to heaven?"

"Of course, Frankie."

"My foster father said my soul is loaded down with sin."

"I don't know much about the sin stuff. I do know that Frankie is one great kid. He's kind and funny and terrific at long division. Enough to get into heaven."

"I worry about the fire and brimstone."

"Forget it. Hell doesn't take kids. You've got to be eighteen."

I rubbed his shoulders with the bath oil I'd brought from home. Little circles, then big circles, just like bath-times at the Mill. Frankie giggled.

"Shhhhh," I warned. "If we wake anyone up, the nurse will get mad at us."

He quieted down and asked for more ginger ale. "What do you think people wear in heaven?"

I held the cup until he had slurped down the last drop. Then, I asked, "What would you like to wear in heaven?"

"Bell bottoms," Frankie responded right away and laughed. It was a huge belly laugh. His whole body jiggled. "I want to wear blue-and-white-striped bell bottoms and a red muscle shirt. What do you think, Doc?"

"Perfect!" It took me a while, but I finally understood—for pants to fit around his huge waist, the legs had to be shortened, and the bell bottoms were cut off.

We sat in the quiet for a while. I'd started to nod off when Frankie asked, "Do you remember when you came to my house? Where I lived with my mother?"

"Yes, why?" Who could forget him curled up in that cocoon of dirty clothes with his mother passed out on the floor? I had hospitalized him. Foster care came next.

"I miss her."

"I bet you do. She loves you, Frankie." I pulled my chair closer. "You know that she's had a really hard time taking care of herself and you."

Frankie nodded like a solemn Buddha. "That's what Dr. McChesney said too."

When the ward nurse came to get his vital signs at four in the morning, I shook my head no. She nodded and moved on. We both knew the drill: Don't disturb the death watch. I was grateful for the privacy and the darkness and the quiet. Frankie's breaths got shallower and shallower. Saliva was beginning to collect in his throat. I fell asleep to him gurgling as his breath bubbled through the fluid.

It was around seven when Dr. Mac squeezed my shoulders and woke me up. "Morning Sunshine," he whispered. "Time to rise and shine. And let him go." I turned my face into the sleeve of his suit jacket and sniffed. He patted my head.

Frankie died later that morning. His mother didn't make it. I was in clinic, but Dr. McChesney was with him. He never woke up.

At the funeral, when the foster father prayed for Frankie's soul, I focused on Frankie's blue-striped bell bottoms.

And his red muscle shirt.

· 14 ·

Settling into Leadership

Fall 1972–New Year's Day 1974

By our second winter at the Mill, the focus was planning the perfect garden and sledding, snowmen, and snowball fights on weekends when it snowed. Sundays, we debated who would drive into Foods of All Nations for the *New York Times.* The ceasefire in Vietnam was so overdue that we hardly talked about it, but I was ecstatic and a bit incredulous when the Supreme Court handed down the *Roe v. Wade* decision in January 1973. The Department of Obstetrics and Gynecology immediately protested. Dr. Mac shook his head in disbelief. At Thursday meeting, Dr. Thurman modeled a quietness I couldn't fathom. At C&Y, we tried to figure out pathways for our patients and their families.

It was time to decide what to plant in the garden that spring. Kaki wanted more little peas. Beverley collected the best office supplies, matte pencils, and quality pens. I commandeered one of her lined accounting journals to function as my garden planner and putting-up ledger. Asparagus grew wild by the well house, so in late February Alan added more asparagus crowns. Kale and spinach followed in March. We argued about white potatoes versus sweet potatoes and decided on both. We'd failed in our efforts to grow cantaloupe and celery, but Alan remained determined. "We just need deeper troughs."

"And sand for the melons. Shade for the celery," I muttered.

Even with the black snakes, the rats, and the extended family of groundhogs who scavenged the garden, the Mill was our home. In early spring, daffodils bloomed amid the rocks, and later Mr. Gilmore's orange daylilies popped out by the snowball bushes along the road. The twenty-minute commute into town made the Mill both a retreat and a destination. The distance only became problematic when I forgot the milk for cereal or when Yvonne had a crisis.

Usually, it was a black snake crisis.

We discovered that each day by noon, the black snakes were stretched out to sun themselves on the deck outside the kitchen. Not until the sun started to dip lower in the sky would they slither, one by one, down to the creek. If the snakes hadn't vacated by the time Yvonne arrived, she refused to get out of the car.

"Snakes! Snakes! Send Doc home!" Yvonne screamed at Clariece from the public pay phone at the Crossroads store. If I happened to be out in one of the rural clinics, Yvonne would go back up Route 29 to Neve Hall for Erla's intervention.

I stomped my feet and hollered a lot. If the snakes didn't leave, I'd use the broom to ease them off the deck toward the creek. The kids laughed and cheered and jumped up and down. Alan regularly reminded the family, especially Yvonne, that black rat snakes were important for the environment. He even suggested the snakes were afraid of us. Yvonne would have none of it.

When a snake came into the kitchen, Yvonne climbed up on the table and screamed. I had no choice. I got the broom. I was the resident grown-up during the week.

On weeknights, either Yvonne or I were stationed at the stove getting supper. The rocking chairs were usually occupied by somebody. If Beverley wasn't trying to teach Dee how to handle a football, she was pouring herself a Scotch. The Danes stayed clear of Kaki when she set up her horses in the middle of the kitchen floor. On the weekends, Alan and I did the *New York Times* crossword or played cribbage while the kids napped. Alan cheered when I sometimes went barefoot and braless.

The Mill became the safe place I'd never known growing up.

Peter visited less and less as he prepared for the transition from his UVA fellowship to his cardiology practice in Nashville, but he promised to return for Thanksgiving and the Blessing of the Hounds. Patty was regularly camped out in the guest room. When UVA denied Ray tenure, they had moved to Philadelphia for his appointment at Temple.

Patty still consulted with the C&Y Project and was completing her PhD dissertation at the Curry School.

Maybe it was my change in night call or the spaciousness of the Mill, but we started having a steady stream of out-of-town visitors—friends from Vermont, Beverley's brothers, one by one, from Florida, and Alan's DC work friends who were glad to leave Watergate behind. The kids thrived on the attention, and Alan recruited the extra hands for his weekend projects. I regularly served supper to a full house on Saturday night.

Alan even managed alone on the weekend I went to New York City with Nellie for a cooking contest. The cookoff was at the Park Lane Hotel on Fifty-Ninth Street. I didn't comment when she competed in a white uniform, apron, and duty shoes with her hair tucked into a net. Her egg salad with chopped spinach and carrots on whole wheat bread was the national winner in the sandwich contest. I did not invite her to the Mill.

Our holiday rituals were established. Thanksgiving was getting the turkey in the oven and the kids bundled up for the Blessing of the Hounds in Cismont followed by Bloody Marys and dinner with all the fixings. Alan had to make the pie crust if he didn't want a graham-cracker crust on the pumpkin pie. Sometimes Beverley made her mother's tomato aspic, a Southern delicacy, with homemade mayonnaise. If I collected the ingredients, I could count on her for the cranberry and orange relish from a Julia Child recipe.

Alan attributed his commitment to cutting down our own tree and putting it up on Christmas Eve to the solstice rites of his Druid ancestors. As he told the story, he'd identified as Druid when he entered the US Coast Guard and experienced several psychological interviews before he was finally commissioned.

Making popcorn garlands and baking cookies became part of our tradition. No caroling or Midnight Mass. We even had visitors drop by—callers, as they say in the South. Jan brought homemade Swedish meatballs—she insisted you had to marry into the family for the recipe. AV shared tins of English toffee. On Christmas morning, Beverley sectioned pink grapefruit and Alan made French toast and bacon. Yvonne was home in Palmyra. Alan demanded that we all eat breakfast at the table before we could open presents—and then he insisted we take turns.

I finally had a rhythm at work. I loved being part of all the C&Y teams. Each one was distinctive. Was it because of the staff or our families in that area? Sometimes we lost sight of our role as part of a national intervention. President Johnson's War on Poverty legislation in 1964 had established two C&Y Projects in each state, one rural and one urban, with each site responsible for uniform data collection, which was analyzed and presented to Congress.

In August 1973, Dr. Thurman delegated me to attend a national C&Y conference to review the program's cumulative impact on health outcomes. The conference was located outside of Salt Lake City. I would get to visit Gioia. Beverley and Yvonne teamed up to cover childcare while Alan went back to DC.

Gioia managed to coax her wheezing station wagon up the mountain to Snowbird, an alpine resort surrounded by wildflowers and empty ski lifts. Stevie, almost two years old, delighted in running and tumbling in the fields. It was a glorious afternoon, but Gioia looked weary. Big Steve was stationed in Greenland. When I inquired, she reported a network of women friends in Ogden. I thought about Alan with Kaki and Dylan back in the garden at the Mill. I think it was the first time I considered that Alan was Stevie's grandfather.

Three months later in November, I headed to Washington, DC, for a national conference on sickle cell screening programs. The commissioner from the Thomas Jefferson Health Department (TJHD) had approached Dr. Thurman to consider a joint venture. By 1973, Virginia, and the rest of the United States, had established mandatory neonatal screening for phenylketonuria (PKU) and hypothyroidism. Both diseases were treatable. Although we understood the genetics of sickle cell anemia, we had no treatment. I was surprised when Dr. Thurman didn't brief us. But neither did I do any reading or research on my own to prepare.

I traveled to the conference with two others. We were an odd threesome, in no way a team. Mary was a White public health nurse in her late fifties. She'd grown up in Charlottesville, graduated from UVA's School of Nursing, and started working at the health department when her youngest kid started school. Louise and I were in our early thirties. Louise was a new faculty member, a medical social worker on our C&Y team.

Louise was Black.

I don't remember if we referred to Louise as Black or African American, but certainly not as Colored or Negro. How did Louise refer to herself? Had we ever talked about it? I doubt it. During her interview process, Louise and I traded stories of growing up in the country—she described her mother curing fresh ham in Southside Virginia, and I talked about stealing field corn, but we hadn't yet worked side by side in clinic.

I worried that Louise might not be welcomed at the conference hotel. Just three years before, twenty nurses and I were turned away at Farmington Country Club's front door because one nurse in our party was Black. We had no celebration of UVA's first neonatal nursing course. No certificates by Dr. Thurman, no speeches, and no after-dinner toast to Mr. Jefferson.

Someone eventually reassured me about the hotel, "Don't worry. DC's a Black town."

The drive to DC was awkward. Mary was eager to start screening in the schools. She wanted us to start strategizing. Right then, in the car, before the conference. I was curious about the practical stuff like timing, permissions, and tracking strategies. Mary persisted, but Louise made it very clear that we were *still learning* about the possible impacts on the screened children and their families. She deflected Mary's attempts to jump-start the project before the conference even started. I stayed out of it. I hadn't considered the rationale or guiding principles to initiate such a program.

At the conference hotel in downtown DC, Mary wore her white nurse's uniform with white lace-up shoes and service pins on her lapel. Louise and I dressed in street clothes appropriate for representing the University at a national meeting. The audience of maybe five hundred community and healthcare workers came from across the country. The presenters on the first day were White. I wouldn't have expected anything different. That was the norm at UVA and my experience at national meetings.

They lectured about hemoglobin, the genetics of Hemoglobin A and Hemoglobin S, and the etiology of sickle cell disease. Most people in the United States have Hemoglobin A (Hb AA), but approximately 8 percent of African Americans carry one mutated gene and have sickle cell trait (Hb AS). If a baby inherits a mutated gene from both parents, she has sickle cell disease (Hb SS). If only one mutated gene is received, she has sickle cell trait (Hb AS).

Children with sickle cell disease present as infants with episodes of devastating pain called pain crises and are susceptible to serious infections. They might die before adulthood. Sickle cell disease was a terrible disease with no cure. In my experience as a young pediatrician, sickle cell trait was what we called an incidental finding. It was not a health concern.

Sickle cell trait was not associated with disease or disability, yet some speakers suggested, with little or no data, that excessive exercise (physical education, team sports, or even exuberance on the playground) *could possibly* be associated with decreased oxygenation. It was suggested that young people should be aware of their Hb S status and *should* seek genetic counseling before making reproductive decisions. The unspoken goal of screening programs seemed to be the eventual elimination of sickle cell disease.

I took care of children with sickle cell disease and understood the physical anguish of the patients and the toll it took on their families. Lamarr, my infant patient from internship, was now nine years old. Superthin and already behind in school, Lamarr was becoming dependent on opiates. His father had long since left the household. Lamarr's family lived in public housing and struggled financially even with assistance from welfare and food stamps. His mother couldn't keep a job because of caring for Lamarr, the ER visits, and the frequent hospitalizations.

During the afternoon session, discussants introduced the pros and cons of creating screening programs for sickle cell trait. Many of the proponents didn't seem to understand the distinction between the disease and the trait. Screening theoretically would identify healthy African American children with sickle cell trait in grade school and, I guessed, direct them to later genetic counseling—to encourage someone with the trait not to have a baby with another person with the trait. Screening proponents expressed enthusiasm for action. For them, doing something seemed preferable to doing nothing. No one addressed the consequences to the patient or the family.

The second morning was different right from the start. We sat up straighter as we listened to stern words of warning. I was startled by the strong emotions expressed by the speakers, many of whom were Black. They were not only healthcare experts, but sociologists, ethicists, economists, civil rights leaders, ministers, school leaders, lawyers, and actuaries. They spoke forcefully. They argued passionately. They opposed screening programs. The auditorium became eerily silent.

I was surprised at such stridency expressed at a scientific conference. I heard feet shuffling, deep sighs, and even some under-the-breath muttering. Speakers used terms like "witch-hunts" and "targeting" and "Jim Crow." There were even comparisons to the Nazi concentration camps and ethnic cleansing.

"I've got a terrible headache," I said, massaging my temples.

"I bet you do," Louise said and exhaled slowly.

I fled the auditorium and retreated to my room.

Louise probably anticipated the articulation of these perspectives long before we departed Charlottesville. She understood why my head ached even if I didn't. I was unable to identify the source of the pounding in my head. Much later, I wondered if it was avoidance, embarrassment, or shame?

I took two aspirins and lay down, but I couldn't fall asleep. I gave up and joined Louise and Mary for the afternoon session.

The afternoon session featured testimonials from Blacks who had been identified through screening as having sickle cell trait. They described job loss, withdrawal of life insurance, impossibly high health insurance premiums, and mortgage foreclosure. The consequences they described seemed so extreme that I began to wonder about the veracity of the speakers. I had never experienced this restrained anger, the just-below-the-surface rage. I was getting uncomfortable.

I started thinking about my interactions with Black people when I wasn't working at the UVA Hospital or the clinics in Charlottesville. One summer waitressing at Lake George, I danced late into night at the New York City Musicians' Union meeting next door. That was fun, certainly out of the ordinary, maybe even exotic because the musicians were all Black. As an acting intern in Rio Piedras, I visited the home of my patient with sickle cell disease. When Alan was doing harbor development in Jamaica, I met him not at a fancy resort on the touristy

North Coast but in gritty Kingston. We drank Red Stripe beer, ate curried goat on the street, and went clubbing. We were the only White people. Pregnant with Dylan, I'd shimmied under the limbo bar in St. Thomas the night after I interviewed for a position in public health. In those interactions with Black people, I'd never felt uncomfortable or unwelcome. It seemed that everyone was having a good time.

This conference was different. I felt out of place, ill at ease, maybe even an intruder. I sat stiffly between Mary and Louise. Mary couldn't sit still. She shook her head side to side and muttered under her breath. Finally, she pulled out *The Odessa File,* opened it to a folded-down-page, and stopped listening. Louise sat upright with rapt attention. She followed the speakers with head nods and sighs. My headache gained momentum until I was nauseated and saw bursts of scattering light. But, by then, I realized that I had no escape.

At supper, Mary was visibly agitated. As we sat down, she complained that we should have left at noontime, that the afternoon session was a disaster, a disgrace. Louise excused herself and walked to the cash bar for two white wines and a beer. A Budweiser for Mary. Same as the night before.

"We've got what we need," Mary persisted. "Target grade school, probably fourth or fifth grade before team sports and puberty. Do it in the spring. No colds, no flu, no bulky clothes to deal with. I'm ready." She folded and unfolded her napkin. I watched as she struggled for the right purchase in the chair, glaring first at me and then at the nearby tables.

"What would we accomplish?" I said slowly, feeling my way along. "We're not going to identify new cases of sickle cell disease." I thought for a minute. "And I doubt we'll prevent new disease. Even if there was an interest in premarital counseling, we don't have access to genetic counseling—"

"Come on!" Mary interrupted. "You thought this was a great town-gown collaboration."

"I know I did, Mary, but I'm not sure anymore."

"Well, I'm going to recommend that the TJHD start a pilot project in fifth grade, a model for the Commonwealth." Mary paused to accept the Budweiser from Louise. "Where do you stand, Louise? Sharon's not sure anymore. She's got cold feet."

Louise sat down, glanced at me quizzically, and pushed her untouched dinner plate aside. Her attention was focused on her wine. The din of the dining room rose and fell as the three of us sat in silence. People at other tables argued, some loudly and angrily. A few fists of defiance were raised. Others, like us, sat in uneasy silence.

Eventually, Louise swallowed her last sip of wine, placed her glass on the table, and looked at us.

"It's not always a bad idea to plan a prevention program for a specific population," she said and paused. "But we heard today what happens when a program is implemented without adequate input from the targeted group *and* when the health outcomes don't make a significant difference."

Mary frowned and shook her head in disagreement. Louise ignored her and continued. "Today, we heard about the *unintended* consequences that cause emotional, economic, and social harm to the very people we're trying to help."

Louise held us in the intensity of her gaze for a few beats before she continued. "Have either of you considered that the negative consequences described today may have been intended?"

Mary stood up, threw down her napkin, and slammed her chair. "Today's rabble-rousing has no relevance to Charlottesville and Albemarle," she said and glared at Louise. "*We're just trying to help your people.*"

I couldn't make eye contact with either of them. I considered putting the napkin over my face or crawling under the table.

"I thought you were different," Mary said and shuffled her things together. "*Not like the uppity Negros from the North—not knowing their place, stirring up trouble.*" Mary stormed off.

Louise returned to the cash bar. Two glasses of white wine.

"We'll have plenty of time back in Charlottesville," Louise said to me as she sat down, "to examine the origins of your headache."

She swirled her wineglass in deliberate circles and studied the patterns. We drank our wine slowly and in silence. Silence was never easy for me, but that evening I couldn't begin to summon the requisite words for conversation.

We were the last ones to leave the dining room.

At the elevator, Louise shrugged and gave me a wry smile. "At least," she said, "you knew enough to come back to the afternoon session."

I dreaded working with Louise in the clinic, but the awkwardness soon passed. I paid attention when she offered an opinion or made suggestions about our patients or the families. Later, Louise invited me to her family place in Chatham. Everyone lived within a stone's throw of one another, an enclave. We drove by the Black school Louise had attended. She explained that White people lived in Danville, the Black people in Chatham. Even when Louise pointed where the road surface changed from paved to dirt at the boundary, I didn't recognize the example of what we now call systemic racism. Did I think then that the separation represented preference? *If so, whose?*

The Thursday after the conference, Dr. Thurman wasn't surprised when I said that we recommended against collaborating with the screening project. "I'll take care of the commissioner," he said.

When I got up to leave, Dr. Thurman handed me an envelope. "This was delivered while you were in DC. Let me know if you need anything. Don't let it ruin Christmas." It was a subpoena to appear in Juvenile and Domestic Court on December 28, 1973.

Which is why, on Friday, December 28, I was seated in a third-row seat at the Regional Juvenile and Domestic Court. I nodded to the bailiff and the court stenographer when I took my seat. I regularly found myself in front of Judge Ralph Zehler, testifying as a friend of the court for the C&Y patients and families. Usually they were cases of truancy, child abuse, custody, or misdemeanors. Less often, rape or incest.

Today was different. I had been summoned to appear before Judge Zehler as the defendant. The charge was contributing to the delinquency of a minor.

In medical school, they made fun of me for my detailed chart notes, a little long perhaps, written in beautiful cursive, legible, and often with accompanying diagrams. I would have made a fine monk in the days of delicate calligraphy and illuminated manuscripts. My notes in the medical chart detailed our clinical conversations, the multiple sessions of counseling, including my repeated recommendation of abstinence, and finally the sit-down with Eileen and her boyfriend.

The unprotected sexual encounters continued between these two young lovers, both responsible college-bound honor students, for four months of documented counseling of abstinence. I prescribed oral birth control. That was a year ago. They were still together, campus tours completed, college essays composed, and applications submitted. They were terrific young people.

Just before Labor Day, Eileen let me know that her mother had found the birth control pills. Her parents were threatening to throw her out of the house, withhold college funds, and arrest the boyfriend. Eileen refused my offer to sit down with her parents. I documented that conversation, too.

Sitting in court, I did some quiet breathing and tried to settle down. The nausea passed, but my heart rate was still ramping up. I was a hellion growing up. I had forged Nellie's signature more than once, but I'd avoided real trouble, like legal trouble. I'd never shoplifted or gotten a speeding ticket or even been stopped when I'd had too much to drink.

The father showed up and sat across the aisle. A dour guy on a good day, he was in his mid-fifties, tall, and a bit humped over. He had a five o'clock shadow and a permanent scowl. I'd never met him, but I knew he was a professor. When he filed this suit against me, I figured out who he was by sight. His daughter was my patient in the private clinics.

"All rise!" boomed the bailiff as the black-robed Judge Zehler swept into the nearly empty courtroom and assumed his position at the raised bench. Dr. Thurman had said I wouldn't need a lawyer, but I was beginning to panic. I sat upright, eyes straight ahead, my hands clenched in my lap. I struggled with how I would defend myself against the father's charge of contributing to the delinquency of the minor named Eileen. My patient.

Judge Zehler read the charges and directed Eileen's father and his attorney to approach the bench. He glanced over at me as they spoke in whispers. They returned to their seats. Zehler stood up behind the bench. When he had everyone's attention, he announced, "The statutes of the Commonwealth of Virginia clearly permit the prescription of birth control by a licensed physician for a child between the ages of thirteen to eighteen within the confidentiality of an established doctor-patient relationship—*without parental knowledge.* Case dismissed."

I was grateful so few people had been in the courtroom and that neither Eileen nor I was called to testify. Out on High Street, the court stenographer hugged me, wished me a Happy New Year, and handed me a note—"Please meet Dr. Thurman in his office at four o'clock Tuesday.

He'll be returning from New Orleans." Tuesday was New Year's Day, the day of black-eyed peas and cornbread for many Virginians. I was so relieved that court was adjourned and so eager to spend the long weekend with Alan and the kids at the Mill that I wasn't concerned about Dr. Thurman's summons. Not initially.

"Happy New Year, Sharon," Dr. Thurman said. His voice didn't match his words. I sat down and willed myself to be still.

He shuffled papers around on his desk. Eventually, he looked up at me and said, "I have a great opportunity for you."

I wasn't seeking any more opportunities. My gut started to churn.

"I need you to move out to the Children's Rehabilitation Center as the medical director. Maybe, it'll be co–medical director with that pediatric orthopedist—"

"Never," I interrupted. I flashed back to August of my internship—the hostile head nurse, the disinfectant odors, the funeral home next door. "No way!"

"You have strong leadership skills. C&Y is thriving. The Center needs a leader." He shifted uneasily in his seat. "And the Department needs your help. There's a regular war going on between Orthopedics, Neurology, and Pediatrics. The Curry School and ENT are skirmishing on the sidelines."

"I hate that place," I interrupted again. "The staff are snobs. They're mean to our C&Y patients. Read their reports. Stuff like, *Johnny failed paper cutting.*"

"Stop it, Sharon." He raised his voice. "This must happen or the Department will lose a place to train our students and residents. We need to develop specialty clinics for patients with genetic disorders and behavioral issues. Inpatient competencies to take care of children with cancer, teenagers with trauma."

"No."

"This is not a discussion, Sharon. You'll move out there by Monday, January 14." He paused. "Take Dr. Merrill's office off the lobby."

What the hell had I done wrong? I was close to screaming.

This couldn't be happening. With Beverley's and Yvonne's commitments, I finally had some semblance of a schedule. Alan was in Washington or North Carolina now, no longer traveling around the globe, and most weekends he was with us. Kaki and Dylan were thriving. The Mill was home.

"This is NOT about you. It's a strategic move for the department. The Center needs to be a star in our crown. We need the patients for training and research." I didn't understand for years that Dr. Thurman had been clairvoyant about the future direction of children's healthcare.

"Why not someone else? Why me?"

"Sharon," he interrupted. "It's New Year's Day. I want to get home to my family, and you need to get back to Alan and the kids."

I was about to bawl. I didn't understand why everything was so urgent. Then the dam burst.

Dr. Thurman slid the Kleenex box across the desk.

"Stop crying, Sharon. *Promise me that you will not repeat this to anyone.* Not Alan. Not Beverley. Not Clariece. *Can you promise me that?"*

My shoulders shuddered with sobs, but I lifted my face out of the wad of Kleenex and nodded.

"I've accepted the position as dean of the School of Medicine at Tulane. Officially, I start late spring, but I'll start commuting to New Orleans by the end of January." He explained that UVA would conduct a national search. Tulane would announce his appointment the same day UVA announced the Search Committee for chair. Tentatively, on January 15.

"My family doesn't know yet, not for sure," he said. "Not until I get home."

I couldn't imagine the department without Dr. Thurman. Who would run morning resident rounds? Who would show up in the middle of the night when a sick kid crashed? Who would be Kaki and Dylan's pediatrician? Not only did I have to get moved, but I also had to organize the C&Y clinic schedules and close out the budget with Denby. He promised to explain the Center dynamics and something about promotion and tenure.

Dr. Thurman pulled himself to standing. The meeting was over.

I shook my head. I had stayed at UVA because of Dr. Thurman.

What the hell would I do?

· 15 ·

You're Beautiful and You're Mine

Spring and Summer 1974

Alan helped me pack up my C&Y office on the Corner. The Children's Rehabilitation Center, which we called the Center, was slightly more than a mile west of central Grounds, but it felt like Outer Mongolia. It was dark when I stacked the boxes on the floor of the assigned office off the lobby. I'd spent the day seeing patients with the C&Y team at the Keswick railroad station. And saying goodbye. It was 7:00 p.m. on Monday, January 14, 1974. I'd met Dr. Thurman's deadline, but I had little interest in unpacking my boxes.

The next day, Dr. Wilton Bunch, the pediatric orthopedist, invited me to his office, poured sherry into the Murano stemware he stored in his desk, and toasted our "shotgun wedding." We both understood it was a farce. Neither one of us was interested in being co-director, co-leader or co-any-damn-thing. We both preferred the role of king, but the decision was not ours. Despite the awkwardness of that first meeting, and the stark divide between everything from our medical to our religious orientations, we would become productive sparring partners—for decades.

I learned right away that the Center's warring factions were intent on maintaining the chaos. It was nearly a month before the nursing supervisor told me that the clinical supervisors from Physical Therapy, Occupational Therapy, Speech and Hearing, Psychology, Social Work, School and Recreational Therapy met weekly with Dr. Bunch at a time when I was dependably out of the building—attending pediatric grand rounds at the main hospital. The next week, I arrived early, well in time to greet them one by one.

Much to Dr. Bunch's surprise, I appeared each morning for his inpatient rounds with the orthopedic residents. I learned about the inpatients, their mobility goals, and the surgical procedures planned, but I also discovered unrecognized genetic syndromes, hearing and vision problems, and developmental delays. I became determined to fulfill Dr. Thurman's aspirations for the Center as a model of care for children, a place to teach students, and a setting for clinical research. I had a lot to learn, but my most important lesson was recognizing the social impact of disability.

I missed Clariece. I missed Helen. Most of all, I missed our patients and their families. Jan and AV regularly popped in at the Center. When Dr. McChesney called me for consultation, I recognized it was an excuse to maintain contact. Beverley knew how isolated I felt, and she invited me out to lunch at the Mousetrap, an unheard-of luxury in the middle of a workday.

Those first few weeks out at the Center, I did nothing but whine at the Mill. Complaining made it worse. Alan was quick to offer alternatives like selling the Mill and living on the houseboat near the shipyard in North Carolina. I stopped complaining.

Red Hill Elementary School was less than a mile from the Mill, but from the very onset, Alan was opposed to the kids going there. Red Hill was distinguished for having the lowest funding per pupil in the county. On both Erla's and Patty's recommendations, we applied, were interviewed, and pre-enrolled them at a private school in town. Eventually, I learned the accepted lingo—it was a child-initiated curriculum of experiential learning in a socially respectful setting.

I loved the freedom my kids had to wander around the Mill, but I worried about their easy access to the creek. So I recruited graduate students to teach Kaki and Dylan to swim. Louise decided to sign up, too. Black kids never had access to the public swimming pools in Virginia, so Louise had never learned to swim.

At the Center, I learned that most of our patients didn't attend school in their local communities. Children with special needs were not welcome. It was not until the following year, 1975, that Congress would pass the Education for All Handicapped Children Act, which required public schools to provide education for all kids with physical and mental disabilities in the local schoolhouse. It would be years, sometimes decades, before there would be serious attempts at implementation.

One of the many interests competing for power at the Center was the Curry School of Education. They were trying to organize an inpatient school. The faculty needed access to children with disabilities to train their student teachers. The Center was a potential lab to prepare the workforce needed for public schools everywhere.

Next door to my office, a PhD student, as part of her dissertation project, ran an integrated kindergarten with a group of five-year-old kids from Charlottesville who came every morning. *Integrated* disabilities meant her pupils had blindness, deafness, cerebral palsy, cystic fibrosis, autism, and giftedness. I became a frequent observer, a cheerleader in the classroom, and a staunch supporter outside of the classroom.

While Dr. Thurman guided me through the politics of the department clashes, I shared what I learned making rounds at the bedside, attending therapy sessions, and sitting in on the kindergarten. I made a glossary of the endless, seemingly eclipsing terms—special needs, disabled, handicapped, chronically ill, neurodevelopmentally challenged, sensory impaired. I initiated meetings with the chairs of Neurology, Orthopedics, ENT, and Neurosurgery. I took notes as I listened to their concerns about recruiting patients for teaching and research, improving residency training, and the future of the Center.

One evening as I ranted about all the conflicts, Beverley got out one of her huge pads of white paper and drew charts and graphs, arrows pointing this way and that. All I knew about organizational models was what I'd later learn was called "command and control," a vertical communication pattern that only went from the top down. She pressed me to describe the patterns of the meetings, who talked with whom, who had informal influence. Beverley encouraged me to listen and to identify the recurring patterns.

Beverley insisted that I needed a better grasp of the economics of the Center and suggested that I focus on how the funds flowed for the inpatient service. That line of inquiry quickly led me to the Division of Crippled Children's Services and the Virginia Department of Education. Deciphering the complex bureaucratic state systems was frustrating at first. I was battling for the children who still lived at home or in back rooms without services. Identifying the enemy focused me and gave meaning to my efforts.

That spring, I met the doctors' wives who volunteered at the Center and learned why they volunteered—empty nests for some, meaning-making, and grief work for others. It turned out that the wife of the chair of Surgery, the one who had fussed about my heels and flesh-colored hose when I was an intern, spent one afternoon a week writing thank-you notes to our donors. Another mother shared that she had a son at the Lynchburg Training School, committed directly from the nursery with Down's syndrome. She was tearful when she told me that she had never held her baby. I flashed back to my role in court as an intern when I participated in the commitment of a newborn with Down's syndrome to the Lynchburg Training Center. I cringed, remembering how I had pointed out the single palmar creases to the judge only to learn that both Dr. Thurman and Dr. Birdsong had single creases.

I learned from the UVA Hospital administrator that healthcare was considered big business. Hospitals, pharmaceutical and insurance companies, even doctors, needed to make a profit. I had a flashback to an economics class at Middlebury, when I'd objected to the professor's inclusion of medicine as a business. The administrator explained the concept of a loss leader in business, then gave the example of pediatrics as the hospital's loss leader. I couldn't believe it. His bottom line was that I couldn't count on insurance companies or hospitals to fund altruism but that there were creative ways to raise funds. I needed to sort it out.

I learned to appreciate Dr. Thurman's genius for raising money to fund his dreams. Early on, I realized the financing strategy would be like stitching a patchwork quilt. No single source would ever be sufficient. From the C&Y experience, I realized that I'd have to compete for federal monies. Patty coached me through the paperwork of the first federal grant application, but Dr. Thurman coached me on how to hone the story. Once I began to understand the children's needs and their families' dreams, telling the story was the easy part.

My Thursday meetings with Dr. Thurman continued when he was in town. He transferred information as fast as he could, but his attention was increasingly in New Orleans. He warned me that I would probably be summoned by the Search Committee for the new chair. I should be at ease, take my time to explain the outreach activities. He still brought breakfast. I secretly wished that Dr. Thurman would recruit me to New Orleans, and I was disappointed when he didn't.

He didn't talk about promotion and tenure except to say he'd prepared my packet for the new chair to submit. That turned out to be a major omission.

As a junior faculty member, I had to apply for and receive tenure, or I would be fired. I didn't understand that process until it became a full-blown disaster.

When I received a Dean's Office summons to the Department of Urology to meet with the committee, I had no idea what to expect.

At the appointed day and time, the secretary led me into an office lined with bookshelves and diplomas. Seven men in long white coats stood up from the circle, nodded, and, one by one, shook my hand.

I was taken aback when the most senior member opened with a rant about the current state of affairs in the Department of Pediatrics. Deplorable, he said. It didn't take me long to recognize the rhetoric from the law faculty cocktail party that Labor Day of internship year—the ranting about the abandonment of medicine's core mission for social activism, the recruitment of social scientists and misfits as faculty members, and the solicitation of grant monies from the federal government for what amounted to political agitation in the community. When he finished, the others harrumphed and nodded in agreement. Beverley had cautioned me to listen for the question and only answer the question, nothing else. But no questions were asked. I sat still, which wasn't easy for me to do. After additional tirades without inquiry, Dr. Stu Howard, a pediatric urologist, invited me to talk about the C&Y Project, why it was relevant, and what role I played.

I think the group was surprised when I framed the public health status with supporting data, the premise of the local demonstration project, and how it compared to its peers nationally. Patty had coached me with our local data and her observations from the University of Pennsylvania.

Eventually, they did ask questions. What was the purpose of the big orange van they saw driving out of town in the morning? Did we really examine patients in the Keswick railroad station? What about the protests from the dental society? Was it true that Dr. Thurman appointed a *Negro* woman to the faculty?

In the meantime, I kept trying to make sense of the Center. I sat in the therapy gym and watched as the therapist worked with a child to increase range of motion or decrease muscle tone. I observed in the preschool as a four-year-old burn patient played the same scene again—the doll house was on fire, the fire engine came with sirens, and finally the ambulance. The ambulance never arrived in time to save the dog. I watched adolescent girls get fitted for braces with close attention focused on their scoliosis, with no concern for their modesty. I even went bowling with recreational therapy and learned about adaptive devices and how getting a strike can be such fun to a kid in a wheelchair. I signed up to see patients in all the clinics—from cystic fibrosis to cerebral palsy. Patients became my best teachers.

I didn't do so well with the parents. I dreaded the sight of Mrs. Stilfried waiting outside my office. She was determined that her son, Franz, with fragile bones, should be allowed to swim in the Center's indoor pool. The pool was solely reserved by Recreational Therapy for sessions only with the inpatients.

"Why can he swim in the pool if he sleeps at the Center, but not if he sleeps in his own bed?" she demanded. She was not impressed by my references to the Center rules. "Who makes the rules? Don't you?" Mrs. Stilfried ignored my cautions about taking four-year-old Franz to the Outer Banks. Of course, Franz was knocked down by the waves, but he screamed in delight in spite of his broken bones. Franz would become an important mentor for me, explaining that a certain level of risk-taking was necessary to be alive.

Jan, the speech pathologist at C&Y, helped me understand the tensions between ENT and the Speech and Hearing Therapy program at the Curry School. ENT needed audiologists for training their residents, referrals for rarer diseases like tumors of the auditory nerve. Curry needed the hearing-impaired children for training the speech therapists to work in the schools. What they had in common was they were both committed to the best possible patient care and ensuring that their training programs had the requisite patients for clinical learning. The conflict was much more complicated than an argument about the hearing-aid business as I'd initially thought. More than ninety different genes were involved in hearing. There was major conflict about teaching children to communicate by signing, which was relatively easy, or learning to speak, which was a very long, difficult, and frustrating process. We couldn't imagine a future with cochlear implants. We added a Division of Speech and Hearing at the Center, put Jan in charge, and encouraged the many collaborations. It was one of my early victories.

After my meeting with the Search Committee, I had no further involvement in the process of finding the new chair. I heard after the fact that a few candidates had visited UVA, but I never was invited to meet with them. It felt a lot like when I was back on Vernon Street playing with the neighborhood boys. I'd spend all afternoon in center field shagging balls down to the creek, but I never had a chance to bat. Although I felt increasingly alienated from the faculty in Pediatrics, I reassured myself that I was becoming part of the Center team.

By early summer of 1974, the dean announced the new chair—Dr. Robert M. Blizzard, a pediatric endocrinologist from Johns Hopkins and reportedly the world's expert on growth hormone. Five years before, Dr. Thurman had recruited Dr. Ann Johanson from Hopkins as the division chief of Pediatric Endocrinology, and she had three faculty now. Did we really need another endocrinologist?

I'd spent six months at the Center. We still had our controversies, but we'd begun working out the solutions together. The inpatient teams were engaged and optimistic. The outpatient clinics were coming along, except for the Child Development Clinic (CDC).

The CDC was a federally funded project designed to demonstrate a process of interdisciplinary assessment of children with combinations of diseases, disabilities, and learning styles. The newly recruited CDC staff were legitimately cramped for space in a building that was designed for inpatients. The Center had an indoor, heated swimming pool, but the school principal sat at a desk at the top of the stairwell.

The problem wasn't that the CDC didn't have a highly competent team. Each discipline was committed to perfection. The problem was that they didn't trust themselves to negotiate overlaps with their colleagues in other disciplines, so they duplicated assessments that had already been done by other disciplines. My goal for the CDC was to assess more than one patient each week, preferably five; to create a single interdisciplinary summary to share with the local community; and to share the findings with the parents and to provide them with a copy of the report. The team opposed me on all points.

My solution was to invite them to an all-day retreat at Big Meadows in Shenandoah National Park. By mid-August, they received their invitations. I would accept no excuses, no exceptions. I sent out the agenda with data and our goals for the day. We would begin at 8:30 a.m. that Tuesday, September 11, and head back down the mountain by 4:30 p.m.

The week of the retreat was complicated for me. Kaki's birthday was the weekend before. The following Wednesday was the first day of school for my kids. I asked Erla to keep Kaki and Dylan that Tuesday, so I could leave early for Big Meadows, an hour away. The Center's head nurse invited me to ride with her. She thought we could use the time in transit for planning. I laughed, accepted her invitation, and suggested that the return trip would be our chance to debrief. As it turned out, we never had that chance.

To celebrate Kaki's sixth birthday, we found a table upstairs at the Mousetrap and ordered our cheeseburgers and french fries. It was early, and the band was just warming up. Kaki was the star in her long, red-and-white-checked Granny dress with puffed sleeves and ruffles, a white apron tied with a big bow in the back. By the time we finished our cake and ice cream, the place was swinging. Alan walked over to the band, made a request, and invited Kaki to dance.

All eyes were on them as Alan twirled Kaki around to Ringo Starr's "You're Sixteen, You're Beautiful and You're Mine." The crowd started to clap and sing the lyrics. *Peaches and cream, ribbon and curls, eyes that sparkle and shine.* By the last chorus, Alan and Kaki were alone on the dance floor. He scooped her into his arms for a few fancy moves. "*You're six, so beautiful and you're mine.*" The music finally ended. Alan bowed to Kaki. The room was silent as he led her back to our table. The drum roll started low and slow. The crowd stomped and cheered. Encore! Encore!

Little did I realize then how many times I would replay the scene of Alan and Kaki dancing at the Mousetrap on her sixth birthday. Alan and Kaki never danced together again. I would cry for years remembering that dance.

The next day we set out first thing Sunday for the Blue Ridge Pool. Dylan didn't like to dunk his head under the water, but he loved to splash everyone around him. Kaki could dog-paddle across the pool with her head arched out of the water.

Lunch was fried chicken and red potato salad straight from Foods. The kids curled up on the grass and fell asleep, still in their bulky orange swim vests.

I lay next to the kids, but I wasn't napping. Alan sat cross-legged next to me. I was drifting in and out of the woodsy silence. I wasn't fidgeting or making a list. I think it was the last time I would feel totally relaxed for years.

But out of the blue, Alan launched into his distress with our life, the weekly commute from DC to Charlottesville each Friday, and back to DC each Monday morning, week after week. My call schedule. My working on Saturday mornings. His voice was low, but intense.

He reminded me of my reluctance to move to New Zealand after medical school. My resistance after Kaki's birth to finding a farm in Nova Scotia like his Dimock ancestors had done, where we would tend apple orchards in the Annapolis Valley along the Bay of Fundy. My refusal to pack it all in after Dylan was born to live on a sailboat, drifting from port to port in the Caribbean. Or moving to North Carolina to live on a houseboat after Peter Johnson and he bought the shipyard on the New Bern River.

He wanted us to be a different kind of family, a family who began the day together at the breakfast table, committed to one another and to exploring the world. Routines to share together at supper and bedtimes, maybe star gazing. I was stunned as Alan continued in his soft, pressured voice. Maybe, he suggested, since I had rejected living on a sailboat, maybe we should consider homesteading in West Virginia or some other wilderness. I concentrated on listening. Maybe. I took a few deep breaths, but I didn't interrupt. That was unusual.

I don't remember what I was thinking as the kids napped by the pool and Alan spun out that dream of his, only that I was surprised, taken aback, maybe even annoyed. I remember asking if there would be a hospital in that wilderness of his. I reminded him that I was a pediatrician. I'd need a place to treat my patients.

The spell was broken when the kids woke up. As we loaded up, I whispered to Alan that I wasn't Patch Adams in disguise.

Monday morning was chaotic as usual. The kids were finishing up breakfast at the kitchen table. I was packing up their lunches. Alan hugged me from behind and rubbed his beard across the back of my neck. He kissed the kids on the tops of their heads, worked his way through the Danes, and went out the kitchen door.

That was our routine: Alan would leave on Monday and return on Friday. There was no reason to think this week wouldn't be the same.

· 16 ·

The Man on the Phone

September 8, 1974

It was late Tuesday morning. The retreat was way behind schedule, but the conference room at Big Meadows was finally quiet. The CDC staff arrived already on the edge of rebellion. They resisted my direction to move the chairs into circles. They shuffled the case summaries from one hand to the other, not reading them. They refused to talk to one another. We were way behind, but at last they did begin to talk to one another—maybe, I hoped, about the cases.

The door opened, and the lodge manager motioned me into the corridor. I had an urgent call in the lobby. The lodge had only one line. It was a long-distance call.

Who was the man on the phone? Why was he calling me?

I listened to the man's voice on the telephone in the lobby of Big Meadows Lodge on Skyline Drive. I didn't know who he was, the man on the phone. I didn't know his name. I didn't recognize his voice.

The man on the phone said he was a colleague of Alan's at OSE. But really, who was he? Why had he interrupted our retreat at Big Meadows? I stood in the lobby and leaned against the counter. Why was the manager standing so close to me? Was he trying to eavesdrop? Did he think I'd steal the phone?

"Are you listening?" asked the man on the phone. He said he was worried about Alan and Bob. Had anyone tried to contact me? The man thought Alan and Bob were on Eastern Airlines Flight #212. The flight that crashed before it made it to the runway at the Charlotte, North Carolina, airport. At 7:32 a.m. this morning. Crashed in a cornfield.

Who was this man on the phone? Why did he call me at Big Meadows? Why was the manager so close to me? Eastern Airlines? Charlotte?

He kept talking, the man on the phone. He said that Alan and Bob had checked out of the Holiday Inn in Charleston, South Carolina, at 5:30 a.m. and returned the rental car to the Avis agency at the airport. Eastern Airlines hadn't released the passenger manifest. Eastern Airlines weren't answering their phones. Not in Charlotte or in DC.

The manager touched my arm, asked me if I needed anything. What I needed was to know who the man on the phone was and why he kept talking. Did Alan fly Eastern Airlines that day? I doubted it. We flew Piedmont Airlines.

The man on the phone said the radio announced eighty-nine dead and nine admitted to the hospital. He wanted to know if I knew someone who could check the names on the admit list at the hospital in Charlotte.

I was at the end of my rope retreating with the damn clinic staff—the team of prima donnas who could see only one complicated patient a week. What the hell? One patient a week?

The man on the phone wouldn't shut up. Did I know someone who could access the admission list at the Charlotte hospital?

Yes, I told the man on the phone, I knew someone who could find out who was admitted to the Charlotte hospital. Who was the man on the phone? Did he really know Alan? Did Alan fly on that Eastern Airlines flight that day?

The Big Meadows Lodge manager granted me permission to make a long-distance call. I got to hang up the phone. The man finally stopped talking.

I called the UVA Hospital operator, identified myself, and asked to be patched in directly to John Harlan, the hospital administrator. Instead, it was his secretary who answered. It seemed Mr. Harlan couldn't be disturbed—he was chairing the Hospital Board Meeting. Emergency, I told her. I had to know the names of the passengers admitted from the Eastern Airlines crash in Charlotte. I whispered that Alan might have been on the flight.

I held the phone, leaned against the counter with my back to the lobby, and waited. I heard the CDC group whisper as they went into lunch. The manager waved them away. I waited and waited. It seemed forever. The manager was still next to me. What did he want?

"Dimock—NOT on the admit list. Synder—NOT on the admit list. I'm sorry, Sharon." It was John Harlan. "Did you know I was the student administrator when Piedmont crashed here in 1959—"

I hung up. My whole body started to shake. The manager let me use his office. He brought me the phone, shut the office door, and sat down with me.

I had to get to North Carolina to find Alan, but I didn't have my car. I called and called, but I couldn't locate Beverley.

I called Clariece. I called Jan. In desperation, I called Dr. Mac. He knew where Beverley was—she was in the private clinics. Dylan crashed his wagon going over the stone wall at Neve Hall. He was getting stitches, 107 stitches, above his right eye. Dr. Mac told me to stay at Big Meadows, promised that Beverley was on her way to pick me up.

The phone rang, and the manager handed it to me. It was Alan's colleague Pete Johnson, his boatyard partner. "I'm on my way from DC to Charlottesville."

"Meet me at the Charlottesville Airport. I'm going to Charlotte. I've got to find Alan."

Beverley drove me to the airport in Charlottesville. Piedmont Airlines had no flights to Charlotte, but they suggested a charter. I wrote a check for $450, more than I had in my checking account, and asked them to hold it for a week or so. They knew Alan and me, and by then, they knew that Eastern Airlines had crashed in a cornfield. Pete arrived, and the three of us flew to Charlotte. The kids stayed overnight with Erla. She promised not to turn on the radio and to keep them home from school the next day, the first day at the new school.

Eastern Airlines had not released the manifest for Flight #212.

No one was at the Eastern Airlines counter in Charlotte. The sign said CLOSED.

No one would take us to the cornfield where the plane had crashed.

No one would let us into the hangar where the National Guardsmen were unloading black plastic body bags from the cornfield.

I couldn't find Alan.

· 17 ·

Where Is Daddy?

September 9–13, 1974

I awoke to the roar of a plane taking off outside my window. It was barely light out, and, for a moment, I was irritated. Then I remembered. I struggled to breathe. It felt like I had a heavy vault on my chest. I gasped and let loose a full-throttled scream. Eastern Flight #212 had crashed. Alan missing, maybe still alive, but probably dead. Dead in a black plastic body bag in the airport hangar.

I was at the airport Holiday Inn in Charlotte, still in the clothes I wore to the retreat at Big Meadows. That seemed years ago. When we got in the night before, I tried to get into the hangar to identify Alan, but the National Guard wouldn't let me pass, even when I explained I was a doctor.

Maybe Alan wasn't in a body bag. Maybe he and Bob stopped for coffee, missed the flight, and decided to drive back to DC. Maybe he'd come home on Friday like always. Alan and Bob might not even know about the crash.

Denial was nearly impossible when the body lay in a hospital bed—pulseless, cold to the touch, and stiff with rigor mortis. Denial was easier without evidence like a name on the manifest to prove that Alan boarded the flight. Denial was a whole lot easier without a body.

A wake of vultures swooped into the Holiday Inn—the undertakers of Charlotte arriving, commissioned by Eastern Airlines as a service for the families. No manifest with the names of passengers on Flight #212. It was now more than twenty-four hours after the flight had taken off from Charleston and crashed in Charlotte. No contact from Eastern Airlines.

I didn't know or care how many funeral parlors there were in Charlotte in September 1974, but Eastern Airlines must have hired them all. Apparently, Eastern guaranteed all the burial expenses. The mortician salesmen maintained appropriately morose miens, belying any excitement at the unexpected boom in business. They went door to door with brochures—photographs of caskets padded with satin pillows and lined with lead.

I remembered the undertakers for Uncle Tom, Pa, and Hop back in Rutland when I was a kid—the shame of choosing the cheapest casket, the open caskets in the living room, and the hypocrisy of last rites with burial plots in and out of consecrated grounds.

I asked the first vulture to leave in the middle of his obsequious spiel. I interrupted the second to show him to the door. He'd persisted in pointing out there was no cost, no need to hold back, no limits at all. Eastern Airlines was honored to foot the entire bill. I was ready for the third one. I didn't let him even start his pitch. I told him I wanted to discuss cremation only, no ceremonies, no burials. Send the ashes to Charlottesville. He nodded, opened the color brochure, and suggested perhaps a simple cherry casket? I clarified that I had no interest in burning the casket, just the body. He stepped back, turned pale, and reminded me about the sensitivities of the crematorium workers. How would they feel pushing a body in a cardboard box into the fire? How the hell did I feel thinking that it would be my red-bearded husband in the cardboard box?

I didn't know it then, but it would be weeks, even months before Alan's body was identified. There would be no red beard left.

The confrontations turned out to be therapeutic, a way for me to vent my rage. I didn't really believe Alan was dead. I considered it a theoretical exercise. However, Pete and Beverley convinced me that I needed to sign a contract, even if it was only theoretical. Then, there were the laws about crossing state lines. I called Dr. Mac for help.

"Hill and Wood, downtown on First Street," he said without hesitation. "Charlotte and I send our love to you and the children."

I don't remember how we got back to Charlottesville, but I think Pete must have paid the charter pilot to stay overnight in Charlotte and fly us back. There was another scene with the National Guard when I demanded access into the makeshift morgue. Pete grabbed my arm and pulled me away. He warned me to keep moving. I turned back to look at the clutch of reporters shouting questions, but Pete never slowed down.

It was midafternoon when we landed in Charlottesville. Pete went back to DC, and Beverley took me to the Center to get my car. I thought about what I would tell the kids as I drove to the Mill. Yvonne was sobbing in the kitchen. *Was Mister Dimock really on that plane?* I didn't know what to say.

I sat on our bed and gathered Kaki and Dylan in my arms. The dogs leaned against my legs. I told them Daddy had been in a plane crash, a terrible crash in North Carolina. "Where is Daddy?" Dylan demanded. "Why isn't Daddy here?" I started to cry. Dylan alternated between hitting my arm and the pillows. Kaki became strangely quiet. She leaned into me with her arms around my waist, then she grew pale and her whole body shook. That triggered the dogs. Max laid his head on my lap and nudged Kaki with his nose. Mattie, even more high-strung now that she was pregnant, crawled up on the bed and stretched out. She growled when Dylan punched anywhere near her.

Where was Alan? I wanted to know where he was, too. I didn't believe in angels or heaven, but I was tempted to spin that magic. Maybe I should have taken them to Sunday school. Then we might have had a prayer to share. But I didn't. I made up something about Daddy always living inside our hearts and our memories. Even I thought that was weak. It didn't seem the right time for ashes to ashes, dust to dust.

The night before, Beverley had called Harry, her father, in Florida, and he was on his way to Virginia. I'd called Patty and Ray in Philadelphia for help. Patty called. She had arrived in Charlottesville and had stopped at Foods for provisions. Could she use the charge account?

AV was the first one through the kitchen door with two eye rounds of beef, a platter of bread, butter, horseradish, and mustard. The chief resident delivered a bouquet of flowers from the pediatric residents. Warm biscuits and honey from Helen. Cuban meat pies from Jean, the head nurse at the Center, the one who had driven me to Big Meadows. I couldn't imagine what we would do with all that food, but AV knew the Southern rituals of calling. Yvonne labeled the casseroles, but she kept sobbing and praying loudly for Mister Dimock. I worried that her references to the streets of gold might confuse the kids, but they didn't pay any attention. Beverley set up a bar.

Patty arrived and took command. She put on a bibbed apron and tied her hair up in a kerchief. She settled the kids and me in the library with sandwiches and Kleenex. The dogs stayed close. She assigned Beverley the wall phone by the kitchen door and gave her a pad and pencil. Take messages, don't answer questions, write everything down. Patty stationed Erla at the front door. It was a siege of flowers, food, and sobbing visitors—friends, colleagues, and strangers.

The phone never stopped ringing. Pete Johnson checked in, told me he would pack up Alan's office, and asked if I had a key to the apartment. The *Daily Progress* wanted information about Alan's education, the ages of the children. Dr. Blizzard reported he'd taken care of things at the Center and wanted me to call him back. The *Washington Post* asked about the Eastern Airlines manifest. One of Alan's buddies demanded payment, immediately, of a ten-thousand-dollar loan he'd made to Alan ten years before. I was furious when I heard. He never offered condolences to me or the kids. Beverley recorded the messages on her pad, sipped her Scotch, and made no promises.

It was after ten when Yvonne and I got the kids into bed. I couldn't believe it when Patty announced a planning meeting. I needed a shower. I was beyond tired. Beverley had drunk a lot of Scotch. Patty wanted us to strategize about the next days—had I called Alan's older kids? His ex-wife? Yes. His parents were dead. I'd call his brothers. What about Nellie? Oh, dear God, not Nellie here.

When Patty said we had to plan a funeral, I started to perseverate about whether Alan was really dead. Where was he? What would he think if he showed up and we were in the middle of a funeral? First thing in the morning, Beverley would try to reach Eastern Airlines about the manifest. Patty would ask Ray to think about a ceremony, some kind of celebration. Not a funeral and not in a church. Alan was a Unitarian, but I didn't really know what that meant.

When I finally got into bed, I couldn't get to sleep. I floated on the edge of nightmares. I thought about Alan's yearning to be free—to immigrate to New Zealand's South Island, to sail around the world, to grow apples in the Annapolis Valley along the Bay of Fundy in Nova

Scotia or, even last weekend, to go homesteading in West Virginia. The wonder in his eyes and in his voice as he described the exotic women in Jamaica, their graceful bodies, their skin the color of latte or café au lait or espresso. The vibrant women in indigo and jade he bartered with in the night markets of India. Could Alan have missed that flight on purpose? I had totally tuned out his meanderings about homesteading last Sunday at the pool. Maybe he had had enough of UVA, medicine, and me. Bob Snyder was older, married, and, I think, had adult children. I didn't know his story. Maybe they just disappeared. It happened. I'd read about it once.

The next morning, the kids crawled into my bed. Their snuggling brought me to consciousness, and I smiled. But then I remembered, and I felt like I'd been sucker-punched. Eastern Airlines crashed. Alan was dead. Alan wasn't coming home. Not this Friday. Maybe never.

I worried that Yvonne might not come back, but there she was at the stove frying chicken. She wondered about taking Kaki and Dylan into their new school in town. They'd already missed their first day, but I wanted them close by, safe, or maybe to comfort me.

The chaos began anew on Thursday, but Patty remained in charge. No news from Eastern meant no manifest. More calls from people I didn't know. Patty's husband, Ray, was on his way from Philadelphia. Beverley checked on airline schedules. When I called Dr. Blizzard back, he told me my place should be at home with the children. What the hell did that mean? Where did he think I was? I didn't understand that he meant for good.

The siege of phone calls, flowers, and food continued. Patty tried to keep the kids, the dogs, and me out of the kitchen and away from the door. Beverley, Yvonne, and she would maintain the perimeter. Every so often, Dylan asked where Daddy was. Kaki looked at me and shook her head. Dylan didn't understand. But neither did I.

Thursday afternoon, Mary Stamp came to call. She was the wife of Dr. Warren Stamp, the chair of Orthopedics, known in faculty circles to be independently wealthy, allegedly an oil heiress, and the reason they lived in a stately mansion in Farmington with their three boys. Mrs. Stamp offered her condolences, then suggested that she could review my financial portfolio with me. I was confused.

"There are important and time-sensitive decisions you must make," she explained. "I am quite knowledgeable. I may be able to assist you in getting things organized. Let's take a quick look at your holdings."

I shook my head and stammered. I don't think she believed me when I reported that I didn't have a lawyer or an accountant. We had no portfolio of investments, just the outstanding mortgage on the Mill. No, Alan did not have life insurance. He'd had the opportunity. He'd turned it down.

Just six months before, Alan reported a new OSE perk—a life insurance policy instead of the annual cash bonus. Alan laughed and said that I was young and beautiful. If he were to die, the suitors would be lined up the next day. I'd be married within six months. He took the cash.

Mary Stamp didn't ask about Alan's will. I didn't volunteer that he didn't have one. I would learn later that since Alan died intestate, one-third of his estate would be apportioned to his widow and two-thirds to his six children. I would have to buy back the books from our library, including the ones inscribed to Alan from Sharon, but I didn't know that yet.

By late afternoon, Ray arrived from Philadelphia and took up residence in the library. Dylan ignored the comings and the goings. He concentrated on constructing massive, complicated structures that used every Lego piece. Then he smashed his creations and started over. Kaki and Max were never far from my side—quiet and watchful, never in the way, almost ghostlike. Mattie got excited when Dylan destroyed his buildings, but mostly she stayed by Yvonne's side and guarded the kitchen door.

It seemed strange to plan a funeral or a celebration of life or whatever we were calling it without confirmation that Alan was on the flight that crashed in the cornfield.

The Mill continued to be under siege with flowers, food, and people. Well-meaning people like Mrs. Stamp, people from work, and the Black preacher from down the road. When someone arrived, they insisted on bypassing Yvonne or Beverley or Patty to find me. As soon as they spotted me, they started to cry and reached out to touch me. One by one, over and over, it was the same ritual—they shared the circumstances, time, and place when they heard Alan was on the Eastern Airlines flight that crashed. Then they shared the details of some remarkable experience they'd shared with Alan—collecting black walnuts at Beau Pré, planting pepper plants at the Mill, sailing on the Chesapeake. They sought comfort from us, whether it was a hug, delight at the shared story, or gratitude for a casserole. It was confusing, like I was a prop in someone else's play. We were the ones who were still denying that Alan might really be dead. The ones who hadn't acknowledged our own loss. The callers seemed to know all the details of the plot when we didn't have a clue.

By Thursday night, I'd glimpsed some newspaper images of the crash scene, the broken-off tail of the airplane, the rescue workers carrying black body bags. I worried then that Alan might be alive, but unconscious in one of the bags. I left a message with Alan's height and weight, the description of his distinctive red beard, and the engraving on his wedding band. It was a relief to consider that he might not have been on the flight in the first place, even if it meant he had purposedly disappeared, abandoning us.

When I was awake at night, I could hear Dylan talking in his sleep—loud, but mostly unintelligible. Max stretched out in Alan's position on the bed, his huge head on the pillow next to me. When I cried, Max keened right along with me.

Friday morning, the call finally came from Eastern Airlines. The names of both Alan Dimock and Bob Snyder were on the manifest for Flight #212. They had boarded the plane in Charleston. The man on the phone requested Alan's dental films and X-rays of past fractures. I called Pete at OSE, Peter in Nashville, Gioia and Dorothy, Bob Synder's wife in Florida. Beverley organized flights, airport pickups, and places to stay. Ray suggested we call the funeral a celebration of life, create a program, and ask Peter Kaplan to speak. Ray cloistered himself in the library. Patty reserved the University Chapel for Sunday.

Patty, Beverley, and I sat in the kitchen with Yvonne to talk about plans for the ceremony. Yvonne would be a member of the family, a mourner, not a staff person. Yvonne made sure that we had her favorite single-malt Scotch and that she could share the bed with Max and me.

The kitchen was empty when I came down to make coffee on Saturday. As I passed through the common room, I heard a chair rocking. I glimpsed what I thought was the back of Alan's head and caught my breath. Alan was alive.

Once in the kitchen, I could see the rocking chair was empty. I sat down in the other chair and wondered if I was losing my mind. Saturday morning was the first time I had been alone. It was the first time I felt frightened. How could I live without Alan? How could I raise the kids? How would I manage the Center and the Mill? And what the hell was I going to do with Mattie's puppies?

Patty was working on the complicated logistics for the next day's ceremony. Harry, Beverley's father, arrived from Florida and took over the airport shuttle. Yvonne tended to what the kids would wear. I had phone duty.

Harry took orders from Beverley. Dorothy arrived from Boston, Gioia and Stevie from Salt Lake City. They were staying with one of Beverley's social work colleagues. Peter was driving from Nashville. It would be a late arrival, so he'd sleep in the library.

Yvonne and I were at the stove when I recognized the raspy, two-pack-a-day voice. Nellie was at the kitchen door. She was hollering at Mattie, "Get away, right now, you damn dog. Don't push me."

"Where's my luggage?" she snapped at Jean, the nurse who'd picked her up at the airport. "I'm staying here at the Mill. I packed for a good long time."

"The Mill is full to the rafters," I said. I tried to smile, but I was furious. "You're staying with Jean and her husband. The luggage can stay in the car." I took a breath and lowered my shoulders. "Jean said y'all are cooking Cuban tonight—it'll be fun. Have some lunch and you guys can get going. We're flat out here."

"I thought you'd need me around," Nellie whined. "You know how Hattie came after Hop died and stayed with us on Vernon Street. I think it was a year or so." I thought to myself—and that is why you are not staying in Virginia any longer than the service. I was ready to punch her out if she said another word. The last thing I needed then or ever was Nellie around me, the kids, or the dogs.

Patty intervened and invited me into the library, saying Ray needed my advice on what to say at the ceremony. Later, I realized I should have paid more attention.

The next day, I was seated in the front row of the Chapel as planned. As the sun brightened the indigo blue of the stained-glass window above the altar, I began to fret. How would Alan, the Unitarian, feel about his family sitting here at the feet of Christ to celebrate his, Alan's, life? The Chapel had been a practical choice, certainly not a religious decision.

I heard the whispers around us. Whatever will she do? The children are so young. Does she have tenure?

A faculty member from the Music Department played "Greensleeves" on the harpsichord as people congregated. Why had I insisted on "Greensleeves"? It was beginning to sound maudlin. And the kids were getting restless. I thought about getting up to leave, but then Ray called us to order, and the program began. Peter clenched the podium as he struggled to make meaning from Alan's commitment to grow asparagus at the Mill, build a circular staircase from a telephone pole, and carve Kaki's cherry cradle by hand. Peter hesitated, started to choke up, and the Chapel became still. As Peter sobbed at the podium, Dylan erupted.

"Where is Daddy?" He twisted in his seat and got up on his knees to scan the crowd. "Where is he, Mommy? Where is Daddy?" His face crumpled, and he started to howl.

I leaned over, murmured, and kissed the top of his slicked-down, parted blond mop. I wondered who the hell had combed his hair.

Dylan fidgeted and twitched against my side. His four-year-old legs dangled from navy-blue shorts over the edge of the pew and kicked into the air. We were in the very first row, Dylan had no target, but he kept kicking into the emptiness. Kicking had been a primary activity those past few days, when he wasn't building and destroying Lego towers. Beverley and Harry blocked him on the other side.

Kaki sat stiffly on my right in her favorite strawberry dress. She stared straight ahead. Her hands twisted and untwisted the rolled-up goldenrod program. Her eyes focused somewhere near where Peter stood up front. Kaki was so solemn that it was hard to imagine that she'd turned six just one week before. I closed my eyes and remembered Alan twirling her around and around on the dance floor at the Mousetrap.

Next to Kaki loomed Yvonne. She sniffed loudly into her linen handkerchief, blessed Mister Dimock, and praised her Lord. Then came Alan's older daughters—Dorothy in her green wraparound dress and her big sister, Gioia, with Stevie on her lap. Patty was at the end of the aisle. She was a column of black, crowned by a hat with a black veil. Patty was Italian American and a lapsed Catholic. She understood my childhood anxieties about last rites, consecrated ground, and getting stuck in purgatory. But by this point, we both might have preferred the anonymity of a High Mass.

Ray, scholar of French medieval love, chaired the program. It was not a religious service, even though the stained-glass image of Christ dominated the space. I didn't feel celebratory. I wished I had some element, however tiny, of a fairy-dust conviction in angels or streets of gold or a venerable St. Peter–like concierge checking Alan into heaven with an "Ahoy Mate." Not that I didn't harbor flashes of Catholic guilt that Alan, like Hop, had missed out on the last rites. Yvonne was a born-again evangelical, enthusiastic about Jesus Christ, and convinced by the promises of paradise in the next life.

I thought of Dylan's still asking, "Where's Daddy?" Good question. Two days earlier, Eastern Airlines had confirmed that Alan's name was on the manifest, but even with dental records, his body had yet to be identified.

As the service continued, I imagined that I would spend the rest of my life searching for Alan in the masses at train stations in Asia or at a bar in Bergen singing about cockles and mussels with some Viking slut, or, perhaps, on a beach in the Seychelles, building sandcastles with someone else's kids. I was already scanning crowd scenes in newspaper photographs, looking for Alan. Would it be like when my tiger cat ran away when Nellie brought home a second cat? Disappearing and then, months later, showing up the day after Nellie's cat was run over. And what did that mean?

I was aware that Ray was talking, but I wasn't paying attention to what he was saying. For the past week, I'd been rational during the daytime. Intellectually and emotionally, I'd understood the necessity for a public event to deliver the message that Alan was no longer alive. But I was far from rational at nighttime. I had night terrors, and I was imagining things—Alan rocking in the kitchen, Alan sliding into the pew with us, Alan laughing at all this falderal.

The ceremony served as a ceasefire, an end to the chaos at the Mill with the never-ending stream of visitors, casseroles, and tears. We had declared Alan dead. We celebrated his life that Sunday, September 15,

1974. Of course, we would fail. Alan had thoroughly imprinted our neurotransmitters, our ways of being, and the very ways we processed the world. The private and public mourning of his death would continue for months and years, lifetimes.

I needed to pay attention. Alan was not going to show up. I knew that, but what the hell was Ray talking about? I tuned back in and realized that Ray was reading quotes from Alan's library. I drifted off again, remembering the day we, mostly Alan, built the circular staircase for the library from a used telephone pole. We'd had so many magical days.

I tried to focus, but soon I was running the numbers. Counting, trying to decipher patterns, find meaning. Pa was 72, Hop was 36, and I was 12, and now Alan was dead at 42 when I was 34 and Kaki was 6 and Dylan was 4, almost 5. Did the sequence 72, 36, 42 predict 21 for Dylan, which was way too soon? Must I lose the men I loved? Did 104 for Gram somehow protect Kaki? What about me?

I felt the kids squirming against me. I wanted to scoop them up and run away. Hide somewhere. The bed covers hadn't worked. I forced myself to pay attention, but Ray kept going on and on about books. How were books going to protect us? The answer was in the numbers. Ray was talking about the ancient Vikings. Maybe it was the runes, not the numbers, that predicted life expectancy.

I wondered when it would be over. Ray recited a sea chanty about a dead man and a dead horse. Then, it was Ecclesiastes, "*A fixed time for everything, a pre-destined hour for everything that occurs under the sun. A time of birth and a time of death.*" It had to be the end.

I squeezed the kids to me and whispered, "Just like we practiced at home. Eyes straight, keep walking, don't let go of my hands. NO STOPPING. Just walk down the aisle and out the door and down the steps. Peter will be waiting."

Ray's tone of voice changed—less solemn, lighter. He was picking up speed. He must be finishing. I wondered why I'd refused to wear black. Patty protested, but I wore a white-lace Mexican wedding dress. It was embroidered from neckline to hemline, white threads layered into flowers and leaves on the thick linen. I was only thirty-four, too young for widow's weeds. Was I protesting?

I made out a definite guffaw, a gasp or two, and then full-throttled giggles. Polite, embarrassed tittering. What the hell was going on? Ray was concluding with a passage from the lyrics of the musical *Hair.* He said it was for me:

I got my life, mother
I got laughs, sister
I got freedom, brother
I got headaches and toothaches and bad times, too, like you
I got my hair

The congregation was taken off guard, entranced by Ray's recitation. As I registered Ray's booming "*Got my tits.*" I stood up and took the kids' hands in mine.

By the time Ray reached "*Got my ass,*" we were on our way up the aisle. I sensed the shuffling of feet as people stood up in response to my leaving.

I got my guts
I got my muscles
I got Life

We hustled. The kids kept pace. I avoided eye contact. I registered some laughter, some tentative clapping. My focus was on getting the hell out of there. Over the subsequent months and years, I would hear many descriptions ranging from disbelief to delight about that afternoon in the Chapel.

We kept going. I held a firm grip on Kaki and Dylan. We slowed for President Edgar Shannon and his wife, Eleanor, to hug us.

Peter was parked at the curb in his latest Mercedes sedan. He got out to open the passenger door for us, and then he slid in behind the fancy wooden steering wheel. He was still sobbing.

"Daddy didn't come," Dylan said.

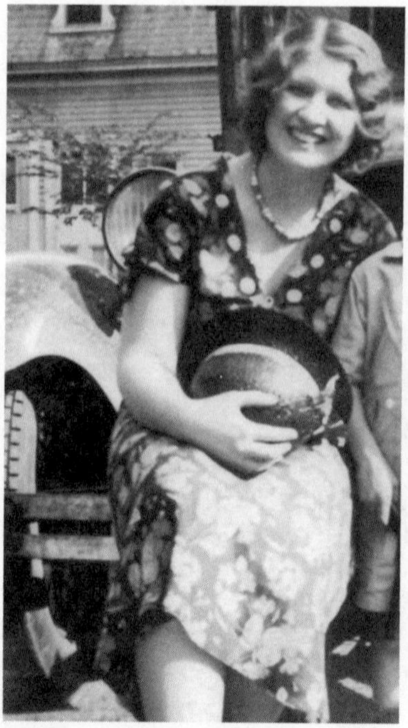

My mother, Nellie, 1939

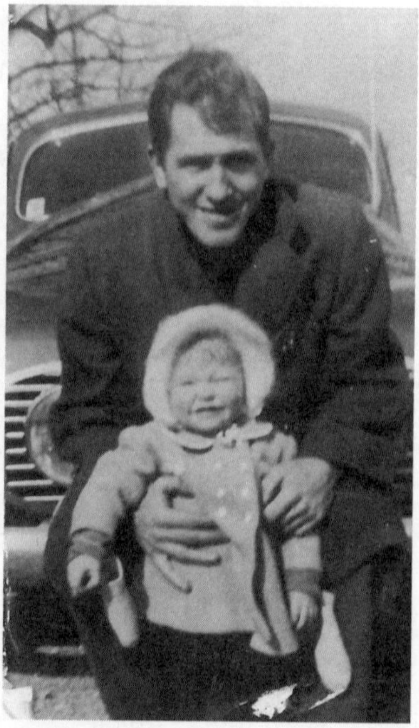

Hop Hostler with me as a toddler

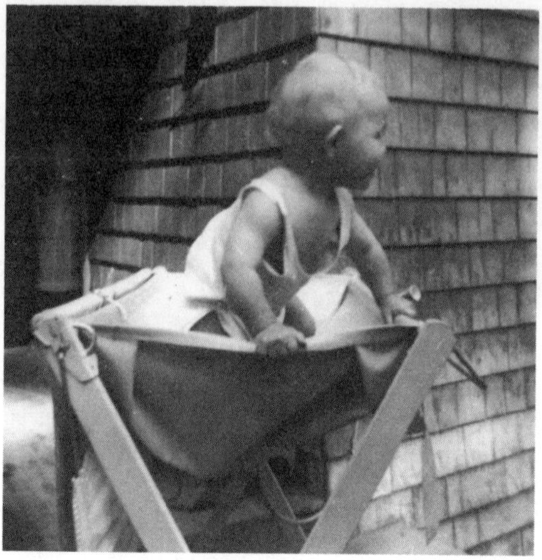

Me at twelve months, 1940

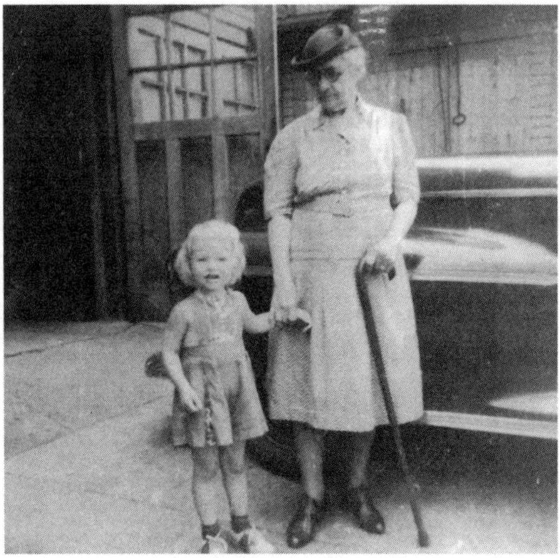

With my maternal great-grandmother (Nellie's father's mother), Whitney, ca. 1941

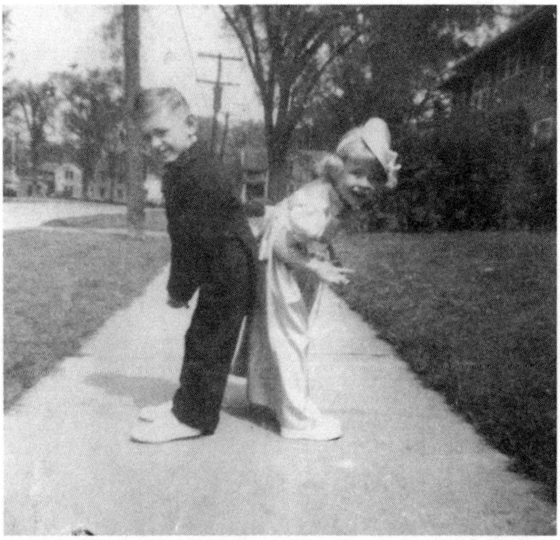

Age three, dancing with our neighbor Steven Foster

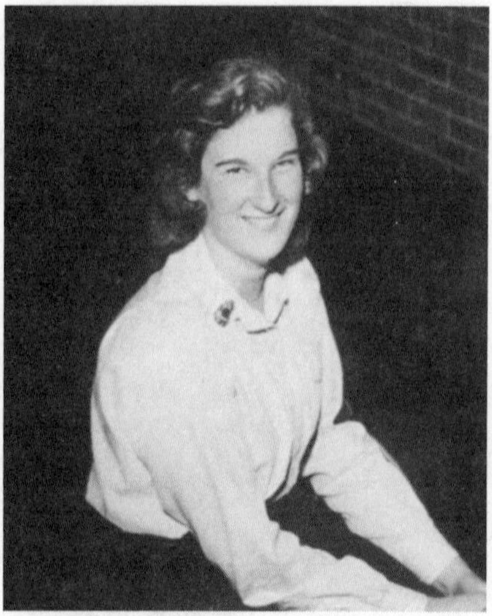

My best friend, Susan Smith, 1957. (From *The Talisman* yearbook, Rutland High School)

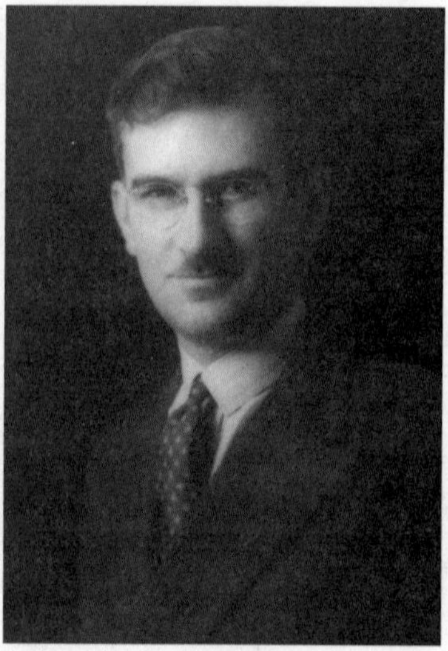

Dr. Gordon B. Smith, ca. 1945–50

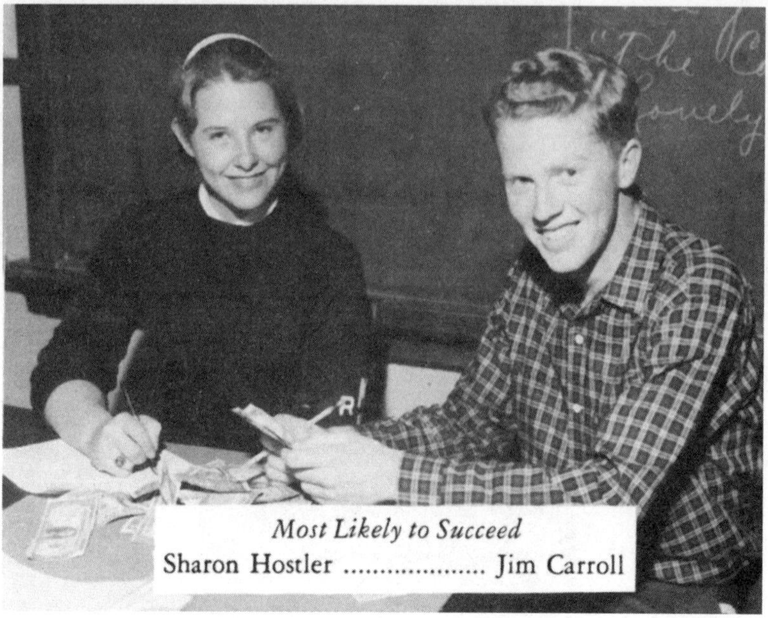

At Rutland High School, 1957. (From *The Talisman* yearbook)

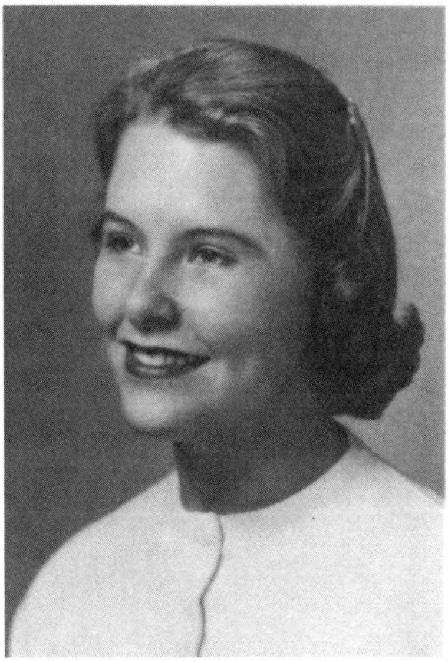

As a Rutland High School graduate, 1957

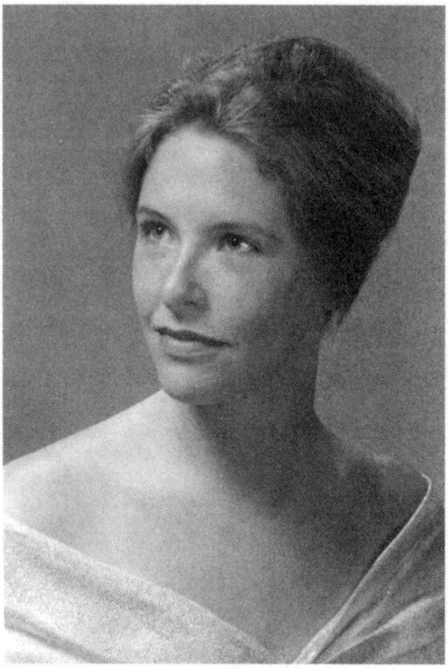

As a Middlebury graduate, 1961

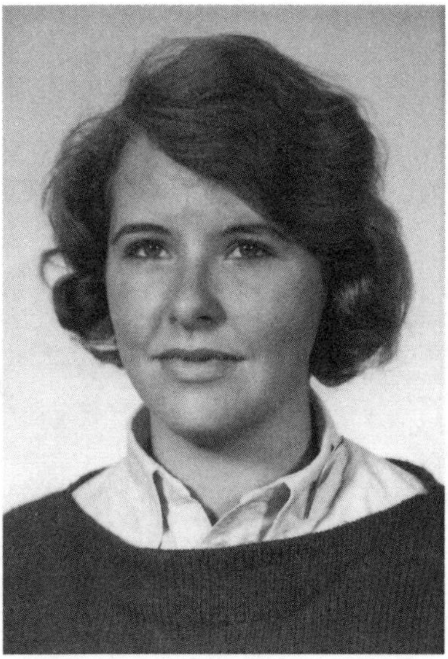

As a University of Vermont first-year medical student, 1962

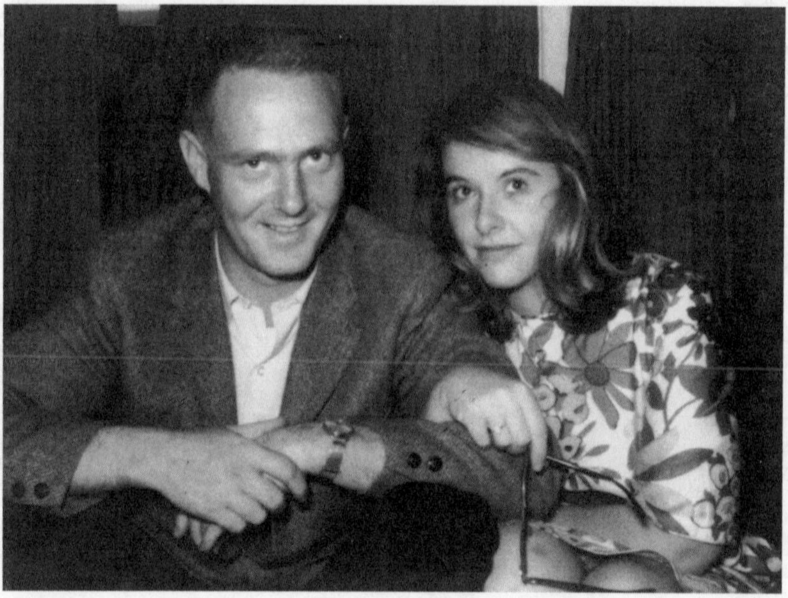

With Alan, 1966

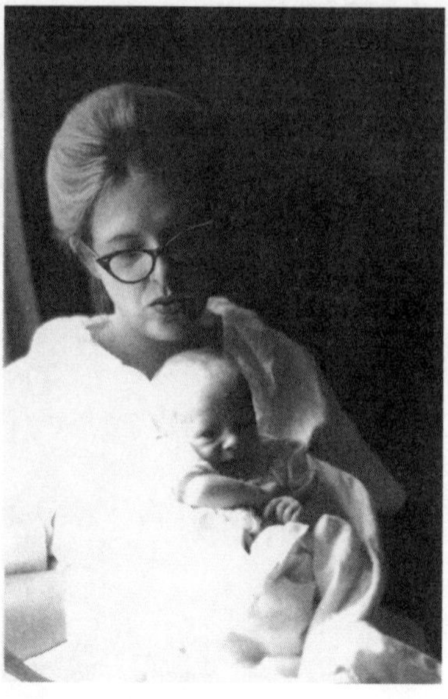

With Dinky as an infant, 1968.
(Photo courtesy George Erlanger)

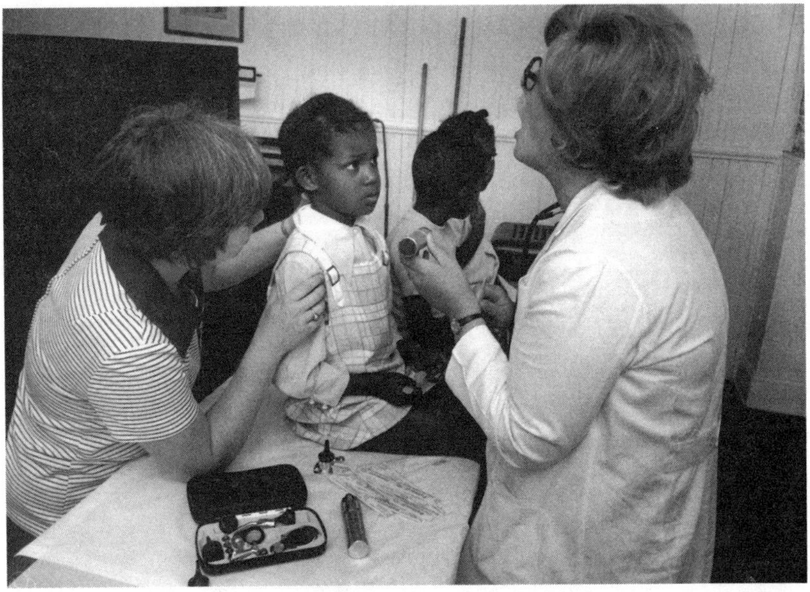

In Keswick clinic with Beverley, 1969

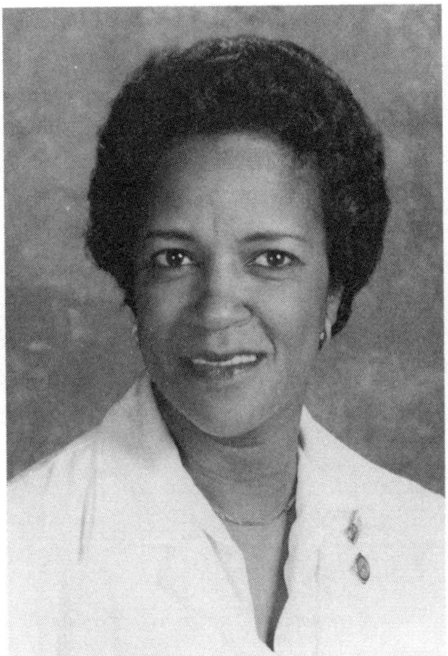

Clariece Harris, LPN at City Children and Youth Clinic, 1968–79

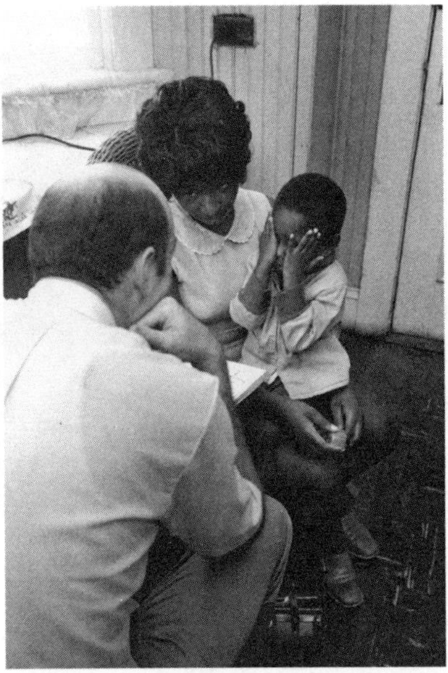

Helen Wright, LPN at County Children and Youth Clinic, 1968–79

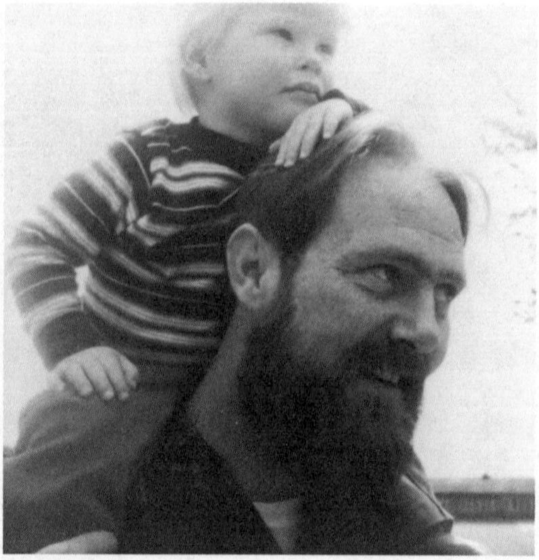

Dylan and Alan, 1970

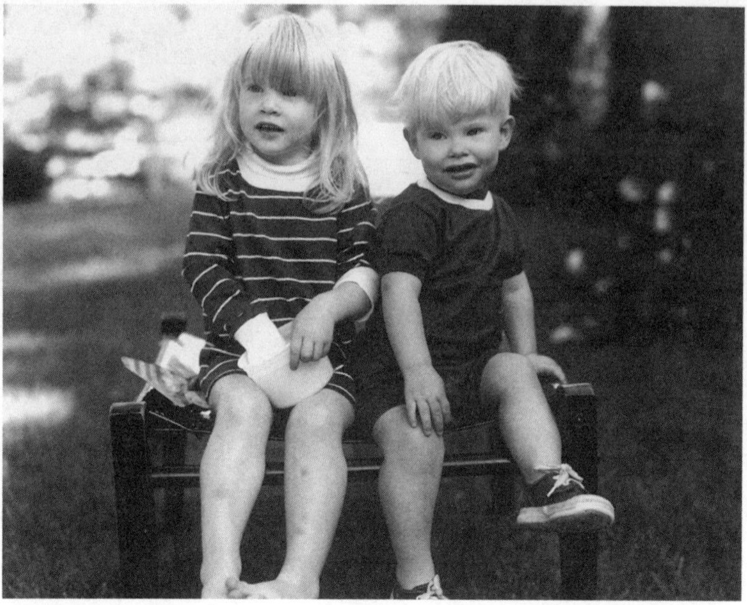

Kaki and Dylan, on the move to the Mill, 1971. (Photo by Paul Huyffer)

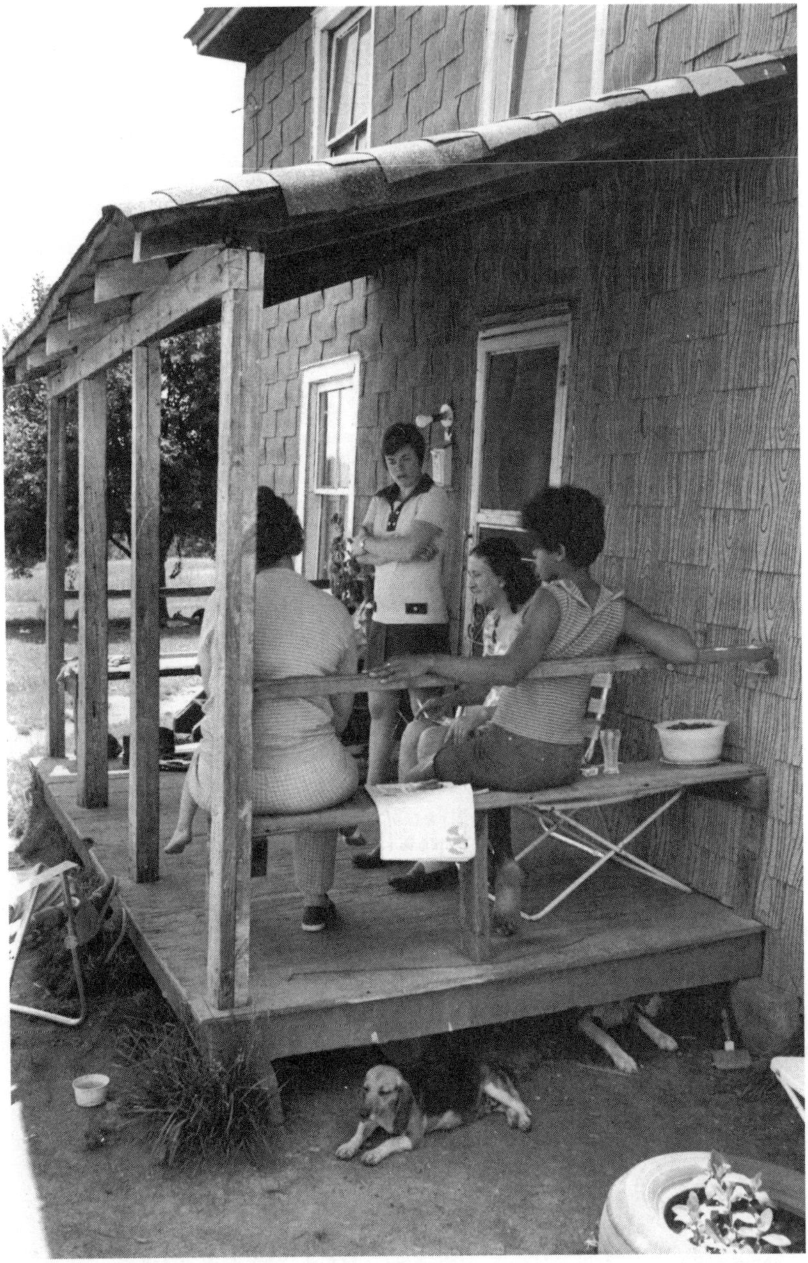

Children and Youth Project social worker Beverley B. Butler on a home visit

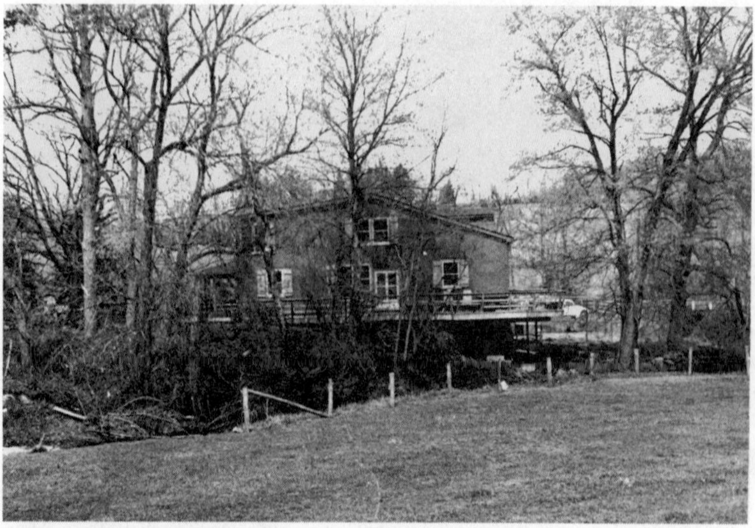

The Mill, from creek side. (Rip Payne Photos)

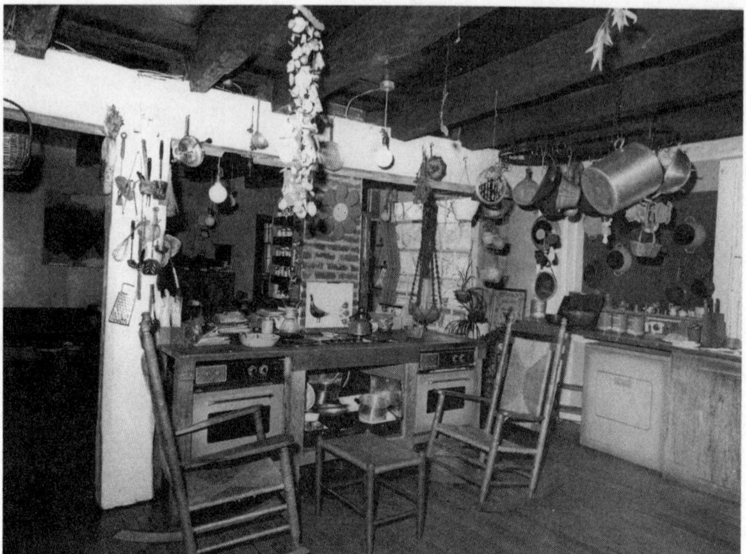

The kitchen at the Mill. (Rip Payne Photos)

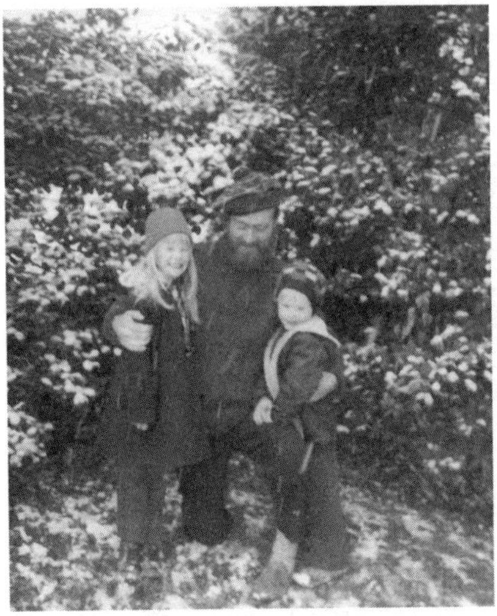

Alan with Kaki and Dylan at the Mill, January 1974

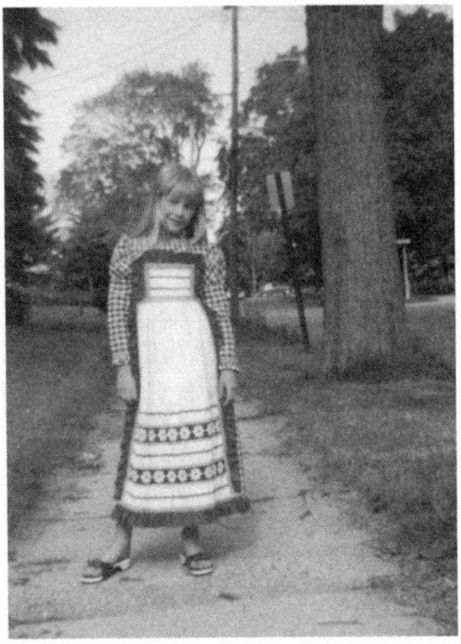

Kaki on her sixth birthday in her favorite red-and-white-checkered granny dress, September 1974

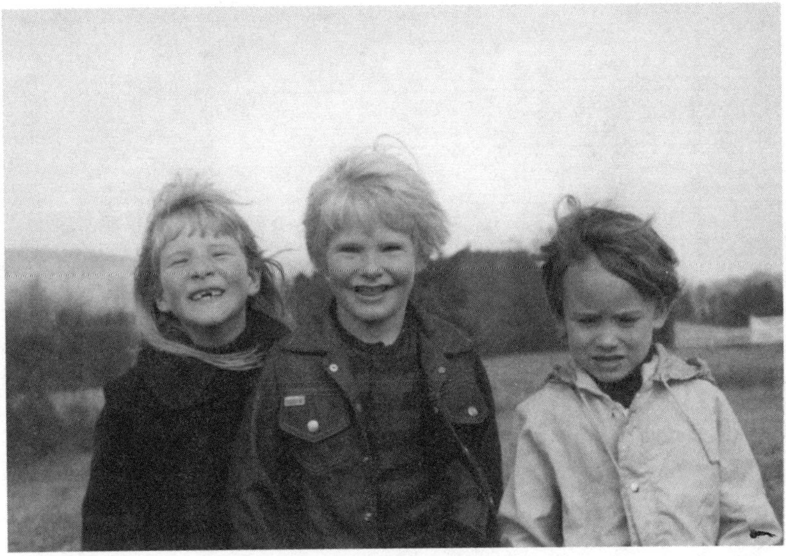

Kaki, Dylan, and our grandson Stevie, 1975

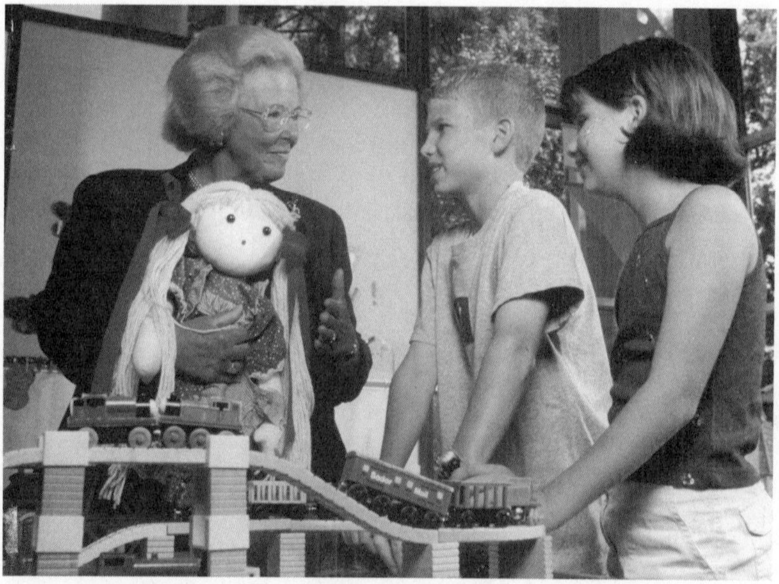

At the Children's Rehabilitation Center with patients

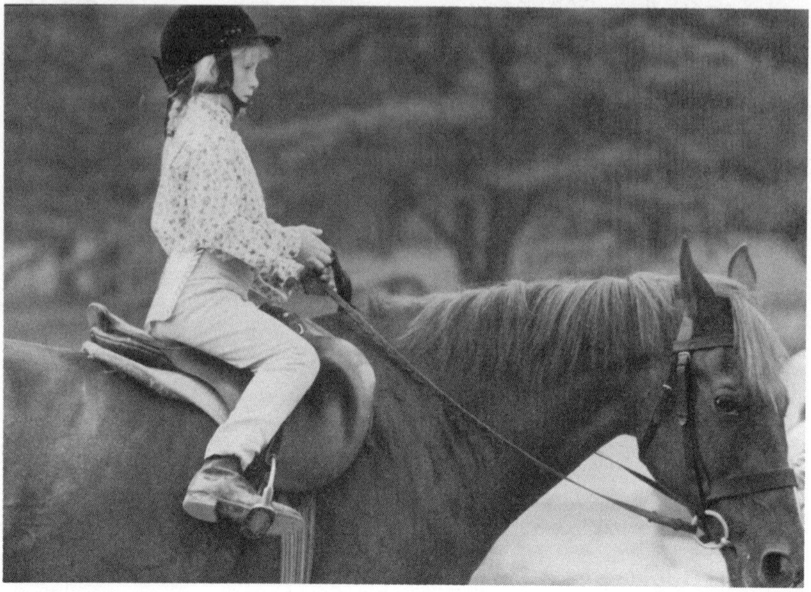

Kaki on Prince

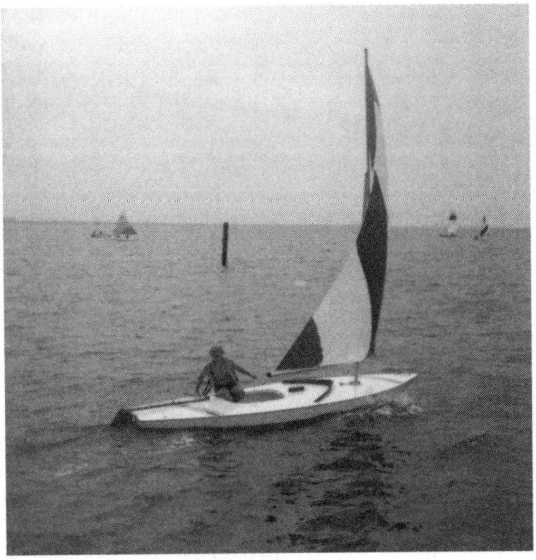

Dylan on Bogue Sound sailing a Sunfish

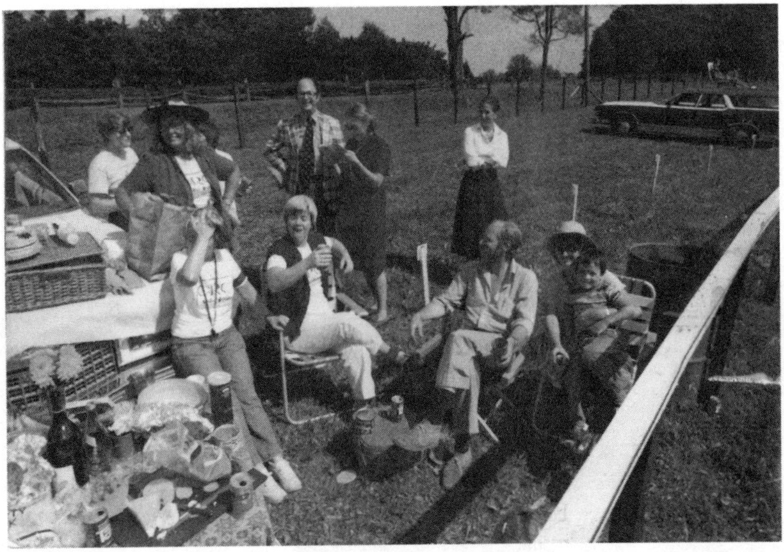

Beverley (seated, in the vest; I'm wearing the hat) with her enablers

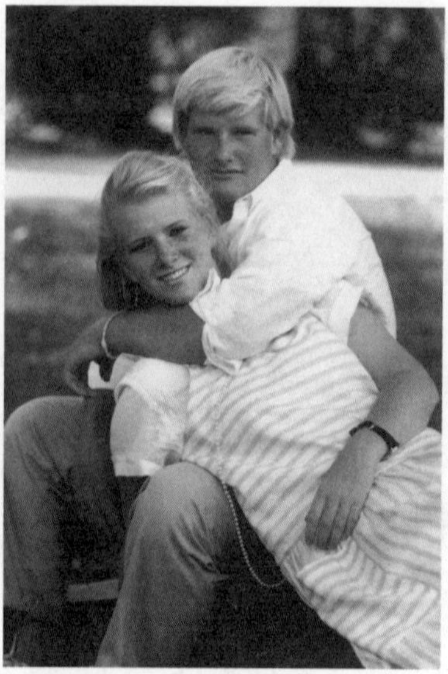

Kaki and Dylan, 1984. (Photo by Dan Grogan)

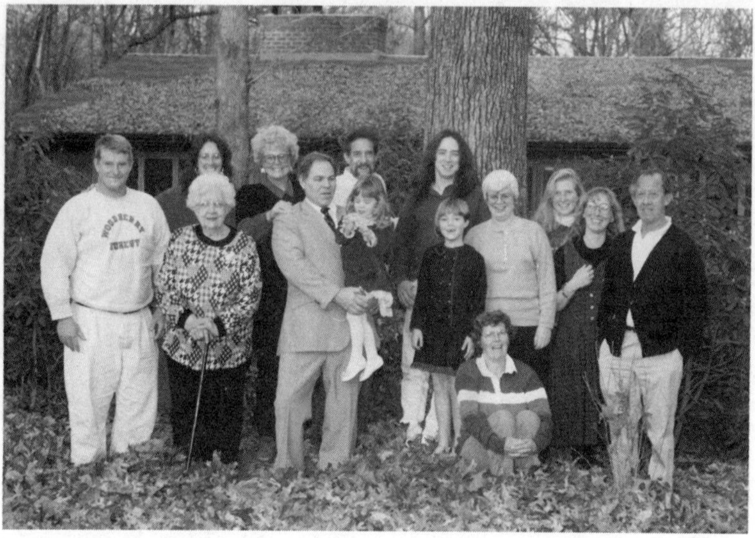

Thanksgiving 1986. Front row: Dylan, Nellie, Richard MacNamara holding Sara, Becca, Beverley, Kaki, Gioia, and Joe. Back row: Dorothy, Sharon, Peter, and Stevie. Jean Eisenhart (my Middlebury roommate) is seated.

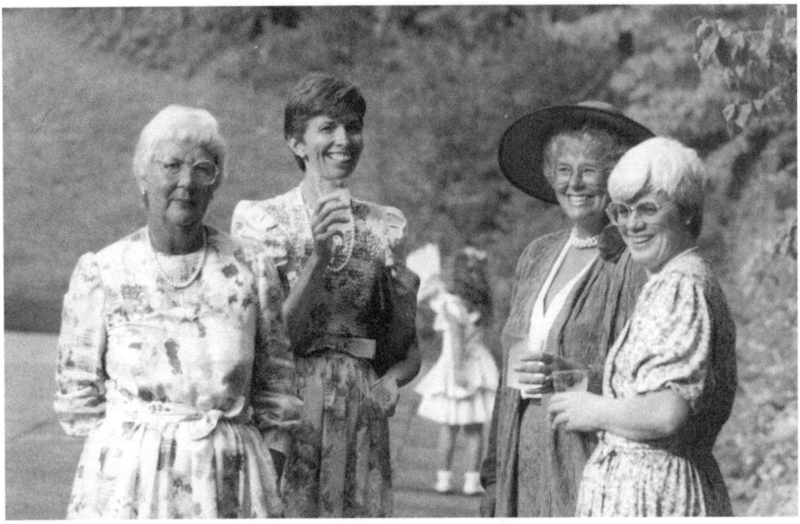

AV Sullivan, Jan Allaire, Sharon, and Beverley Butler, 1979

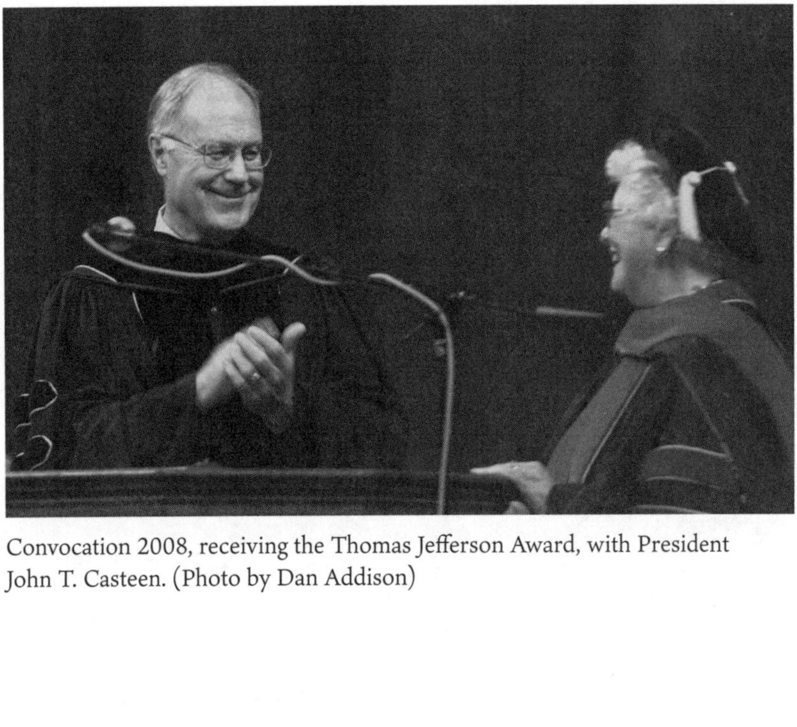

Convocation 2008, receiving the Thomas Jefferson Award, with President John T. Casteen. (Photo by Dan Addison)

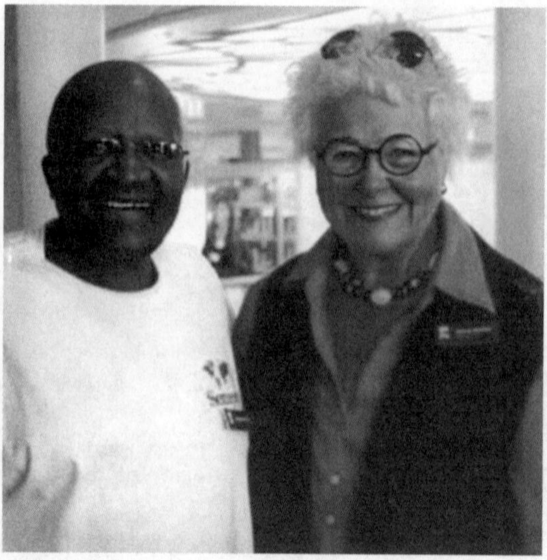

With the Reverend Desmond Tutu, Semester-at-Sea, January 2013

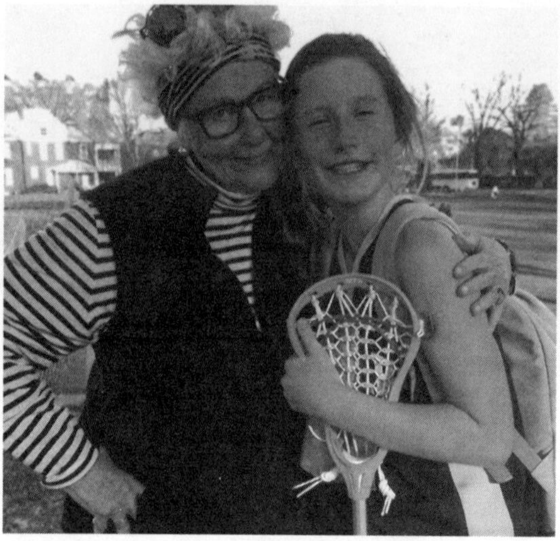

With Lucy at a lacrosse game, Raleigh, North Carolina, 2019

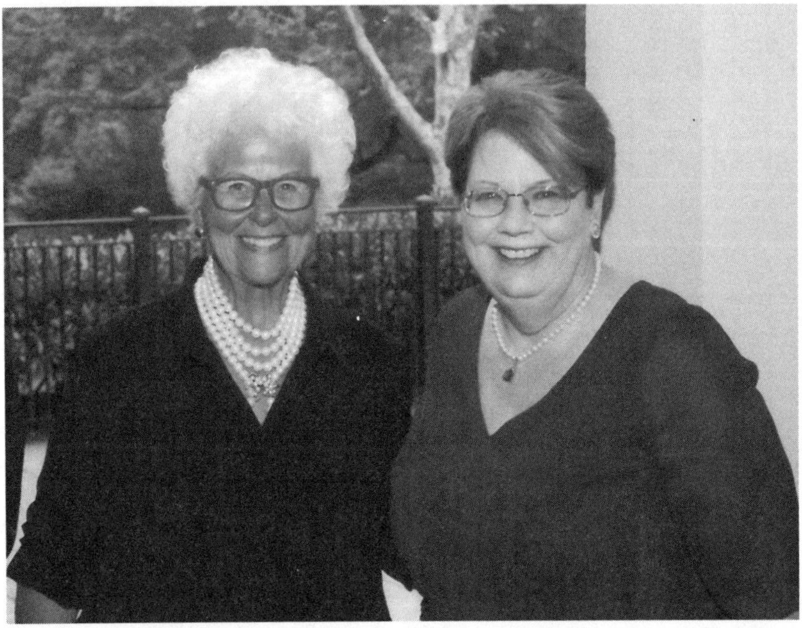

Retirement celebration with President Teresa Sullivan, 2016

· 18 ·

Mourning at the Mill

September to Thanksgiving 1974

Monday was the day of desertion. I kept the kids home from school. Beverley shuttled folks to their morning flights and went to work. Patty reviewed the master list with me, pointed out the labeled casseroles in the freezer, and untied her kerchief. "You know I loved him, too," she said and drove off in tears. Yvonne went home after lunch. She was still praising the Lord.

There were more flowers. More phone calls. No one came to the door except the mailman with a sack of sympathy notes. I stashed them in the basket Patty had designated on the dining room table. We flowed through the Mill as a single organism—Kaki, Dylan, Max, Mattie, and me—alone and afraid. Dylan asked again where Daddy was and then we were all crying. The dogs nosed us onto the couch in the living room.

We were still huddled on the couch with our piles of Kleenex wads when Beverley walked in with more flowers, her overnight bag, and pizza for supper.

Dr. Ruth Weeks called during supper to announce she would join us for dinner the next day. She was a faculty member, a child psychiatrist, the one who'd become my advocate around the child sexual abuse cases my internship year. "Okay, thank you for letting me know," I said in surprise.

Ruth Weeks was a legend. The next night, Dr. Weeks swept into the kitchen, taller than her usual six feet in high heels, asked for a Scotch, and took charge. She was a major presence—even the Danes were cowed. I later learned that, at eighteen, she and five other women in her troupe of entertainers had crossed the Atlantic on a transport ship carrying eight thousand enlisted men. She had entertained the Allied troops during World War II as a member of the Canadian RAF.

"So, are you seeing Alan?" she asked. "You know, around the house?" I hesitated a beat. Beverley and the kids stared at me, waiting for the answer.

"Of course, you are," she answered her own question. "Absolutely normal. You're not crazy, Sharon. You're normal. Don't worry about it."

I sighed. Kaki stared at me, waiting. Dylan jumped right in and asked Dr. Weeks if she knew where his Daddy was and when he would come home. When she shook her head and asked Dylan what he thought, Dylan knocked his chair over and stormed out. Kaki got up, stood next to me, and leaned in.

Dr. Weeks asked Beverley for another Scotch and told us the story of her husband's death. That was when she decided to be a doctor, even though she was already forty years old.

As Dr. Weeks gathered herself up to leave, she looked at each of us, one by one, and commented that all of us would need counseling. "You," she pointed at me as she closed the door, "will need to do some serious work." She said it kindly, but I felt a rush of anger. Who had asked her opinion?

Later that week, I went back to work, and the kids started their new school in town. Yvonne rolled her eyes and grumbled—she didn't like the new school. I was too distracted to register that Yvonne was the only nonparent and the only non-White person dropping kids off at the private school. When I remembered to ask about school, the kids were silent, even Kaki. Erla eventually convinced me to let Kaki go to the barn with her kids and learn to ride. Soon Kaki was carrying her riding helmet with her everywhere, wore jodhpurs to school, and seemed happy at the stable.

Dylan kept asking for Daddy. On Friday nights, he waited at the kitchen window for Alan and sobbed when he didn't come. Kaki and the Danes were never far from me. Beverley drank a lot of Scotch and kept pouring wine for me. And I drank it. Yvonne talked to Alan—Mister Dimock—in the front hall closet and prayed for his soul. Such was our new normal.

The last week in September, I was surprised to get a phone call at work from Dr. Paul Van Ostenburg. He had been a pediatric dentist at C&Y but left to join the faculty at the University of North Carolina, one of the guys whose salaries had eclipsed mine when I'd started as the medical director. Paul was tearful on the phone. It seemed that he was part of the forensic team at the crash site in Charlotte and recognized Alan's name on the manifest. He knew Alan from parties at the Mill. Paul promised to look out for Alan and keep me informed. I reminded him that Alan had a full red beard. Why was it so hard to identify my Viking? Maybe he really hadn't been on the plane.

Where was Alan, anyway? I felt more and more like Dylan every day. In the mornings, I saw Alan in the rocking chair, but at night, I saw him injured and abandoned in the cornfield or regaining consciousness in one of the black body bags stacked in the hangar. Driving into work, sometimes I conjured him up on a beach in the Seychelles and got furious about being abandoned.

I tried to work, but it was godawful awkward. The Center staff weren't sure how to respond. Some felt I shouldn't be at work. Dr. Bunch headed that faction. I wondered where they thought I should be. Wearing widow's weeds and on my knees fingering the rosary beads, or just out of sight? A few staff were sympathetic, wanting to be helpful, but not comfortable talking about the tasks at hand. Most amazing was the group that believed that I should just get on with it, buckle down, and get to clinic. The CDC team was ambivalent. They resisted the changes I'd introduced, but their presence at Big Meadows made them somehow complicit, maybe feeling responsible for me. If they were confused, so was I.

It took only a few weeks before Dr. Bunch confronted me. No sherry in fancy glasses this time. He said that I had to do something, see someone, take drugs. That I looked and behaved like a zombie. I did as he suggested. I took the prescribed antidepressants, the muscle relaxants, and the sleeping pills, but I still cried at odd moments on rounds, saw Alan in the rocking chair, and had night terrors. And struggled with the inevitable medication-induced dry mouth.

In early October, not even a month after the crash, Beverley's father had a fatal heart attack. Harry Butler was only sixty-one. He'd visited the Mill, sat at the kitchen table, and was an honorary grandfather to the kids. I went with Beverley to Florida for the funeral.

A week later, Yvonne called me at work. She sounded frantic. She'd heard a fracas and found Mattie convulsing in the whelping box. I went home, but even the two of us couldn't pick Mattie up. She weighed almost 150 pounds and was still seizing. Improvising a rug as a sling, we managed to scoop her out of the whelping box and get her to the vet.

Mattie had preeclampsia. She required IV magnesium sulfate to stop the seizures and lower her blood pressure. By the time we got Mattie back to the Mill, she was in active labor. It was too early. Beverley and the kids and I kept vigil next to the whelping box as Mattie delivered ten tiny preterm puppies. Only two pups made it through the night. I failed to save the other eight, despite Kaki's frantic exhortations to do something.

The two tiny puppies latched onto Mattie and nursed. They were survivors. Mattie stayed in the whelping box even though it was crowded. When we were home, we were up and down the circular staircase checking on Mattie and her puppies. We had a focus, something concrete to do, and it was a relief.

That is, until the night Beverley fell down the stairs and broke her leg. It was Halloween. Kaki held Beverley's hand and tried to comfort her, but Dylan's body shook with his sobbing. I called 911 for the rescue squad and got some ice and a pillow. Then I paged Dr. Bunch, the pediatric orthopedist, to meet Beverley in the emergency room. It was nine o'clock. I explained that Beverley's blood alcohol was sky-high, and I was concerned she'd get the DTs. He promised to titrate the opiates.

I don't remember exactly when Paul called me to let me know that Alan's body had been identified, but I do remember it was a bizarre conversation. I didn't understand why Paul was the one in tears. He had been the one who made the forensic identification of Alan's body. I ended up comforting Paul. My belief since the crash was, if Alan had indeed been on that plane, that Alan and Bob and all the others had died on impact. That their deaths had been sudden. No suffering. No consciousness. That the passengers never knew what happened.

Paul assured me he would call over Thanksgiving to deliver the autopsy report and debrief me. Did I thank him? Did I think a visit was strange, excessive? I don't remember. I do remember that I felt the heavy weight press on my chest while he was talking on the phone—

just like when I first heard about the crash and like I felt every morning when I woke up, took the first breath, and remembered. All over again.

At the parent-teacher night at the new school, the conversation focused on Dylan's activity level. How he never sat still. How he didn't join the circle. And what did I think about medication for attention deficit disorder? No way, I said. He's a boy and he's not even quite five years old, and his father was just killed in an airplane crash. They shook their heads in disbelief when I reiterated that there would be no medicine, not even a trial. I was a pediatrician, for God's sake. Almost as an afterthought, Kaki's first-grade teacher reported that Kaki spent her free time in their little library, all by herself, crying. Every day. I thought then that I should let Kaki spend all her days at the barn. She seemed content there.

It was at that parent-teacher meeting when I first remember being angry at Alan. The school was his damn idea, not mine. Child-centered learning indeed. Where the hell was Alan? Where the hell was Alan on Friday nights at the Mill? Or when Harry died? Or when Mattie had convulsions? Or when Beverley fell down his damn circular stairs? And where the hell was Alan for these parent-teacher meetings?

Thanksgiving rolled around. Peter was sleeping in the library. Beverley was in the guest room. Gioia and Stevie bunked in with Kaki and Dylan. But where the hell was Alan? Thanksgiving was his holiday. I had no family tradition of Thanksgiving. Over the years, Alan had shaped our rituals, selected the seasonings, and set our family's standards. And there I was—standing all alone at the kitchen counter with Max, Mattie, her pups, the twenty-pound turkey—trying to orchestrate the day to Alan's expectations. I couldn't risk any foggy thinking. I skipped the antidepressants.

Joy of Cooking provided explicit directions for the perfect roast turkey. The early-morning mist streamed up from the creek. The state of my mind was a lot like the mist, shapeless and shifting behind a scrim. Maybe I could shower once I got the bird in the oven. I thought, once again, that I really had to get it together. Not the turkey. My life. *Joy of Cooking* wasn't much help.

Gioia and Stevie had arrived from Utah two days before. In the kitchen, Dylan climbed up on the stool at his end of the long red table. Stevie started toward Kaki's end, but I plunked him down on a stool in the middle. Stevie was antsy around the dogs. He was only three.

I plopped down glasses of milk, crayons, and a coloring book from the catchall basket under the table. "Be quiet until I get our Tom Turkey tucked into the oven. If all the forces in the universe work in my favor, we'll sit down by three or four o'clock."

Neither of them could tell time yet. I was coaching myself. Mattie and Max wound around my feet. The tiger cats perched on one of the rocking chairs and cuffed at the puppies.

"Mommy?" Kaki appeared at the counter in bare feet, a blue-striped sweater pulled over a nightgown and new beige jodhpurs. Her towheaded hair going every which way. Even at six, Kaki had a quiet presence, watchful and wary. Vigilant.

"Beverley needs help on the stairs," Kaki said.

"Okay, Kaki, I got it." I ruffled her hair. She shrugged when I suggested she might like to take off her nightgown.

I fixed a mug of black coffee with lots of sugar and gave it to Kaki for Beverley. "Use both hands. Tell Bev to sit tight for a few more minutes."

I finished the apple-and-sausage stuffing, packed it in Tom's thoracic cavity and his bottom hearing Alan's voice coaching me, "Don't pack it too tight. Stuffing needs space to expand." I put the leftovers into a Pyrex dish with bacon strips on top and recalibrated. By then, it was 8:45 a.m. The turkey required thirty minutes at 450°. I had to cover the breast at 9:15 a.m. and turn the temperature down to 350°.

I realized then that no matter what I had promised Peter, there was no way I could get that brood fed, dressed, and delivered from the Mill in North Garden to the Blessing of the Hounds at Grace Episcopal Church in Cismont. Not by ten o'clock.

Kaki was back. "Beverley says if you don't come soon, she's going to slide down the banister." Kaki imitated Beverley—wrinkled her forehead, pursed her lips, and made a big frown. Then she grinned. "She wants to know if you've started the Bloody Marys."

I turned away from the counter, squatted down, and wrapped Kaki in a great big, happy hug. Dylan and Stevie cheered, but it was not because of our hug. Mattie had slipped behind me, stood up against the counter and, with her front paws stabilizing the bowl, slurped up my sweet potatoes.

"BAD DOG! BAD DOG!" Kaki wagged her finger, hands on her hips.

We heard a creak as the library door opened and Peter appeared in full costume. Dressed in an ensemble *Town and Country* might prescribe for a day in the English hunt country. Plaid wool slacks, burnt-orange velvet vest, pinstriped, buttoned-down shirt with cuff links and a Princeton ascot. He had his blazer, leather gloves, and orange knit scarf over his arm.

"Who's ready for the Blessing of the Hounds?" he asked.

I glowered first at Mattie and then at Peter. "You might just make it, if you leave right this minute. Make sure you bundle the kids up and give them potty breaks."

"Sharon, I wouldn't abandon you."

"You mean that you're not competent to deal with these kids without me? But if we plan to sit down for Thanksgiving dinner before midnight, I need to stay right here in the kitchen. Though I may take a break to get dressed."

The kids watched the adults face off. The dogs settled under the table. The kitchen was quiet.

Peter eventually harrumphed, turned away, and fiddled around with some lemons on the counter. "I'll start the Bloody Marys. Where's Beverley? We have a lot of Alan toasting to do today."

"Daddy?" Dylan asked. "Is Daddy coming home?"

Kaki glanced at the ceiling, slid down to the floor, and sat cross-legged under the table with Max and Mattie. Stevie whimpered. When I tried to pick Dylan up, he pushed me away.

"I miss Daddy," he said and sobbed.

"So does Mommy." I bent across the tabletop to hug him, positioning my back to Peter.

"Good God, Sharon!" Peter said, "You've put on the pounds—just since September. You can't just let yourself go."

The oven timer went off. I slammed the knob and gagged back the rising bile. Let myself go? If I had my way, I wouldn't ever open my eyes. Wouldn't allow the creeping consciousness when sleep fades, wouldn't remember again and again that Alan was dead.

I jerked the roasting pan out of the oven, used tongs to drape the buttered-soaked towel over the golden turkey breast, and slammed it back in the oven. I turned down the temperature, set the timer for the basting interval, one hour, and squared my shoulders.

I vowed to myself and maybe Alan that we would have a goddamned, beautifully roasted turkey on the table.

"Peter," I said, "go upstairs with Kaki and help get Beverley down the stairs."

As Peter started out of the kitchen, Stevie hollered, scrambled up onto the table, and pointed. A big, black snake was slithering out of the pantry. Very slowly.

"Keep going, Peter. I'll get the broom." Max and Mattie made a barricade, nose to tail, between the kids and the black snake. The cats arched their backs and puffed out their tails, but they stayed put.

I cracked open the outside door and prodded the snake with the broom. The boys clapped and cheered when I slammed the door. The snake could find its own damn way back down to the creek.

Alan claimed that the black snakes kept the water rats away. "Rats or snakes?" he'd asked. As if that were a rational choice to be made by all families in their homes.

I decided to set our table at one of the round tables and lay out the food buffet-style on the other. I couldn't tolerate the formality of the dining room without Alan at the head of the table.

When I got upstairs, Gioia glared at me. "I can't believe it. Doctor Hostler, with all your hoity-toity talk about medical ethics and the importance of your medical license to make a living. All the carrying-on about Dotty and me—as if *our* smoking dope under the bridge affected your job."

What the hell had upset Gioia? I was ready to roll over on the bed, cover my head with a pillow, and stay there. Let them fix their own damn dinner.

"Look at you." She pointed at me. "You're a zombie. You're slurring your words, you're drugged!"

Gioia was right, but I was still angry. The antidepressants made my mouth feel like hay drying on an August afternoon. I had to focus on making sufficient saliva to make it through an entire sentence. It was awful on morning rounds.

"I flushed them all—the Valium, the antidepressants, the sleeping pills. You're going cold turkey."

I giggled. Turkey day seemed the proper day to go cold turkey.

"Sharon, it's not funny. You can't take this crap."

I laughed. "I agree with you, Gioia. I hate the way it makes me feel—slow and stupid, especially at work. I didn't take it this morning because I needed to keep my wits."

"Why do you even have it?"

"At work, they want me to focus, to stop being sad. The new chair and the orthopedist at the Center. What they really mean is to stay at home with the children. Take leave." I sighed. "Preferably, go back to Vermont."

Gioia sat down on the bed next to me. "I'm sorry, you really scared me."

I put my arm around Gioia. We sat for a moment in silence. Gioia took a deep breath and said that things weren't going well with big Steve. She wondered if Stevie and she could stay at the Mill. She paused, then started to laugh. "Probably not, not after I flushed your pills down the drain."

"Gioia, do you know what I'm thinking? About the Woods Hole jail when your father was out at sea."

"When you bailed me out."

"Go downstairs," I said. "Baste the turkey and monitor the Bloody Mary consumption. You've got drug rounds today."

When we finally sat down for dinner, it was late, almost dark outside. Beverley offered a string of toasts to Alan, but Peter had to do a few more. It sounded like a cross between an Irish wake and New Year's resolutions.

The adults consumed a lot of wine. Everyone had seconds, even skinny Peter. In the moments of quiet, our thoughts were of Alan and why he was not at the table. How could it be Thanksgiving without Alan?

Peter stood up, "Happy Thanksgiving to Sharon, Kaki, Dylan, Gioia, Stevie, Max and Mattie, Puppy #1 and Puppy #2. Dimocks one and all." He clinked his knife against the wine glass. "Officially, I hereby declare that from this day on, Beverley and I are honorary Dimocks."

We raised our glasses and cheered.

We'd survived the first holiday. Alan would be disappointed that we'd missed the Blessing of the Hounds, but he'd be pleased that Gioia and Stevie were coming to live at the Mill. He would not have been surprised that Peter and Beverley hung in with us. Would he have imagined Max as my blue velvet guardian?

And then a car pulled in. I'd totally forgotten that Paul Van Ostenburg had said he would drop by.

I introduced Paul to Peter and explained Paul's role in Charlotte. He remembered Beverley. After I tucked the kids into bed, Paul and I settled into the vacated rocking chairs. Eventually, Paul handed me a manila folder. Stomach acid was at the back of my throat. Finally, I folded out the flap and reached inside. I retrieved an official copy of the autopsy report and a plain gold band. Alan's wedding ring.

Eventually, Paul started to talk. And talk and talk. He seemed to need to share the precise details of the horrendous weeks in Charlotte, day by day, hour by hour, moment by moment. Memories from more than a month that he spent as a member of the forensic team. I was a bit surprised by his tears, but, of course, Paul had known Alan, been to parties in the Mill's kitchen.

Over and over, I had learned one important lesson since the crash. Each mourner had to tell his own story. How they found out. Where they'd been when they heard. Who was where. And always, the details of the last time they remembered being with Alan. Once again, I wondered how I became the designated listener.

Paul insisted on reading the autopsy report out loud to me there in the kitchen.

I wondered why Paul felt it was so critical to share all the details. I couldn't make sense of the words. I watched his face. I tried to pay attention, but eventually I stopped listening. At some level, I understood what Paul was trying to tell me, but I couldn't hear it. I became completely dissociated. And after a while, I started to wonder what the hell Paul was doing in my kitchen. It was Thanksgiving.

At last, Paul folded the autopsy report precisely along the original creases, returned it to the manilla folder, and ceremoniously placed it on my lap.

Here is what I learned that night in my kitchen that still smelled of sage and cinnamon. Alan was alive when Eastern Airlines #212 crashed into the cornfield in Charlotte. He was alive when the right wing of the McDonnell Douglas DC-9 clipped a tree and continued careening in the air until its left wing sheared a stand of pine trees and crashed into an open field surrounded by dense woods and underbrush. It skidded another 995 feet into a ravine before stopping.

Alan had not been killed by the impact of the crash.

Alan had been alive and trapped as Eastern Airlines #212 burst into flames.

My red-bearded Viking had not died suddenly and painlessly.

Alan had burned to death.

· 19 ·

Christmas Without Alan

Christmas 1974

I was determined to follow the Dimock rules for Christmas: festivities on the solstice, homemade gifts, and tree-trimming on Christmas Eve. At the last hour, I recruited AV's sons, VG and Mike, to make it happen.

Our bountiful Norwegian spruce was fifteen feet tall. We pruned stray limbs and balanced the tree in the stand, but after a few minutes the tree first tilted and then fell over. There was jingling and jangling as the boughs strung with sparkling white lights, icicles, and ornaments landed on the couch and the floor lamp tipped over. The Danes barked and ran around in excitement. Dylan cheered, but Kaki sat on the floor in tears.

How did I think I could do Christmas at the Mill without Alan?

Last Christmas Eve, the tree lights were sparkling, the kids were long asleep, and we were sipping champagne. How had Alan done it? My first happy holiday ever had been with Alan at Beau Pré—I'd arrived home at the end of a week on inpatient call to find champagne, a fire roaring, and a tiny tree covered in lights and gold-wrapped packages tied with black ribbon. Magical.

So different from the Christmas when I was six living with Hop and Nellie in Pa Hostler's house on 72 Library Avenue. Christmas morning, there were presents under the tree and a goose hanging by its neck on the back stoop—but no grown-ups. When Pa got home, he described the accident. Hop had been driving the taxicab, drunk. Nellie was badly injured, in surgery.

Hop had run off with Rosalie. Pa died four years later; then Hop died two years after Pa. Some holidays, Nellie managed a bedraggled little misfit of a tree, but she'd be passed out by the time I got home from Midnight Mass and hungover mean in the morning. By college, I was "regular" Christmas staff at the Lake Placid Club, serving the same laughing, heavy-tipping families year after year.

Over the past decade, Alan had nurtured our expectations of Christmas magic. That first Christmas without him, I tried to follow his example, but even with the help of Beverley and AV's sons, I didn't come close.

It was almost two thirty in the morning when VG and I finished wrapping presents on the kitchen table. "Be careful driving home, guys. Your mother would never forgive me if anything happened." Both were tall and handsome, varsity lacrosse players. Red-haired Irishmen with twinkly eyes. I didn't want them to leave. "We'd never have gotten everything done without you two. Stringing up that damn tree was nothing short of brilliant."

Mike laughed, "More like desperate."

"Sharon, let them go," Beverley said from the kitchen door. "AV will be sending out the sheriff."

I stood out on the stoop with Max and started to cry as the truck's taillights faded. It hadn't been very long after Alan's death when Erla set some boundaries. "No more hugging Jim," she'd said. "I understand that you lost Alan, but don't think that I am sharing Jim."

Christmas morning was early and noisy. "Santa came. Santa came," Dylan hollered as he ran circuits between the living room and the kitchen. The dogs stayed out of Dylan's way.

"Don't touch the presents—not until after we have breakfast," Kaki said. "Daddy's rules."

Kaki realized that I hadn't filled the stockings, took them down without a word, and tucked them away in the pantry. Even at six, Kaki was sensitive to the feelings of others and didn't hesitate to intervene.

I took the warm croissants out of the oven, poured myself a mug of coffee, and sat down at the head of the dining room table. Kaki settled next to me, unfolded her napkin on her lap, monitoring my face. Beverley brought a plate of bacon and glasses of milk for the kids. The three of us sat quietly, hands in our laps, and waited.

Dylan stopped handling the presents and glared at me. "Why are you in Daddy's place?"

"Dylan, you know Daddy's not coming for breakfast," I said very slowly, very softly. I clasped my hands together in my lap and pressed hard. What I wanted to do was to scream at Dylan, "NOT NOW, NEVER! NEVER! NEVER!"

Beverley got up, hugged Dylan, and tried to slide him into his chair. Dylan shouldered himself away from Beverley and stood in the doorway. "Daddy is coming. Daddy's coming for presents. I know he is."

"No, Dylan," I said quietly. "Daddy is not coming. Not for my warm croissants. Not for presents. Not even when we all want Daddy to be here with us right now." I paused, "Please come sit down."

Kaki slid out of her chair and stood next to me. I could feel her lean against my side. Dear God, don't let Kaki start to cry, I thought. I reached my arm around her and snuggled her to me, but I kept my eyes on Dylan.

"Daddy wouldn't miss Christmas."

Beverley scooped him up in her arms and handed him his folded napkin. Dylan pushed it off his lap and onto the floor.

"Daddy is dead," Kaki whispered. "He isn't ever coming. Not even for Christmas. Isn't that right, Mommy?"

There were only fifteen months between them. I couldn't fathom how Kaki seemed to grasp the meaning of death and dying but Dylan could not. I was beginning to realize it wasn't just Dylan's refusal to understand that Alan had been killed in a plane crash. I had shown them a newspaper photograph of the airplane, Eastern Airlines #212, crashed in the cornfield. Not the images of the plane on fire or the body bags, but shots of the broken plane on the ground. But Dylan still expected his Daddy to come home every Friday night. Of course, he would expect him for Christmas morning. I struggled with why a span of fifteen months made such a difference. Was it because he was a boy?

Gioia was gone, and I was relieved that Beverley decided to stay at the Mill for Christmas rather than go home to Florida with her widowed mother and two brothers. Beverley was off the crutches but not back to normal. Moving around was a challenge, her leg ached at night, and she was worried about Dylan's behavior, which was worse without Stevie around.

The real Christmas miracle at the Mill was that our tree was still upright by noontime. There had been some swaying, but the tree stood.

Beverley took responsibility for stuffing the crumpled wrapping paper into a black garbage bag, but the corner of the living room was still piled high with all manner of glittering debris. I rolled the rescued ribbons and stashed them in sandwich bags for future festivities. My Gram, the one who lived to 104, used to iron the leftover paper. I restricted myself to the ribbon.

The puppies were sound asleep in the corner of the sofa, usually not allowed but overlooked today. Kaki wore her riding helmet and sat cross-legged on the braided rug from my medical school days. She was directing a horse show. She arranged the ponies in a ring, stacked Dylan's Legos as fences and oxers, and announced the events. Then she swept the braided rug and started over. It was like a ritual, a doing and undoing.

Dylan tossed handfuls of Legos higher and higher, not aiming at the Christmas tree but gradually coming closer and closer. Louder and louder. More and more frenzied. Angrier. His distress far exceeded even his usual cycle of painstaking, elaborate Lego construction, which sometimes went on for hours, followed by his wild destruction of what he had built. How was I going to contain him?

Around the tree, piles of presents remained unopened. I had a roast that Frank the butcher from Foods of All Nation had prepared, a little chateaubriand. I put it back into the refrigerator and turned off the oven. Instead, I returned to the living room with a glass of sherry and a plate of crackers and cheese from the kitchen. Plus, fresh oranges and chocolate chip cookies for the kids.

Beverley was telling the kids about her Christmases in Bradenton. "When I was growing up," Beverley said, "we got underwear and socks in our stockings."

Dylan eyed her warily. "Santa brought you underwear?"

"Yep."

The puppies started to whimper.

Dylan beamed a Lego directly at them. They howled. In an instant, Mattie trotted in from the kitchen. Her ears were up. She positioned herself between Dylan and the puppies.

"Stand up slowly" I said, "and tell Mattie you're sorry. Then, walk over to the sofa and pet the puppies. Very gently."

"NO!" He stood up to face me directly. "I won't." He put his hands on his hips.

"I want my Daddy." I picked him up and tried to comfort him, but he refused to be cuddled. He turned his face away and stiffened in my arms.

"We all miss Daddy, Dylan," I said. "We all love Daddy."

The image of his burned body, the flames consuming his skin, muscles, and bone flickered in my mind. Every morning when I awoke, Alan died all over again.

"You know," Beverley said. "I miss my Daddy, too. You remember when we all played football by the garden and drove the dogs crazy?"

"Harry's in Florida with Alice," Dylan said.

"No, Dylan. Harry is dead. He died the month after your Daddy died. Remember?" She started to cry. I asked Kaki to get her some tissues.

I'd had it. I was done with the charade. Done with pretending to be a regular family on Christmas Day. Tree dangling from the spike in the beam. Legos underfoot. Presents untouched. Too much drama and too little sleep. I understood that each of us was hurting in his or her own way, but I couldn't console anyone. I was helpless.

"Naptime!" I decreed and shepherded the kids through the dining room past the breakfast debris. "Upstairs into your rooms. No dogs. No playing. Doors shut. No getting up until I knock on your door. Not a goddamned sound! Do you understand?" My voice got louder and louder as I hurried them up the stairs. Even the dogs got the hell out of my way.

Beverley curled up on the sofa with a fresh Bloody Mary, her box of tissues, and the puppies. I did the dishes, stowed butcher Frank's fancy chateaubriand in the freezer, and took out some boxed mac and cheese. And turned off the Christmas carols.

"Christmas is over for today!" I declared in my most authoritative, commanding, pediatric ward–attending voice. No one was listening.

Fragile ornaments shifted ever so slightly on the branches. The room was fragrant with the bouquet of evergreen. Beverley nodded off and started to snore. The dogs were asleep on the couch, a velvety heap of Danes. I hoped against hope that we would get through supper and the kids would sleep through the night. I preferred being at work where I was competent, but tomorrow would be more of the same. I worried how I would manage next week, when Gioia and Stevie moved back into the Mill full-time.

As I ruminated about how very disappointed Alan would be on this Christmas Day, I curled up in my chair, tucked the afghan around my knees, and focused on the tree.

It was elegant—sparkling with lights and icicles. Lisa, a nurse practitioner from the Center, had created many of the most delicate ornaments by quilling, making paper filigree. She'd shown me how she selected strips of thin paper to roll, curl, and shape into snowflakes. All of them were elaborate, elegant, and different. Nellie had sent clunky creations with photographs of the kids. Other balls were wrapped in beads and gold braid. All in all, it was a gorgeous tree. And remarkable, dangling from that chestnut beam. Upright.

We had plenty of food and drink, an abundance of presents, and a magical tree in the living room.

Santa had come.

But not the one who really mattered.

· 20 ·

Despair

January–June 1975

Winter was long and dark. No family arguments at the kitchen table about what seeds to order for the garden. No building bookcases for Kaki's room. And no relief from Friday nights without Alan. Beverley located homes for Mattie's puppies, who were then well over fifty pounds. Yvonne grumbled about the kids' private school. Even the excitement of Gioia and Stevie moving into the Mill didn't lift the gloom. I would have insisted that I no longer needed the antidepressants, but when I stepped on one of Dylan's Lego pieces in my bare feet in the middle of the night, I wailed like a banshee. Only when I recognized the terror on Kaki's face did I quiet down.

Work was a relief. I had resisted when Dr. Thurman assigned me to the Center the year before, but I was settling in. Most of the Center's patients were between three and thirteen years old. I focused on how to recruit infants and toddlers for diagnosis and treatment, assigned a therapist to the Neonatal Intensive Care Unit (NICU) follow-up clinic, and received a federal grant from Maternal and Child Health. The grant monies supported a home-visiting program for families of newborns with special needs. At first the Center staff resisted working with children under two years of age, but their attitudes changed when they met the new mothers and their swaddled newborns in therapy.

I'd loved dealing with difficult adolescents at C&Y. Despite their acting-out behaviors and grand hyperbole, they taught me important life lessons. At a clinic for migrant workers the previous fall, I'd argued with a fifteen-year-old boy who needed minor heart surgery. I'd suggested he stop picking apples, leave the migrant team, his family, and graduate from high school in Charlottesville.

He soon tired of my tirade and invited me to visit Carter's Mountain. That was why I found myself walking with him and his family to the orchards in the early morning. The group was maybe thirty-five to forty strong—women with burlap sacks gathered under their arms, men carrying ladders, and everyone with a thermos of coffee. Sleepy-eyed kids straggled along behind, munching their breakfast biscuits. Without a spoken direction or an obvious first note, I was aware of a quiet humming, soft at first, but building into a rollicky chorus. The workers staked out their trees as sunbeams cut through the mist.

The men climbed their ladders, and the women spread out the bags below. Their singing seemed to dispel the morning mist. My young host waved goodbye, beamed a wide smile, and started picking. Their singing faded away as I drove down the mountain. What hubris to suggest he abandon his web of love and labor to sit at a desk indoors.

The adolescents at the Center taught me a lot. Danny was a thirteen-year-old in Cerebral Palsy Clinic who got my attention when he mistook wet dreams for a new kind of seizure.

Patients with disabilities often identified the normal changes of adolescence as just one more pathology. The inpatient nurses resisted any shift in their own thinking and continued to "tsk-tsk" the guys about early-morning erections. Gradually I gained traction, introducing small changes. First, I hired three men in their twenties to work on the inpatient ward as patient advocates—a returning Vietnam veteran, a conscientious objector, and a performing mime. Then I recruited a small subset of staff committed to patient independence and autonomy. That team of teachers, therapists, and psychologists were excited to work together and led the movement toward adolescent autonomy. Without my noticing, that team coalesced not just together but around me.

It was easier to effect changes in the inpatient setting than in outpatient clinics. The adolescent boys in the Muscular Dystrophy Clinic were my most challenging. Held on the third Wednesday of the month, it was a grim clinic. Not only were those patients losing their physical independence, they and their families understood the progression to total dependence and death. To make matters worse, the funeral home next door received its scheduled deliveries from the Batesville Casket Company on the same Wednesday every month.

One Wednesday, a loud knock on the exam room door interrupted my examination of Jerry in Muscular Dystrophy Clinic. Without waiting for a response, Dr. Blizzard, my department chair, stuck his head into the room. I pulled the sheet up over Jerry's naked body, apologized, and prepared to step out.

Jerry would not be ignored. "But, Doc, you said we could talk this visit." He struggled to catch his breath. "I'm running out of time—we need to talk."

"Later," I said and pulled the door shut. I glared at Dr. Blizzard. "Sir, I'm the clinic attending—"

He ignored my protest. "Meet our guest from Johns Hopkins," he started. "One of my boys, a medical geneticist, an MD-PhD. He's here for a tour. Call my secretary when you're done," he said as he walked away, "she'll pick him up."

We made a quick loop through the clinic, ward, and therapies. He exhibited no interest, asked no questions. I skipped the hospital school and the pool. We waited in my office for his ride. He inspected my bookcases, Kaki's framed finger painting, and my Raggedy Anns and Andys. "Way too small," he said. "Totally unsuitable for a director."

I stormed back to clinic, apologized to Jerry, and promised to meet next time undisturbed in my office. It wasn't until my drive home that it dawned on me that it had been the new chair who had urged me to stay home with the children and was now recruiting this MD-PhD guy for my job.

I slammed the kids' supper plates onto the table, piled with fish sticks, fries, and Mrs. Somebody's godawful zucchini sticks. I fumed as I explained what was happening to Beverley.

"Yuck, Mommy," said Kaki.

Dylan joined in, "Yvonne doesn't make me eat the zucchini sticks—"

Stevie stuck out his tongue in support.

"Too bad, kids. Eat up, buttercups. Animal crackers for dessert." I was not interested in supper reviews. My chair had declared war.

Beverley poured herself a Scotch. "Listen, kids, I bought popsicles today. Who's interested?"

"Mommy said animal crackers," Kaki said.

"Both, if you clean your plate," Beverley said.

"Did anyone hear what I said about Blizzard?" I raised my voice. The tiger cats skulked under the table. "Is no one listening to me?"

"Well, what are you going to do about it?" Beverley said as she let the Danes inside. She settled in the rocking chair and sipped her Scotch. "Any ideas?"

"I could call Dr. Thurman, but I don't want to be a crybaby," I said.

"Sharon, war is war. Call Ann Johanson, see what she thinks," Beverley said as she turned to get the popsicles out of the freezer. "Dylan, are you stashing your fish sticks behind the radiator?"

"No, Ma'am."

"Then what is Max scarfing down?"

"Johanson trained at Hopkins in Blizzard's lab before she came to UVA. She's on his team. One of his boys." I was heating up goulash for the grown-ups and trying to find enough leftover greens to make a salad. It was winter. "Where is Gioia, by the way? Is she coming home or spending the night in Stubblefield's darkroom?"

Beverley shrugged.

The kids finished the popsicles and the animal crackers. Beverley wiped the leftovers off their faces and hands. "Thirty minutes to bath time. Grown-ups are eating now."

The boys ran into the family room and dumped Legos on the floor, but Kaki stayed in the rocker. She had an unopened book on her lap. Beverley and I sat down at the table.

"Mommy, there's a Valentine's Dance at school."

I put down my fork and looked at Kaki. "What kind of dance?"

"The first-grade girls get to bring their daddies, the boys their mommies."

The heat started somewhere on my chest and spread up my neck to my cheeks and scalp. My ears pounded. I pushed away from the table, poured myself another glass of wine, and sat in the rocker across from Kaki. Stevie was screaming at Dylan for knocking down his tower. Beverley didn't move. I worked at a crocodile kind of smile for Kaki.

"Maybe, you and I will go. What time does it start? Do you remember, Kaki?"

She sunk her face in her hands. "NO substitutes. The teacher told the whole class, but she looked right at me."

"Damn all!"

"I'm sorry, Mommy."

"It's not your fault, Kaki, that Daddy died—" I picked her up and snuggled her onto my lap. She tucked her head into my neck as we rocked back and forth. My heart eventually slowed down, and Kaki stopped crying, but I was still crucifying the first-grade teacher in my head. That was the final blow: We were switching to public school in September.

Beverley took charge. "Call Ann Johanson, it's only eight thirty. Dylan and Stevie, pick up the Legos. All of them. Kaki, come help me get their baths ready."

Kaki nodded. I gave her a great big bear hug, kissed the top of her head, and patted her bottom. Mattie followed them upstairs. Max stayed with me as I made the call.

The next day, I sat in a café on the Corner with Ann. She was over six feet tall, pretty, and had a scarf printed with Van Gogh's *Starry Night* tied loosely at her neck. Ann was the only one I knew in Charlottesville who wore small, round, rimless glasses. Initially I'd thought they were old-fashioned Granny glasses, but later realized they were hip, like John Lennon's.

"Look, I was excited to work in Blizzard's lab," she said. "I would have shaved my head if he asked me to. I was proud to wear the Hopkins baby-blue lab coat. Back in St. Louis, my family proudly sent my brother, Jim, off to orthopedics training, but they objected to my even considering medicine. It took a master's in anatomy, which was a total waste of time, to prove my intentions."

"I notice that Blizzard still wears his Hopkins blue coat."

"I bet his new recruits will don the blue, too."

"Not you?"

"Well, I was tickled when Thurman invited me to come here as division chief of Endocrinology. I had done my lab work and published my scholarly papers, but I was destined to be one of Blizzard's girls for life. Loyal, grateful, you know the drill. There were four women then, but we've all flown the coop."

"And now?" I asked.

"Blizzard will be a good chair for our department. You know, he will increase the national rankings, develop more lab research, and collaborate with the growth hormone guys in adult medicine. But he will still act as the division chief of Endocrine and take over my role." She shrugged and smiled. "He's already hiring faculty for me."

"What will you do?"

"Beat him at tennis every time I get a chance." She laughed. "I'm happy here. I have great colleagues. I love my new house. And I just bought my childhood girls' camp in Wisconsin. Once I get it fixed up, you'll have to visit. It's on Virgin Lake. Honest."

"What about the other women from Hopkins?"

"They all have their own divisions at first-rate places." A few years after that conversation, Ann would leave academia for industry. As medical director, Ann led Genentech through the FDA process to license a growth hormone made by *E. coli* and made millions.

"I am not about to leave UVA," I said, "as much as Blizzard would like me to. I'm not abdicating the Center's leadership for one of his boys."

"In that case, what is the status of your promotion and tenure decision?"

I stopped short and looked at her. "Thurman said he put my portfolio together before he left. All Blizzard had to do was move it forward. I've been so busy, I haven't thought about it."

"You need to pay attention," Ann said. "Call Dr. Thurman. Tenure is time-sensitive."

As soon as I returned to the Center, I called Tulane and left him a message. Then I called Dr. Brunner, my colleague in Internal Medicine who was a year ahead of me. Yes, she had been promoted and tenured.

When I stopped by the therapy pool, it was magic. The kids who otherwise couldn't stand up against gravity could float in the pool and feel empowered. The Center had changed a lot in the ten years since I was an intern. But kids with disabilities and chronic illness were still not welcome in the public schools.

My last and favorite stop was always the hospital school. The kids were making chocolate chip cookies while they learned about pricing of goods, selling shares, and how the economy worked.

Back in the office, I gathered my slides and headed to the conference room with Raggedy Ann under my arm. It was time for my seminar talk on the developmental milestones of babies and toddlers. The next week, I would discuss children's understanding of death. Piaget wrote that kids don't have an adult concept of death, of death's inevitability, universality, and irreversibility, until around ten years of age. Preschoolers called anything that moved alive, like cars or water in the bathtub. All things not useful, like garbage, were "dead."

My patients with leukemia sometimes talked to me about dying. Their siblings asked me about how long fingernails keep growing in the coffin. And whether the dead sibling would hear us singing at the graveside or get cold in the winter.

Jerry, my patient from Muscular Dystrophy Clinic, was eighteen. He was mentally and emotionally competent to make his own decisions. But physically, he was totally dependent on his parents. He couldn't even brush his teeth. But he understood death and dying—he was experiencing it. Since he had set up his appointment to talk to me about time running out, I had prepared to hear his anxieties about dying.

The day of our appointment, he jockeyed his wheelchair through my office door. Jerry looked dapper in a blue-striped shirt and tie. He had enough muscle strength to operate the joystick, but not enough to shake my hand. I squeezed his shoulder in greeting. He sat upright, but the long leg braces poked sharp angles in the knees of his baggy trousers. The space in my office was tight. Too close. I could smell his toothpaste.

"This isn't easy," he said.

"It never is."

"I'm getting worse." He paused to breathe.

"Do you want to talk about it?" I asked. "You know, about dying?"

"To hell with that—I've got it covered," Angry, he took a long, slow breath and glared at me. Then, he grinned, "I've even picked out my tombstone."

"Oh, my." He was way out ahead of me.

"Pay attention, Doc."

"Okay."

"Living's damned limited these days." He was sweating, struggling to breathe. "I don't want to die—"

I interrupted, "Of course not."

He swallowed, took another breath, and continued, "a virgin."

"What?" I must have misheard him.

He looked me in the eye, paused, and whispered, "A virgin. I don't want to die a virgin."

I was not ready for that response, but why not? Jerry was eighteen. I remembered how it felt to be young. I sat up in my chair, crossed my legs, and resumed my clinical persona. "I have a few questions."

"Shoot."

I managed to ask him about masturbation.

He sighed. "Doc, that's not what I came to talk about. Listen to me. Listen."

"Okay."

"My days are numbered, Doc. Numbered."

"I know." I could smell Jerry's body odor. There wasn't enough air in my little office for the two of us.

"You were the one talking about the 'developmental tasks' at the conference. Remember? I was on the panel."

"I remember."

"Well, Doc, I'm ready for the 'losing my virginity' task."

Someone knocked on the door, probably his father. I think we were both relieved that our time was up.

The next morning as I drove into work, I was still thinking about Jerry. I reviewed his request from every perspective—ethically, developmentally, practically, morally, and professionally. I didn't trust my medical colleagues, mostly orthopedists. And I couldn't involve Jerry's clinical team. And not the uptight social worker.

I dialed Johns Hopkins and asked to speak with Professor John Money. I'd heard him deliver a keynote about sexuality and disability at a national conference. I owed it to Jerry.

"Money here."

I presented Jerry's dilemma. "You mentioned medical prostitutes in your keynote."

His voice boomed over the phone. "Only for my transgender clinic."

It was worth a try.

Dr. Money continued, "Any connections with the prostitute community there?"

"I'm a pediatrician, sir. No way."

"For God's sake and with all due respect to pediatrics, use your imagination." He paused. "Get the phone book."

I pulled the local directory off the shelf.

"Flip through the Yellow Pages. I'll hang on."

I was damned sure there were no listings for prostitutes, but I looked anyway.

"You're in a college town. There must be sexual resources. Exotic dancers or massage parlors?"

"Exotic massage?"

"BINGO. Close enough. APPROXIMATE, doctor. Make do. And good luck on a happy ending." He hung up.

I considered the logistics as I went to clinic. By noon, I identified two agents from the patient advocates. My plan would involve use of the recreational therapy van as transport. I judged it to be a necessary breach.

The fact that I wasn't yet tenured and could be easily fired hadn't factored into my plan.

The following week, I opened a letter from the School of Medicine dean informing me that my promotion and tenure decision had been deferred to the next academic year. I never heard anything from my chair, but Ann let me know my portfolio had been submitted late.

Conflict with the chair escalated, but it was not restricted only to me. And it had nothing to do with Jerry's unauthorized night out in the hospital van. That remained a secret.

The monthly meeting of the division chiefs started at five o'clock on Thursdays. In March 1975, almost nine months after he arrived, Dr. Blizzard announced the division budgets would be managed centrally by his department administrator. Blizzard ignored the raised hands, the grumbled resistance, and moved on to the next item. Ann rolled her eyes. The cardiology chief interrupted, "My division faculty generates the bulk of the clinical income in this department. We will not subsidize the low earners. We are academic cardiologists, not communists." The neonatology chief countered, "Now wait a minute. The NICU brings in the lion's share of the budget, not cardiology."

As I drove home, I realized that Blizzard must not know that I managed three budgets at the Center: one for the division; a larger academic budget, which included Orthopedics, Neurology and Dentistry; and another very sizeable allotment from the hospital. I had to get home to feed the kids, and I had to keep control of my budgets. I'd almost forgotten to register the kids for the fall at Red Hill Elementary School. The next day was Friday. I hated Fridays. Also Saturdays and Sundays.

When Alan was alive, the rhythm of life at the Mill revolved around weekends. Most weekends, but not all, Alan came home. In all our years together, nearly twelve in all, we had never lived under the same roof or in the same city. Our biorhythms had adapted to a weekly not a diurnal cycle.

Even six months after Alan's crash, I faced Fridays with dread. Dylan expected his Daddy to show up by Friday bedtime or, certainly, by wake-up time Saturday. Sometimes he spent all day Friday building a monster bridge with intricate towers and fences to show Daddy. We'd have to protect it from Stevie and the dogs. He'd refuse to eat his supper "until Daddy got home." Saturdays were usually busy with grocery shopping, double-feature movies, or visiting Neve Hall to play with the Hagens. Sunday was the worst—interminably long and empty. Each of us carried our own private hurts and losses, and each of us rocked Dylan, hugging and sweet-talking, but nothing soothed his terrifying rages. Week after week.

Beverley decided that we should have a family council. The weekly meetings were scheduled on Sunday afternoons in the living room at four. Gioia was expected to attend, even though she rolled her eyes and shook her head a lot. Kaki was the president. Beverley, the secretary who kept notes. Beverley's template of family function didn't resonate with my chaotic upbringing or synchronize with our various and sundry stages of grief. But we tried.

In one of those weekly meetings, Beverley introduced us to a version of transactional analysis, or TA. The gist was that each of us had our child roles, our adult roles, and our parent roles. Her stated goal was that each of us had to behave like adults, to follow the Mill rules, and to share in doing the chores. And if we did the chores as assigned, no one had to be the parent or administer punishments. TA was not particularly helpful at the Mill, but at the hospital, it was a different story.

I recognized that the principles of TA had potential for my negotiation with the chair over control of the Center budget. Beverley's coaching began in earnest. Ann and I both believed that women faculty would always be perceived as children to Blizzard's identity as parent or mentor or chief. Beverley insisted that TA had the potential to change that dynamic.

Beverley suggested I appear for my weekly appointment with Blizzard exactly at one o'clock. No sitting down to wait. I was to maintain a dominant, upright stance as I waited. I was to walk into his office already talking in a kind, conversational tone, hopefully with him remaining seated at his desk. Keep control by continuing to chat, lightly, but stand tall with him still sitting behind his desk. Smile, exude confidence, maybe even think good thoughts about him. Make a small gesture, preferably maternal or kind.

An early script for that small gesture read like this:

Say, "Bob, I made oatmeal cookies last night and I brought a treat for you." Then hand him the paper plate, smile, and sit down in the designated chair next to his desk. At the end of the meeting, offer him the recipe card.

Success was defined simply. Blizzard doesn't get up out of his chair, he smiles, and he eats the oatmeal cookie during the session.

My second task was to maintain control of a tight meeting agenda and always open with an acknowledgment of his importance, such as, "Would you sign this grant application, please? I can't do it. It requires the signature of the department chair." Or: "You were absolutely right about that reference last week. I shared the article with all our division faculty. Thank you." Keep control of the agenda, smile and nod a lot. Stand up at 1:28 p.m. exactly, hand him the division budget summaries. As you leave, remind him of something fun coming up in the community, like Garden Week.

I was dubious at the beginning, but the dynamic of our weekly meeting gradually changed. Make no mistake, it was hard work. I had to be superorganized, remain nonoppositional, and be attuned to any medical school politics that might affect him. Beverley would debrief me, offer new tasks, and coach me for the next encounter. I didn't know what happened during those Thursday meetings, but things changed.

When I invited Dr. Blizzard to the May Day party at the hospital school, he accepted. Not only did he arrive on time and shake hands with the teachers, but Dr. Blizzard wore a ribbon-festooned party hat without protest. The kids had great fun. Maybe he did, too.

For the remainder of that spring, on the first Thursday of the month,

I presented him with the updated division budget with an additional column showing the funds flow from Orthopedics, Neurology and Dentistry. And quarterly, a summary of the annual hospital budget for the Center, around $250,000. He had full access to my divisional budget, but no control. At the division chief meetings, the rancor continued about financial control. I remained quiet. Occasionally, Ann smiled.

And on each third Wednesday of the month, Jerry found some way to give me a clumsy but clear thumbs-up sign. Sometimes he trailed me down the clinic corridor in his motorized chair. Neither of us said anything, but his grin told me all I needed to know.

· 21 ·

A Horse for Kaki

Early Summer 1975

As Labe, the designated Dylan wrangler for the summer, walked into the kitchen, Dylan pelted him with a raw egg. Labe was a UVA student, highly recommended by my colleague, his uncle.

Dylan laughed and started to run away. Labe caught Dylan and dangled him by his ankles. Mattie growled at Labe. I hollered at Dylan. Yvonne turned her back.

I hadn't paid much attention to Yvonne's reports about the weekday chaos at the Mill. Kaki was contentedly off at sleepover horse camp. Gioia and Stevie had gone to Cape Cod. I dismissed Yvonne's head-shaking assessment that Labe was way more trouble than Dylan ever was. I could be stubborn.

Beverley and I drove to Camp Strawderman, almost two hours northwest of Charlottesville. I was excited to see Kaki, meet her cabin mates, and see the camp in action. She was only six, and two weeks was a long time.

I spotted Kaki first. She was perched on the front steps of Dumpty cabin in her riding boots, jodhpurs, and white T-shirt, helmet in her lap.

"Come quick, to the barn." She took my hand and pulled me along. "Sarah's waiting." Then came the big grin.

"No hugs?" I could smell the barn, sweat, and baby shampoo on her.

She shook me loose. "No crying. That's the rule."

"Well," I said, "if I don't get a great big hug right now, *I* will cry. Loudly."

All barns looked and smelled alike to me. Leather, fresh hay, and manure. Horses, hay, water buckets, kids of all ages and stages in riding garb always busy combing coats, braiding manes and tails, and picking hooves. To be honest, I was afraid of getting too close to the horses, but still, I felt a little weepy watching the easy intimacy between these girls and their mounts. I was never afraid for Kaki. Perhaps I should have been. But she seemed competent.

Sarah strode out of the barn, a trim, confident, no-nonsense young woman in snug riding britches. Tanned, toned, with short, curly blonde hair, and in charge. "Get Snowball saddled up, Kaki," she said, "while I talk to your mom."

We watched in silence as Kaki strode off.

Sarah announced, "Kaki needs a horse of her own. You need to get that arranged by the end of camp."

No social chitchat for Sarah.

I thought of Mattie growling at Labe in the kitchen. The two Great Danes easily exceeded my capacity. Who was this woman? What kind of dream state was this? Kaki needs a horse?

"How much would a horse for Kaki cost?" was what I said.

Sarah's face lit up, and she smiled for the first time. "Not a problem. She just needs a little hunter who likes to jump. Kaki will do the rest."

"How much?"

"Well, as much as you've got, really." Sarah laughed, put her hands on her hips, and scuffed her riding boots a bit before she added, "I mean it."

"Ballpark?"

"Five hundred would be a solid start," Sarah said. Of course, she didn't mention the cost of the tack, the shoeing, the stable fees, the vet bills, and the sundry other costs I would learn about later. Not where to stable said starter horse, not how I would transport said horse or that this single decision would inevitably lead to sending Kaki and her horse to boarding school. I wouldn't have believed it, anyway.

I nodded my head. No one was going to shame me over five hundred dollars. All my life I had said "no thank you" or "maybe next time." Poverty prevented me from accepting invitations to visit Bermuda on spring break, to join the family skiing trip to Glacier, or to sail on my roommate's ketch to South America the summer after Middlebury graduation. No more shame over money. Five hundred dollars for a horse for Kaki? Done.

At that point, I was either too stubborn or didn't know how to ask for Sarah's help. I was way too proud to reveal my complete ignorance of all things equestrian. All around me there were excited conversations about foxhunts or dressage trials or the next steeplechase that might as well have been in Japanese. I had no clue. To ask a clarifying question would risk blowing my cover as someone who belonged. As someone who knew when Kaki was ready for a horse of her own. And would know how to find the right one.

Eventually, it would be Beverley who remembered Felix Neusch as the Swiss guy who stabled his horses at Beau Pré. Felix not only brokered Prince the high-stepping parade horse but also found him a barn.

Kaki would turn seven on September 8, was a rising second-grader at Red Hill, the local public school, and had been a camper for just two weeks. But she already commanded her own Greek chorus.

Parenting was more complicated than I had ever imagined. I was relieved that both kids were reading and writing. Who the hell knew about horse shows and T-ball when they got pregnant? Yvonne had to teach me to holler, "Way to go! Get a slice of it!" at Dylan's Little League games. It was Beverley who remembered what gear he needed to pack for practice. The face mask, the glove, and the special cup when he played catcher. And Kaki had to decode the hunter-jumper judging criteria for me.

I struggled to avoid thinking how Alan might have reacted to Sarah's mandate. But Alan wasn't there. And I was.

We drove away slowly. Kaki stood in the middle of the driveway, waving until I couldn't see her in the rearview mirror.

"You've got to make a decision soon," Beverley said.

That was all it took for the knot in my stomach to tighten up, bile to ooze into the back of my throat, and my chest muscles to squeeze the breath out of me. I wished she'd been talking about finding a horse for Kaki, but I knew better. I had to decide whether to accept a settlement or go to court.

"It makes me furious," I said. "Bastards, all of them—from Eastern Airlines to the Safety Board to McGuire Woods. Even Alan for being on that damn flight in the first place."

On May 23, 1975, the National Transportation Safety Board (NTSB) reported its findings on the Eastern Flight #212 crash at 7:32 a.m. on Tuesday, September 11, 1974, in the cornfield 3.3 miles short of runway 36 at the Douglas Municipal Airport in Charlotte, North Carolina. The probable cause of the "nonsurvivable accident" was "the flight crew's lack of altitude awareness at critical points during the approach due to poor cockpit discipline in that the crew did not follow prescribed procedures."

Until precisely two minutes and thirty seconds prior to the impact, the pilot and copilot had engaged "in conversation not pertinent to the operation of the aircraft, including politics, OPEC's control of oil, the effect on car prices, demonstrating strong views and mild aggravation."

The final report included a graph of the plane's descent, annotated with a second-to-second recording of the cockpit conversation: OPEC, the price of oil, the cost of automobiles.

I worried about the other families who lost loved ones, who waited days for confirmation that their names were even on the flight manifest, and who had to send medical histories and dental records for identification of the bodies. I wondered about the funerals and whether they waited for a body or went ahead as we had, weeks before Alan's body was identified. I thought about Lorna Colbert in South Carolina, who lost not only her doctor-husband James, but two sons, Peter and Paul, in that crash. Stephen Colbert was ten at the time, the youngest of Lorna Colbert's remaining children. It would be the college-student Kaki who listened to comedian-commentator Stephen Colbert's interviews and who shared that Colbert's antidote to grief was finding and creating glee. Pure, unmitigated joy was his solution.

I had moments in those early days, very brief, obsessing about the copilot and stewardess who survived the crash. I'd spotted a newspaper photograph taken as they arrived at the NTSB hearing. I wondered how they could sleep at night. How they'd live the rest of their lives bearing the guilt of eighty-nine deaths. Did they have differing degrees of culpability? He was in the cockpit, responsible for keeping the plane in the air. Would he ever fly again? What about her? Did they have nightmares? Did they wonder about the lost lives, the families?

Over the years, I imagined them struggling with overwhelming guilt, the guilt of surviving when so many died. Eventually, I wished them relief from nightmares and painful memories. And years later, to love and be loved.

But it was decades before I considered the same for Eastern Airlines. Later academic medicine developed a review process to address the pathogenesis of serious, often fatal, medical errors. Learning about the matrix of seven distinct levels of missed opportunities to intervene and avert disaster allowed me a measure of cognitive peace. I think Archbishop Tutu gave me the final lesson on forgiveness—and acceptance—decades later, while on the MV *Explorer* for Semester at Sea.

Beverley was right to keep pushing me to make a decision. I was paralyzed in rage. What was a forty-two-year-old man's life worth? How could my own lawyers consider me an unsympathetic witness in court? They disdained a man who didn't leave a will, his working widow who lived in a decrepit old mill with three other adult women, one of them Black, three kids, and two Great Danes. Why didn't they challenge the wrongful death limits set by the Commonwealth of Virginia?

"They've got you hijacked emotionally," Beverley said. "It is doing no good for you to keep railing against all of them."

"It's not fair, damn it." I started counting the cows, then split them into two columns in my mind: the ones lying down and the ones standing up. If more were on the ground, we should expect rain tonight. Counting always helped to calm me down.

The legal processes were punitive. Why the hell did I have to buy back two-thirds of the equity in the Mill and its contents because Alan had no will? Why did I have to pay the appraisers to go through our library books, even the gift books I had purchased and had inscribed to Alan? Why couldn't I waive Kaki and Dylan's rights to Alan's first wife's home on Cape Cod? None of it made sense.

And the damnable hubris of the lawyers' request for photographs documenting us as a regular, happy little family? For written reports from therapists laying out our individual and collective distress? It was an endless assault. I lumped the lawyers in with Eastern Airlines.

How did one monetize the rage and disappointment of Friday nights when Alan didn't come home? When we waited and waited, week after week. When Dylan wouldn't leave the kitchen window and insisted with tears and tantrums that Daddy was coming this week.

I wanted my day in court. I wanted to swoop into the courtroom on a broom like a wicked witch screaming at Eastern Airlines' leadership, damning their shareholders, and cursing the copilot who survived. But why? Beverley reminded me that the only audience would be the suits hired by Eastern, the front men, the corporate pawns.

As we turned off the highway to head down the mountain toward Charlottesville, I announced: "Thirty-five cows in all, nineteen upright. No rain tonight." At least I was certain about something.

I hated the unspoken judgments. Each transaction required my paying someone: the know-it-all lawyers, the assessors and appraisers of our belongings, the clerk of the court, the ad litem lawyers for Kaki and Dylan to protect them from my squandering their assets. All of them privileged members of some Southern male club, some vaguely and some overtly disapproving of me and my decisions to marry a divorced man, to live like a hippie at the Mill, and especially to keep working *in these difficult times when the children needed me.*

"I don't know, Beverley," I said. "I don't think it's morally right for a check to be written in exchange for my silence. Alan burned to death because of Eastern Airlines' incompetence. Pain and suffering beyond imagination. All six kids lost their father. Amy's four and my two. Little Stevie lost a grandfather. I want justice, Old Testament justice, an eye-for-an-eye kind of justice."

"You're going to destroy yourself and everyone around you if you keep on raging."

"If I'm not raging, I'm giving up, crawling back in bed and staying there."

"In the meantime, you're spending money you don't have."

"I know. I know."

"And what the hell are you thinking? Getting a horse for Kaki? Have you lost your mind?"

· 22 ·

One of the Boys . . . or Not?

Late Summer 1975

The summer of 1975 was filled with turmoil—the Watergate scandal, the fall of Saigon, President Gerald Ford's pardon of General Robert E. Lee. Even rabble-rousing feminists were in the news. I didn't identify with the abrasive Betty Friedan's touting the International Year of the Woman. I more readily identified with Gloria Steinem—the stilettoes, the big glasses, and the Playboy Bunny history.

Lessons from Hop and Nellie established early on that men were the ones in charge. At Middlebury College, Professor Hitchcock dictated that women could not be premed majors. President Stratton designated the women students as "calico" or "velveteen." In medical school, Dr. Lucey directed my internship into pediatrics rather than internal medicine by offering me the opportunity to serve as an acting intern at the children's hospital in Puerto Rico. Dr. Thurman shaped my decision to become a fellow in pediatric hematology. Alan's preferences for Coco Chanel, composting, and organic gardening became my own.

There were no women role models in my world.

I never objected to male dominance. I was far too busy trying to be one of the boys to worry whether I was being treated unequally or what choices had been made for me. But I did understand that I needed to be more than just competent. I had to be superior.

I hadn't sought support or guidance from other women in medicine—not in medical school, pediatric training, or as faculty. I thought the nurses supported me because of my commitment to the patients, not my gender. And I didn't give much attention to the women who were supporting me—Yvonne and Beverley at the Mill; AV, Jan, and Helen in the satellite clinics; and Clariece and Patty in the city clinic.

I wasn't my sister's keeper, but I was delighted when 550 women graduated from UVA that May, a direct outcome of the Board of Visitors' decision in 1970 to consider women for admission. UVA had women's varsity tennis, field hockey, and basketball teams due to Title IX of the federal civil rights law.

In 1968, the Honor Committee had written: "Coeducation will hurt the Honor System and thus should not be recommended. The more intermingling there is between men and women, the less peer disapproval there is about honor offenses." The *Cavalier Daily* banner blazed: "WOMEN HAVE NO HONOR." I read the headline to mean that women were incapable of obeying UVA's code of no lying, cheating, or stealing. I missed the point. *Honor* in the South was a masculine construct, its patriarchal history dating back at least to the chivalry of knights.

In 1975, my rage was directed at Eastern Airlines, not systemic misogyny. But I couldn't sustain rage, work, and raise Kaki and Dylan. For everyone's sake, I settled the case with Eastern Airlines. The financial resources that decision brought meant I could send the kids to summer camp, join the Boars Head Sports Club so the kids could swim in the pool, and even fix up the Mill. The bottom line was that I needed to get promoted. I had to maintain my faculty position at UVA to pay the bills and keep the Mill. That meant getting tenure.

I resisted acknowledging that the women's movement had anything to do with me. Not the faculty salary discrepancy when I was first hired. Not the obstacles to the UVA faculty mortgage supplement when we purchased the Mill. Not the commentary by my own lawyers about how I, as a working mother, would have been an unsympathetic witness in a trial against Eastern Airlines. I remained convinced that I was so exceptional as a physician that being a woman, a Yankee, and a working widow would not impact my career trajectory in academic medicine.

I was delusional.

If Ann Johanson was correct—and I trusted her—Dr. Blizzard delayed my promotion materials. Intentional? Maybe. Unsupportive? Yes. Sexist? That thought never crossed my mind.

I had to get promoted. I made it a habit to remain at the hospital until all the surgeons had completed their day. I matched the men, step for step, patient for patient.

That August, Alec Horniman, my colleague from years ago at Middlebury, who had introduced me to the University beyond the School of Medicine by way of Dr. Joseph Fletcher's session on abortion, invited me to his "Executive Seminar" at Darden, the UVA Business School.

The participants, all men, represented lumber, banking, and mining companies from across North America, all industries in acute financial crisis. Professor Horniman invited us to our assigned seats, welcomed us, and laid out the teaching goals. In his opening remarks, Horniman compared the behaviors of the industry leaders to Dr. Elisabeth Kübler-Ross's model of the stages of grief.

Horniman made brief eye contact with me, smiled, and introduced me as a professor from the School of Medicine, someone who dealt with grief and loss, death and dying every day. One by one, the guys in suits turned around to gawk.

The class quickly broke up into small working groups to address the case studies. It felt awkward, a bit like a preschool, but I was stunned by the easy intimacy created as we worked our way through the options available to our study corporation. Of course, I argued for pay cuts and preservation of positions. My suggestion was dismissed.

By the second day, I started to understand that the conference wasn't just about profit and loss. Horniman discussed how organizations behaved in predictable patterns during crisis. I'd never heard the term "organizational behavior" before, but I learned it was a subdiscipline of psychology. He outlined the stages of change occurring as lumber, banking, and coal mining reacted to massive downsizing. How both individuals and organizations experienced loss—markets, profits, dislocation, professional identity—and coped with that loss.

The conference activities had seemed an intellectual exercise without any relevance to medicine or me. But I started paying close attention when Horniman introduced Andersen's theory on the stages of value change. He explained that the first stage was often window dressing—the CEO pontificating in vague terms to the senior managers with no trickle down to supervisors and frontline workers. As I dutifully copied down the slides and the references, I didn't understand how relevant they would be. It was only much later that I recognized how women physicians could use these tools to challenge the hierarchies and processes of academic medicine designed by White men for White men.

Ann Johanson walked into my office, closed the door, and told me she was worried about our colleague Martha Carpenter. "Blizzard has removed her as chief of Pediatric Cardiology. He replaced her with a cardiologist from Hopkins."

I rubbed my sweaty hands on my skirt. Ann was five years my senior, already tenured, and one of Blizzard's trainees at Hopkins. Martha Carpenter was a full professor and at least ten years older than me.

Dr. Carpenter founded the division ten years earlier, developed the catheterization lab, and collaborated with both cardiac surgeons and experimentalists in basic science. She was the only one in our department at UVA besides Dr. Birdsong and the new neonatologist who had trained at Boston Children's Hospital. Boston Children's was my gold standard. Dr. Carpenter was the reason UVA received referrals of babies with congenital heart defects from all over Virginia and the surrounding states.

The men whispered that, *of course,* Blizzard wouldn't want a woman as chief. But, I thought, Ann Johanson and I were division chiefs. Of course, Blizzard hadn't appointed either of us. Dr. Thurman had.

"She's lost control of the cath lab schedule," Ann continued. "Patients are being canceled. It's not right, Sharon, but Martha is making it worse. She's talking back to Blizzard."

I waited. The kids hollered to one another out in the lobby. Spirits were high. The wheelchairs were clanging, but Ann and I sat in the quiet. I hoped for a knock on the door, anything to break the tension.

"I've watched Blizzard over the years," Ann said. "It may take a while, but he will win." I found myself worrying about who might be listening at the door. After all the idealism at Darden, this was gritty reality.

"You have to tell Martha to stop standing up to Blizzard."

Me? I was cornered in my own office. The easy intimacy of the Darden conference seemed far away. "Martha is a tenured full professor; I'm just an assistant professor. She wouldn't listen to me."

"Martha won't trust me! She'll think I'm Blizzard's messenger."

"Ann," I said, "You're the only one who can talk to Dr. Blizzard."

"He won't listen to me. I'm just *one of his girls.*"

"I need his support to get my promotion and tenure action done." My position was getting more precarious. I trusted Ann, but still, she was one of Blizzard's fellows.

In retrospect, could Ann and I have made a difference? For the next seven years, Blizzard tormented Martha: froze her salary, denied her consultations from outside hospitals, and suggested she was less skilled than his appointed guy. Could we have changed that? I don't know.

Year after year, Martha saw her patients, tolerated the abuse, and worked her way through the torturous reporting mechanisms within the Department of Pediatrics, the School of Medicine, and the University. When I was eventually invited to testify at her appeal before a subcommittee of the University's Faculty Senate, I did so. It was easy to answer questions about her clinical competence. By then I was a tenured associate professor. After long and complicated deliberation, the case was found for Dr. Carpenter. She was reinstated as division chief of Pediatric Cardiology, but her salary, frozen for seven years, was not corrected.

I can hardly believe how naïve I was that day when Ann came into my office. I had no awareness that what happened to Dr. Carpenter could easily happen to any of us women.

All my life, I had assumed that when other women were treated badly, they deserved it. Of course, I was different. I would be treated fairly. I was one of the guys.

Dr. Ruth Weeks, my colleague in Child Psychiatry, was next. Ruth had come to the ER on consult when I was an intern in the ER to help me with the twelve-year-old child sexually abused by her mother's boyfriend. Ruth is the one who assured me that it was perfectly normal to see Alan rocking in the kitchen.

When Ruth was denied tenure by the Department of Psychiatry, she left the University. No appeal. No protest. She established a successful private practice in town. Even then, I did not recognize the pattern.

I still identified with the men, especially the men in power. I assumed that women were not as strong or as smart or as effective as the men. I remembered the messages from both Hop and Nellie. *Who the hell are you to challenge the wisdom of the guys in charge?* Along with the

Uncle Tom house slaves, the Stockholm syndrome hostages, and the abused children, I lined up with the abusers.

I did not connect the dots that August 1975. I was mourning Alan's death. I was trying to provide a safe haven for Kaki and Dylan. And yes, I was trying my damnedest to be one of the men. But, as time went on, I found it harder and harder to see the events occurring to my women colleagues as random acts of God.

· 23 ·

Lessons in Las Vegas

September 1975

I would never have planned to be away for the one-year anniversary of Alan's crash. However, when I learned that Blizzard had sabotaged my application for promotion, I turned to my medical school mentor, Dr. Jerry Lucey, about returning to the University of Vermont. His response brought home just how tenuous my situation had become.

"Great idea, Sharon," he said, "But you have to get tenure at UVA first."

If my own mentor, Dr. Jerry Lucey—the professor who recruited me away from internal medicine into pediatrics, the one who sponsored my acting internship in Puerto Rico as a fourth-year medical student, and the one who nominated me for Alpha Omega Alpha, the medical honor society—wouldn't even talk about my coming back to UVM without tenure, then I was truly abandoned.

I couldn't remain at UVA if I didn't get promoted to associate professor with the award of tenure. Up or out, those were the rules of academic life. Since the harsh reality of that conversation, I had accepted every invitation, every opportunity to demonstrate the emerging national reputation required for my tenure.

So, I dove in. I collaborated with infant researchers at UNC, taught the local orthopedists about child development, and signed off on infant mobiles from the Education for Multi-handicapped Infants (EMI) Project. I considered my campaign essential to survival at UVA, not mania or grief.

I had been uneasy about traveling around the first-year anniversary of Alan's death, but I hadn't anticipated that the kids would be so focused on the exact date. I hadn't even heard the term "death anniversary phenomenon" at that point, but I would later learn about the need to focus on the date, to name it loud and clear. To gather the mourners around the table, to make a menu of favorite food, set the table, sit still, and share the stories that helped us slog through the messy work of grieving. That first year after Alan's death, I naively hoped we could quietly slide through the day like a furtive dive deep into the dark underwater.

I was wrong.

Instead, all hell broke loose at the Mill on the eve of the first crash anniversary. "No, Mommy," Kaki said. "You can't fly."

My head was spinning about my countdown for the orthopedic meetings. I noticed she was biting her fingernails down to the quick and tuned in.

"Mommy has to fly to do her work." I took a deep breath. "It's my job, Kaki, to teach at other places. Las Vegas is too far to drive."

"Daddy's plane crashed." She started to cry. The boys stopped fighting to watch.

I knelt to hug her. She sobbed quietly into my shoulder.

Yvonne avoided me. Kaki reported that Yvonne was talking to "Mr. Dimock" in the front hall closet again, asking him about the streets paved in gold. Even Kaki knew that that was just Yvonne's way of grieving for Alan. We all seemed to have our own ways.

My way was to get on that plane.

We were all at sixes and sevens as we gathered around the red kitchen table. Yvonne banged her way out the back door, refusing to take any of her own fried chicken. I was tone deaf to what was going on and tried to drive the supper conversation toward happy stuff.

"Mr. Cutright is going to start work on the Mill," I said. "Next week!"

"The Mill is fine just the way Daddy did it." Dylan shoved his plate off the table. Food splattered everywhere. We sat there in silence. Even the Danes ignored the chicken leg on the floor. They eyed Dylan like they were awaiting further orders.

"Daddy was going to fix the snake holes, Dylan," Kaki said. "He just didn't get around to it before the plane crashed." She slid off her stool to sweep up the mess.

Beverley announced that we were going to Jamaica for Christmas.

"Remember when Daddy was in Jamaica?" she said. "He told us about the magic bay where the water shimmers like an electric rainbow."

Why the hell was Beverley talking about Christmas now? It was only September. Dylan kicked in the air closer and closer to Mattie. She was smart enough to shift toward the pantry.

Beverley was undaunted. "If you guys want a Christmas tree this year, it'll have to be a palm tree."

Kaki looked at me for confirmation.

"That's right," I said. Anything to avoid a repeat of last year's fiasco with the Christmas tree swinging from the beam in the living room.

Dylan hugged my knees and gave me a great big grin. "Daddy will be there, won't he, Mommy?" he asked. I reached out, but he backed away.

Kaki stood in the middle of the kitchen, hands on her hips, and shook her head. "Daddy is dead. You know that, Dylan. He's never coming back."

"Jamaica," Dylan said. "Daddy's in Jamaica."

"Tell the pilot about Daddy's crash," Kaki said. "Explain he needs to be extra careful."

Years later I shared the story of that supper at the Mill with an academic audience before my keynote lecture, "The Child's Concept of Death," at the University of Rochester. It would be there that I first heard about the concept of the "death anniversary phenomenon," directly from the wise professors of psychiatry who first described it in the academic literature.

The invited talks became an opportunity to integrate my ten years of experience with patients and their families. To braid the lived wisdom from my patients dying of leukemia with lessons about children's cognitive and emotional development and my own clinical observations of kids' language and behaviors.

And it was there that I recognized that what I was living and breathing day to day with Kaki, Dylan, and Stevie at the Mill was my personal laboratory of death and dying.

The Center had turned out to be a productive place for me, but it would be many years before I recognized Dr. Thurman's wisdom in assigning me there, out of the fray of the main hospital. He had understood that I couldn't survive my dogged tilting at the windmills of the hospital's hierarchy.

The Center's structure around interdisciplinary care teams required that my leadership style had to change from the top down, command and control I had learned, embraced, and emulated from my male colleagues. I would have to learn a somewhat more collaborative way to succeed in that setting. My mentors at C&Y had sanded away some of the rough edges, but there were still sharp angles remaining. Those early mentors were all women.

I would not have recognized myself as angry or stubborn. I had worked hard to be just like the men in academic medicine—just as smart, just as tough, and just as focused—even as I resisted their dominance. I would acknowledge being determined, strong-willed perhaps, but always for a just cause: a disabled child or a distraught family. Or so I rationalized. It didn't take much pressure for me to become a bully, just like the guys.

Even though I never played team sports growing up, I was learning to relish the different roles of the physician on the interdisciplinary team, as bedside attending, the consult professor for the increasingly complicated patients, and the creator of exemplary pediatric care models for other academic medical centers. Roles that all involved cooperation, collaboration, and, occasionally, concession.

Third-year medical students rotated for two weeks on the Center's inpatient ward, worked up new admissions, and spent their afternoons in the outpatient area, usually in the Cystic Fibrosis and Diabetes Clinics. Students were supervised by a team consisting of an intern, a third-year resident, and the ward attending. It replicated a rigid hierarchy of power and control modeled by the early Italian universities after some hybrid of the military and the Catholic Church and had remained unchanged for hundreds of years.

When residents complained about the Center, I was unsympathetic. I maintained my emotional distance, the authority of my title, and the respect inherent in my faculty position. I never shared my own stories as an intern assigned to the Center: my terror of the unfixable bodies, the torturous treatments, and the rigid separation of young patients from their families. One-hour visitation on Sunday afternoon was all that was allowed. I hated it, all of it, and I was determined to change it.

No weakness. No soft parts. No vulnerability allowed. Not if I hoped to survive in academic medicine.

The orthopedic residents and faculty grew to value the pediatric presence as part of their rounds and teaching conferences. So much so that the chair invited me as a "distinguished guest lecturer" for two seminars at their national meeting. An invitation I could not decline even it fell on the anniversary of Alan's death.

I arrived on schedule for my talks to the American Association of Orthopedic Surgeons at the MGM Hotel in Las Vegas. I approached the check-in desk through a lobby of slot machines in full swing—bells ringing, coins clanging, cherries popping up. Bawdy red brocade, glittering gold, and shiny chandeliers were everywhere. Show girls in sequined minidresses and big hair sashayed by the wives in their long, billowing prairie dresses waiting as their doctor husbands registered.

The bellman grandly threw open the door, and I gasped. The gaudy suite featured a circular bed swathed in red brocade positioned below a mirrored ceiling, a fully mirrored dressing room and bath. Thick red towels monogrammed with gold MGMs were stacked next to a circular bathtub overflowing with rose petals.

"Serious mistake, sir," I said to the bellman. "I need a different room."

"Sorry, Ma'am. The house is totally booked for the convention, you know, the bone doctors. Sewn up," he laughed at his own joke. "Now, let me show you the minibar."

He opened the bar, "You have unlimited refills. You're a distinguished guest of these guys. Sky's the limit and all that. Here's a complimentary bag of chips for the tables. Have fun."

I couldn't imagine taking a shower with all those mirrors, but my first seminar on infant development would start soon. I managed to squint my eyes almost shut and ignore the multiple reflections of the dowdy, pudgy matron occupying my suite. What had become of the young, attractive blonde? The one wrapped in the red-bearded Viking's arms on Friday nights? What ever happened to her? She was only thirty-four years old.

I stepped up to the podium in the requisite costume—black sheath dress and matching jacket, pumps, and pearls. I aced the first seminar. The audience was mostly men in suits and ties, probably all pediatric orthopedists, but there were a few women, therapists and orthotists.

By then, I had become facile teaching with Raggedy Ann and Raggedy Andy: demonstrating the newborn reflexes, the progression of cerebral motor control over the primitive brain stem. Sitting up with anterior balance at six months, then hands out to the sides, laterally by seven, and finally by eleven months, solid posterior balance. Fine motor competency and then language, first receptive and then expressive.

By one year, I had those dolls not only upright but cruising, saying "*MaMa, DaDa, ByeBye,* and *BaBa*" or some sound for bottle. The crowd was excited when, by two years, my toddler Raggedys started climbing stairs, one step at a time. And we touched on separation anxiety and attachment theories. The crowd, maybe sixty to seventy-five participants, clapped enthusiastically at the end. Babies were easy. Developmental pediatrics was a new field, and the Center was at its forefront.

Late that afternoon, I walked into the second seminar about adolescent development. The room was packed: People were sitting cross-legged in the aisles, leaning against the walls around the edge of the conference room, backed up at the door. What little air remained was charged with testosterone from so many former college football players now bone doctors filling up the space.

The room was buzzing with laughter and multiple side conversations. What was all this energy about?

Sex, it turned out.

As I described the tasks of normal adolescent development, the stabilization of body image, adult sexual roles, separation from family and vocational choices, I pointed out how the various orthopedic interventions for musculoskeletal disorders interfered with body image. Like the Milwaukee brace, which teens were required to wear for twenty-three out of twenty-four hours a day to stabilize scoliosis and, hopefully, to prevent progression of the spinal curve to the point of surgery. Did they make accommodations for breast development in the brace's rigid construction of leather straps and steel?

I heard feet shuffling, a few mutters. I paused and asked for a show of hands: How many of you have a chaperone with the undressed teenager being fitted for braces? How many of you discuss birth control? Suggest condoms?

I had their attention.

I passed out cases for group discussion, took a risk, and invited a few of them to role-play. Sometimes I played the teenager afraid to bring up my squashed breast or my inability to change my menstrual pad in the brace. Someone from the audience played the horny sixteen-year-old, worried about getting out of the braces and into position, worried about failure. The room quieted.

We worked our way through the cases, reached decision points, failed, and tried again. Eventually, we developed creative solutions that none of us had considered.

By the end of the session, there were accolades, expressions of surprise, and promises of invitations as visiting professor. In the back of the crowd, I spotted the sports orthopedists from UVA, the docs for the football and basketball teams, hanging out with the pediatric orthopods from the Center. I sighed in relief that I hadn't seen them earlier.

"Super, Sharon," Frank McCue said. "For a minute there, I thought you were going to ask me to put a condom on a banana." He was Mr. Sports Orthopedist, known nationally and internationally. He operated on players from professional teams and even Olympians. I'd worked with his wife, Nancy, years ago in the Pediatric Clinic. I was surprised that he'd bothered to attend my talk but not at all surprised that Nancy wasn't with him in Las Vegas.

"Let's talk about hormones," Frank said.

"No way, Frank. That's not my expertise. You know that."

"Come on! Join our panel for the sports conference next month and tell us how to do it. Use hormones to enhance performance without screwing up growth and stuff."

I refused.

"Well, aren't you the party pooper? Nancy was right, she said you would be *principled.*"

I was quiet, waiting for what would happen next. I wasn't changing my mind on this matter.

"Alright, then. Come on, Sharon." His tone of voice changed. "Let's go to the tables, play a little blackjack, and get a drink."

I hesitated.

Frank took my arm. "We're in Las Vegas where no one ever sleeps." Frank and his fellow in sports orthopedics swept me out of the gray-carpeted conference area into the razzle-dazzle din of the shimmering red brocade and gold casino.

"Why not?" I said, relieved for the topic change. "But I have an early flight back to Charlottesville."

"So do we! No worries," Frank said. I should have known better.

The hostesses knew our drink orders by heart and kept sliding fresh ones next to our poker chips. I'd been sipping Scotch sours on the rocks, snacking on salty goodies, and slowly growing a fair stack of chips. Then losing them and starting over. Frank and Mike flanked me, raucously coaching, and cheering my successes. I remembered nights like this, being crazy and carefree. So long ago.

How had it gotten to be four in the morning? They'd thwarted my efforts to leave the table. It hadn't taken much. I kept playing. The pediatric guys sensibly departed long ago.

I wasn't so sure about standing up. And I wasn't sure about making it to the toilet to throw up either. But I was damned sure that I had to board the airport shuttle at 5:45 a.m. in the lobby to make the 8:30 a.m. flight east.

"Why don't you stay?" Frank asked.

Why didn't I? Why didn't I stay with the guys? Not just the surgeons, not just the orthopedists, but the sports medicine orthopedists? The jocks? Wasn't being one of the guys what I had been striving for?

I was on the shuttle all alone. I had failed as party girl. I was sure as hell not one of the boys on the wards or at the casino table. But I wasn't that stuffy matron so ill at ease with the bellman earlier. Nor one of the wives, arm candy for the orthopedic surgeons. It didn't matter. I'd been a standing-room-only success as invited professor at a national academic symposium. Not pediatricians, but surgeons, orthopedic surgeons.

I had mastered something maybe more useful: weaving clinical stories to create new learning. Even hungover, I understood. Something important had happened in Las Vegas.

· 24 ·

Raging on the Couch

Summer 1976

It was my first session. I was having second thoughts.

I surveyed the wall of floor-to-ceiling bookcases across the muted Oriental rug and scanned the shelves for Jung, Adler, and Freud. The setting was straight out of Vienna. I'm still amazed I didn't walk out.

After Alan's death, Ruth Weeks, the child psychiatrist and my colleague, had talked repeatedly about my need to "do the work." I had no idea what she was talking about. In college, I majored in chemistry and minored in English literature. No psychology classes. The psychiatry rotation in medical school consisted of completing two intake assessments at the state mental hospital and a month to figure out the correct diagnostic title for the presenting psychosis: schizophrenia or manic-depressive disorder. A coin toss would have been as accurate as my diagnosis.

Ruth endorsed Dr. Josephthal, finagled this appointment, and insisted I commit the time to do the work.

"It is your only way out," she insisted. Out of the debilitating headaches, the nightmares, and my rage and self-loathing. At times I cried, in frustration or anger, but not in grief.

I listened to a clock ticking. "About Alan," he said.

I don't remember what story I told that day—Alan tending goats as a child, Alan sailing the *Kestrel* off Woods Hole, or Alan measuring the depth of the Indian Ocean while Kaki battled chicken pox in Charlottesville, seizing as her temperature rose. I do remember how annoyed I was when he interrupted me midthought: "Time is up for today. We'll continue Wednesday."

It wasn't at all convenient to stop what I was doing in the hospital at precisely 9:45 a.m. on Monday, Wednesday, and Friday each week and then resume that activity seamlessly at 11:15 a.m. Change of day or time was not negotiable. I was informed that I was financially responsible for the sessions whether I arrived late or if, as happened on more than one occasion, I didn't arrive at all.

But talking about Alan was a relief. By then, it was nearly two years since the crash. My friends had grown weary of my repetitive stories and changed the subject. My colleagues simply ignored me and continued the conversation as though I hadn't mentioned Alan.

"About Alan" was initially an approximate chronology, meandering from our first meeting at the Landfall bar through the summer of 1962 in Woods Hole. I described Alan's friends Jerry, George, Cookie, and sometimes Mike at Typhoon Tavern; the Woods Hole Oceanographic Institute; and hamburgers at the Captain Kidd. Alan showing up in Jerry's red Ferrari at the University of Vermont one Friday night that September and our unexpected long-distance courtship. What followed that initial direction when I found out he had four children. Nellie's middle-of-the-night phone calls calling me a slut.

The magic of the summer of 1964 when we sailed on Lake Champlain—dining out on PB&J sandwiches, drinking rum, and sleeping on the deck of a twenty-foot sailboat. Alan moving to Washington, DC, to work for Ocean Science and Engineering while I was an acting intern in Puerto Rico. My last-minute decision to follow Alan south, choosing an internship at UVA. Our wedding at Beau Pré, babies becoming Kaki and Dylan, crazy days at the Mill.

"About Alan" became ranting about the crash, hotshot pilots, Eastern Airlines, the transcripts of the crash, the waiting, his being alive on impact, burning to death, the National Transportation and Safety Board. Alan dead at forty-two. Me, a widow at thirty-four, with Kaki and Dylan and four stepchildren.

"About Alan" didn't include Alan's ghost rocking in the kitchen early in the morning or the nightmares of his body rotting in the root cellar of the Mill. Or Alan's dreams of our sailing around the world or running a shipyard or homesteading or living in New Zealand or apple orcharding in Nova Scotia. Hardly a whisper of my wild fury that Alan might have abandoned me and be on a beach somewhere in the Seychelles. How I searched for his face in airports, railroad stations, newspaper photographs.

"About Alan" settled into quiet, profoundly sad sessions. How it had felt on Friday nights in the kitchen at the Mill to be ensconced in his full-body hugs with his scratchy beard in my neck. Kaki and Dylan pulling on his pant legs, clamoring to be picked up. Beverley and Yvonne laughing. The Great Danes milling around us contently, sometimes a bark but more often just a gruff-gruff or two.

How being in Alan's arms was the only time in my entire life that I felt safe and secure.

Friday nights at the Mill assured me that Alan loved me unconditionally. Like no one had ever loved me in my life. And now, how profoundly alone I was. Scared, too. How I had learned my lesson. I would never, ever trust anyone like that again.

Over six weeks, the Monday-Wednesday-Friday sessions became almost routine. But it was different when I arrived one Friday at ten o'clock in late July.

Dr. Josephthal explained that the past six weeks had been a probationary period to determine if I had loved Alan. He was assessing whether I had a firm attachment to Alan since mourning required a strong bond. What I heard was the shrink suggesting that I might not be an adequate patient.

I had been taking a test without even knowing it. A test I had to pass.

Next, he shared the result, but I was so angry I could barely listen. He assured me I'd passed. I could formally become his patient, and we could begin *the work*. Then he laid down the rules.

"It will be demanding, very intense emotional work," he warned. "There will be times when you will feel that you can't continue. Trust me—that is when the real work begins."

To this day, I am amazed that I remained silent. Was I too stunned to form words? What the hell did he think my last two years had been about? That wasn't work?

"You're a good candidate," he added and smiled. What the hell did that mean?

"As a physician, you know," he said, "that analysts around the world take August vacations. The entire month." I wondered what "real" doctors got to take vacation for a whole month. Not academic pediatricians. The new interns started in July. We needed everyone on board in July and August in the hospital.

"We'll start the real work in September."

Did he remember that September 11 would be the two-year anniversary of Alan's death?

"I'll see you Wednesday, September 1, at ten o'clock." He stood up and opened the door. It was precisely 10:50 a.m.

Normally, I would have called Beverley to meet me at the Mousetrap. But not that day. We were going to visit Dylan.

It was Dylan's first summer at a sleepaway sailing camp in North Carolina. He was six. We had five hours to drive. There would be plenty of time to sound off about this nonsense.

"Can you believe it?" I asked Beverley. "Turns out I required a *Good Housekeeping* seal of approval to qualify for his black magic." I vented on and on, well past the border of North Carolina.

Beverley listened and did most of the driving. She was having a hard time of her own. First Alan's death, then her father's death the same month in 1974, and now her mother's death four months ago.

I navigated the route, read the inspirational messages on the signs in front of the churches out loud, and gradually ran out of steam. The terrain became flat with scrub pine trees, sandy soil in the vegetable gardens, and tiny houses with petunias planted in rotting dinghies. Signs for pulled pork, chicken necks, and collards.

Camp Morehead's term was three weeks. Three terms each summer, drop-off and pickup on Saturdays. No phone calls. No food packages. Visitors were allowed only on the second Saturday after the drop-off. Campers came from all over the Southeast to learn to sail on Bogue Sound.

The next morning, Beverley and I drove through the camp gate the moment it was unlocked. Seven o'clock sharp. Dylan was waiting. I spotted his blond head huddled against the fencing of the tennis courts. He was wrapped up in a Camp Morehead beach towel, grinning, and furiously sucking his thumb. Unlike Kaki, who maintained her distance when I visited Camp Strawderman, Dylan was all about the contact. Body hugs, neck nuzzlings, and, of course, "What did you bring me?"

Dylan's teddy bear was propped against the pillow on his bunk. At the beginning of camp, I bullied Dylan into leaving Teddy in the car, "Big boys don't bring teddies to sleepover camp." The counselors greeted us, grabbed Dylan's duffle bag, and led us into the cabin. Dylan spotted the teddy bears on every bunk, glared, and ran back for Teddy.

His cabin mates walked around us on the cabin steps as I checked out his bruises and scrapes. It was Dylan's choice of the Mommy-thing to do.

"I've been checking in at the camp infirmary," Dylan said.

"Are you okay?"

"Yeah, I just stop by, to check in."

While Dylan and Beverley went off to dig clams, I wandered over to the infirmary to meet the camp nurse.

Brigid greeted me with a huge smile. She sported flipflops with her white uniform, and her blonde hair was braided around her head like a crown.

"Dylan never has a complaint when he drops in." She laughed with her whole body. "But he's become a regular."

"Oh, no!" I laughed too.

"We just chat. Dylan likes to talk about you, the Center, and your 'very special patients.' His words. He is very proud."

I nodded. We stood there looking out at all the sails on the sound. They looked like flickering moths in the water, bouncing every which way. We both knew what this was about.

"The clinic reminds Dylan of you," Brigid said. "It's okay for him to check in. The last thing I'd want is for him to make excuses, fabricate symptoms."

I sighed.

"I like your Dylan. If there are kids in the sick bay, he moves on." She laughed again. "You should hear Cap'n Purcell brag about what a terrific sailor he is—a natural."

When I reached the pier, I spotted Dylan coming about in his Sunfish, alone in the middle of the Bogue Sound. He was fully in control. I thought of Alan and what he was missing.

Sunday morning, Dylan was huddled up at the tennis court, co-

cooned in a camp towel. His sun-bleached hair stuck out every which way. It was not allowed, but I was at the gate for one more hug. Our hugs were tight, fierce. The tears were quiet, but the heaving breaths were not.

Beverley and I drove in silence until we stopped for gas at the border. There were still Sunday blue laws in North Carolina. No sales during Sunday sermons in the South.

"You know," I said, "I don't understand why Ruth thinks it's so important that I see Josephthal. It's a huge time commitment, and it's a lot of money. Besides, I don't see it's doing any good. It's been six weeks already."

We drove a few more silent miles up I-95 North.

"Are you upset," she asked, "about the break in August?"

"Hell, no!"

We drove along in silence, maybe another twenty-five miles.

"Therapy is a process. It's not like taking an antibiotic for an earache."

"Oh, really?"

"It takes time, Sharon, years, even." She sighed. "Don't demean the process. It's hard work." Beverley was always talking about process.

I was a doer, a fixer. Process was the last thing on my mind. Get the chief complaint. Take the history, do the physical exam. Make a diagnosis and treat it, whatever it was. Professionally, Beverley and I argued about these differences, especially around the cases when I insisted a child be removed from the family for abuse or chronic neglect. One weekend, she raced her red Alfa Romeo up Carter's Mountain to reach the trailer park ahead of the county sheriff. She needed time with the grandmother to explain why the county Child Protective Services were taking custody of her nine-month-old grandbaby. The same baby I'd admitted with severe burns from the kerosene heater the night before. The baby left in the crib with only old newspapers for toys. But, as Beverley pointed out, the one who would grow up being passed from one foster-care family to another. She was convinced that living in a consistent, loving environment—however poor, chaotic, and deprived—trumped the alternative of musical-chair foster homes.

"I've been talking about Alan for six weeks."

"I think Josephthal will want to hear about Nellie and Hop, Pa Hostler, Aunt Hilda. Probably, Dr. Smith and Dr. Ryan. For sure, Nellie's wicked stepfather and her guitar-playing dimwit of a half brother, the prime-time predators. There's a lot of process ahead, discovering patterns."

"Oh, for God's sake. That crap is over and done with."

I didn't understand how the process of talking three times a week curled up on his couch could be helpful, but the first week of September I showed up. I continued to resist, and even after the times I stormed out, I showed up for the next session.

Over the first two years at the Center, I was learning about child development. Initially, I was more interested in the neurological dilemmas than the precise language and cognitive milestones. The patients presented a series of never-ending puzzles to solve. Gradually, I learned to listen more, talk less, and function as a member of the team.

One of my early observations was that the Center had no programs for infants or adolescents. The staff focused on preschool children to middle-schoolers. Perhaps it was easier to ignore the developmental challenges of teenagers with disability and chronic illness than to acknowledge them, than to have to engage with body image, sexuality, or even drugs, to say nothing about their odds of achieving independence as adults.

One of the early grants that I wrote at the Center was approved for federal funding as the Education for Multi-handicapped Infants (EMI) Project. The EMI team included therapists, social workers, and infant teachers who made weekly home visits, developed individualized baby curricula, and provided family support. My role was to identify the babies with abnormalities in the nursery, recruit the families, and manage the medical issues. Weekly, I sat with the team to receive updates and listen as they solved problems.

I learned about Chess's work on baby "temperament" from the nursery nurses. We were looking at the newborns differently, trying to identify their innate personalities from "mellow" to "slow to warm." The infant team at the Center introduced me to the concept of the "good enough" mother, Bowlby's work on the child's tie to his mother, and even Ainsworth's early work at Johns Hopkins on infant attachment. Mothers bond to their babies. Babies attach to their mothers. Infant attachment could be secure, insecure, ambivalent, or disordered.

The more I learned about mothers and babies, especially the concept that patterns of parenting were passed from generation to generation, the more I started to think about Hattie and Nellie, Nellie and me, Kaki and Dylan, even their future children. Maybe Beverley had a point; maybe my childhood was a relevant topic for therapy.

I revisited the stories of Hop hollering at Nellie when she failed to deliver a boy, how he abandoned her at the hospital and the nurse chose my name from her detective novel for the birth certificate so Nellie could be discharged. Hop refusing to come for Nellie, sending Pa Hostler in a taxi. The stories of Aunt Hilda coming home from nursing school to feed me when I refused the bottle from Nellie. Hop raging when Nellie miscarried three boys in a row. Hop even bringing home a foster child, a boy. Hop abandoning Nellie and running off with Rosalie.

I realized that with Alan's death, Kaki, Dylan, and I had all lost our singular attachment figure, the one who loved us all unconditionally. I understood at some level that the parenting I experienced from Hop and Nellie must not determine how I parented my children or cared for my pediatric patients.

Ruth and Beverley grasped the many connections and nuances I still had to own and learn to integrate. The task was more than death and dying. More than grieving the loss of Alan. Whatever the reasons, I trusted them implicitly. I now believed that this was critical work for me to do.

And so I was there waiting for the door to open at ten o'clock sharp on the appointed days in September 1976. I don't remember how long—months for sure, maybe years—it took before my rage and fury evolved into profound sadness. Or the day I stopped ranting and began, finally, to cry.

But when I did let my guard down, I couldn't stop crying. I cried on Josephthal's couch. I cried at horse shows when Kaki fell off Copy Cat and when they won the Best in Show satin ribbons. I cried when Dylan hit his first home run in Little League and won the ongoing Monopoly game with his therapist. I cried when I heard Yvonne ask Alan about the streets paved with gold at the Mill. Even on rounds, I struggled with grief, coming close to tears when the intern presented a sixteen-year-old competitive diver with a spinal cord injury.

Late at night in the kitchen at the Mill, I played a lot less Clancy

Brothers and Jacques Brel and a lot more Nina Simone and Lena Horne. Max keened along.

Over the next ten years, I only once or twice—maybe more—stormed out of a session. Furious. Ranting. And slammed the door.

Usually, though, I cried.

· 25 ·

The Death Maven

September 1977

When Dr. O. J. Sahler invited me to present the keynote address for a three-day conference in September 1977 at the University of Rochester exploring "The Child and Death," I was a thirty-seven-year-old widow, mother of two, and a tenured associate professor of pediatrics. I didn't know Dr. Sahler. I'd never been to Rochester. I'd never given that talk, but I accepted the invitation without a second thought. I was an expert.

I never intended to become a death maven, but death was part of my life for as long as I could remember. And when I entered medical school, death became a constant companion. First, the cadavers in Anatomy Lab. The dissecting lab reeked with formaldehyde that made your eyes weep. In my second year, my first patient in pathology class was an eight-year-old girl with cystic fibrosis on the slab in the morgue. She had been alive that morning.

Death, officially, became my personal enemy—to oppose, to fight against, to vanquish. I knew how to fight. I had been fighting since I was four years old and punched the boy on the tricycle, the one with the anchor socks.

Death became the force I would meet on a different battlefield—in the clinic, on the ward, or in the emergency room. If I wanted to prevent second-graders from ending up in the morgue, I needed the scientific knowledge, the wisdom, and the will to defeat death.

Death was no abstract concept. I saw death as it was personified in the bleak, black-and-white films by Ingmar Bergman—a black-cloaked figure, chalk face wrapped tightly in a black scarf, and arm outstretched.

As a resident, I correctly diagnosed meningococcemia in a twelve-year-old girl in clinic, but I missed the pneumonia in the thirteen-year-old with anorexia nervosa admitted to the ward when I was eight months pregnant. When I finally examined her, my tenth admission, she was cool to my touch, and death was in the shadows of the hospital room. Sometimes I saw death behind the boxwoods at Beau Pré when I came home late at night.

During my fellowship years, we fought for a few more days of life for the kids with leukemia. Death always won. Our patients died from bleeding or infection, or even the poisons we gave them as chemotherapy. When drugs were delayed coming up to the ward, I imagined death down in the pharmacy, thumb on the scales, slowing down the operation, delaying treatment. And, in my mind, my struggle with death justified my shouting at the interns, criticizing the nurses, and slamming charts.

After a child died on the ward and the parents sobbed a final farewell, I sensed the invisible presence of death in the room. Some families prayed. Others asked the *why* questions. A parent might talk about the angel of death—halos, wings, and white robes, maybe bright lights and harps, choruses singing. I bowed my head and said amen. Sometimes they blamed themselves for things done or not done. I imagined death listening, face twisted into a grim smile.

I was the one from the team who stayed behind with the family until the nurses wheeled the child's tiny body to the morgue wrapped in a clean white sheet. I held back my tears as the parents packed up the drooled-on teddy bear, the blood-stained comforter. At the elevator, I worried about the parents driving home safely. I missed the dead children, but I also missed their families, and the intimacy we had developed over weeks, months, and even years together.

The hospital had rules for death. The autopsy form had to be signed, a death note entered in the medical chart, and the body transported to the morgue. I respected the rules and usually understood the need for them. But at times, the rules and the authority behind the rules didn't serve the families or the patient, and tension developed between the nurses and the mothers at the patient's bedside.

"You can't take him away," said the Mennonite mother as she covered her son's body with her own. "It's too soon." She started praying.

"It is a hospital rule; we must remove the body," insisted the nurse. She gently tried to lift the mother off the bed. "We need to clean the room and prepare it for the next patient."

As the praying continued, the nurse became more determined. The women gathered at the child's bedside resisted, still murmuring their prayers.

"Wait," I said quietly. "Give us a few minutes." The nurse left the room and pulled the door closed with authority. After the "Amen," I touched the mother's back. "I don't understand what you still need to do."

"We have to bathe him and wrap him in these fresh linens we brought and say the prayers."

"But the autopsy?" I recognized the linens were the death shroud.

"No autopsy. Dr. Thurman understands. No funeral home. Our men are building the wooden casket right now. We will pray until they arrive to take us home." She touched my arm and nodded. "It is our way."

"Two hours," I said, knowing the nurses would have my head. "You may stay in this room for two hours. That is all." I had exceeded my authority, but the head nurse reluctantly agreed.

We all had our own death demons, I think. For much of the staff, our purpose was to heal, to comfort, to relieve pain and suffering. Death became our collective failure. The death of a child on the hospital ward, even if it was anticipated, remained frightening. A shared loss for all of us from the janitor to the chief resident to the faculty attending.

It was unusual, certainly not the norm in our department or others, but Dr. Thurman and I attended the visitations and the viewings if the family lived nearby. We always made it to the funerals, however far away, even on a weekend. On the drive, we would talk about the dead child, share our personal stories, maybe practice what we would say to the grieving families. The parents always welcomed us. We shared their journey. We understood things others couldn't. Over the years, Dr. Thurman and I developed a strange intimacy at the bedside, celebrated our few successes, and faced failure at the hands of the enemy, death.

Dr. Thurman was a great role model and mentor. He knew the words to the hymns, how to greet the minister, and even how to leave the reception gracefully.

I accepted the autopsy as the judge and jury. The morgue was where our treatment decisions were judged, where we saw the effects chemotherapy had on normal tissue, and where we learned whether the cause of death was the disease or our treatment.

Somewhere along the line, I learned to write sympathy notes. I invited the medical students to come with me to visitations, and I taught them how to write a proper note.

Leukemia remained a death sentence for our patients, but the contest we fought with death extended over days, weeks and sometimes years. An international registry was established for children with acute lymphocytic leukemia (ALL). I remember when UVA registered the one-hundredth child in the world to live five years from diagnosis. (By 2019, 90 percent of children diagnosed with ALL were expected to live at least five years. Many would be cured.) We eventually factored in the quality, not just the quantity, of the child's life. How many days in school versus how many days in the hospital, not just how many days alive from diagnosis.

Near the end of my fellowship, Alan and I went to the beach without Kaki and Dylan. The first night away, I was tormented with nightmares. Three or four leukemic children were in the bed with us, all dying, all needing treatment, comfort care, and relief from pain.

"Don't roll over," I hollered, "Willie needs every one of those packed red blood cells."

Alan shook me awake. I was still fussing, "Watch out! Be careful. You're going to pull out his IV."

"Shhh," he whispered, "easy does it." Alan held me tight and rocked me back and forth. When I started to quiet down, he clicked on the light, helped me into my robe, and led me outdoors.

"Tell me about Willie. Start from the beginning," he said when we got to the beach. "Everything, every detail." He took my hand, and we walked in our bare feet on the wet sand.

I told Alan how spunky Willie presented at that first clinic visit. He was five years old with freckles and red curly hair. I described his mother's tears, his father's rage. How the malignant cells looked distorted on the bone marrow slide. I recounted the months of the first remission followed by bleeding, then the second, much shorter remission followed by sepsis. Willie blew out six candles on his birthday cake and made it to the first few weeks of first grade. Then he died.

Alan kept asking questions even after the sun came up. I felt self-conscious in my bathrobe on the beach, but I kept talking about Tommy, Suzie, and all the others who had died. Day after day, that is what we did—talked and walked on the beach. The last night, we both slept through to morning.

Death sabotaged that vacation. I wanted to share the stories of my patients learning to play T-ball, to tie the laces of their sneakers, and to read Dick and Jane. But I had to purge the part of my brain that stored my death and dying files, the memories of lost patients, my failures before I could sleep. Before I could take care of my living patients. Before I could care for my own toddlers.

Death was joined by new enemies when I was named medical director of the C&Y clinics in 1969. I still followed my patients with leukemia, but I no longer took hematology night call, a necessary compromise with two small children at home and a weekend husband. I continued to teach residents. I still went to funerals, now more often held in Black Baptist churches with visitations at Bell's Funeral Home.

The C&Y patients were poor, undernourished, and unimmunized, often undiagnosed with easily remedial or corrective interventions. My new enemies were diffuse and pervasive, the gaping holes in society's supposed safety net. But when the enemy was death, it was likely to be a violent death—a battered child, a house fire, the rape of the fifteen-year-old by her mother's boyfriend, and death from sepsis following a botched abortion.

Death in this population remained the ominous skeleton in a black cloak in the shadows, no longer predictable, but anonymous, impersonal, and often violent. It was almost impossible to strike preemptively.

When Hill and Wood delivered a container labeled "ashes of Alan Duane Dimock," we divided the contents. We—Beverley, Yvonne, Gioia, the kids, and I—hiked to Humpback Rock, spread ashes on the rocks, and said some goodbyes. No prayers. No music. No body. No discussion of heaven or hell. No angels. No Valley of Death. No discussion of how many rooms were in anyone's mansion. When our close friend Peter visited, we tossed the remainder of the ashes into the creek and sang a Woody Guthrie song.

At the Center, death was neither the ever-present concern it had been with the leukemic children nor associated with the violence that threatened the children at C&Y. Death was generally denied and thoroughly ignored by the physicians, staff, and families. No one talked with the adolescent patients about death. However, that didn't mean that our teenage patients didn't worry about their shortened lifespans.

Frequent clinic visits, community outreach, and inpatient "rescue" admissions began to slow the inevitable outcome of genetic diseases like cystic fibrosis and muscular dystrophy, although children with these diagnoses rarely lived past their teens. But we never discussed death and dying, not with our patients or their families, not with one another.

Adolescents with chronic illness seemed to me like slowed-down versions of the younger children with leukemia. Even with all the advances in our understanding of the genetic diseases, we could only slow down the inevitable. Death would win, usually before we transitioned them to the doctors who treated adults. On rounds, we discussed the ethical issues of how to handle parents who refused to allow us to share accurate medical information with their teenagers. In staffing, we considered what it would mean to our patients to be allowed to die at the Center with familiar and trusted staff rather than be trundled off in the middle of the night by the rescue squad to die in the hospital among strangers.

Throughout the hospital and the clinics, I listened and learned from my patients and their parents. Even the siblings. A four-year-old asked me about her sister who had just died of leukemia, "What if the coffin gets too small?"

"I don't understand," I said, leaning toward her.

"She'll keep growing until she bumps her head." She started to cry.

As a faculty member, I was responsible for seeing faculty children in the private clinic. The 1970s were still the days of "professional courtesy" extended to doctors, nurses, preachers, schoolteachers, and UVA faculty. In private clinic, my practice consisted of parents with healthy children, or at least children who did not have a medical diagnosis. I gained a sense of "normal" behavior for the middle class, including decisions to visit Granny in the nursing home in Florida, to take a three-year-old to a funeral, and the protocols for death and dying. My colleagues started to refer families with questions about death and dying to me. I was at ease listening and comfortable helping them figure out these decisions.

A child worried that singing at the grave would wake up her brother. I recognized his magical thinking based on what I learned from my developmental colleagues at our hospital school. Yes, the dead are dead, but not really all the way, all the time. Neither of these children yet had what Piaget described as an adult concept of death—irreversible, universal, and inevitable.

Working with the dying adolescents at the Center, I developed compassion not only for the teens and their families but also for the staff in their denial. I respected the social workers and nurses who stood by for days and weeks and months, even years. I revered the hospital chaplains who comforted team members after the family went home. I hummed along with the hymns at the funerals and said the occasional, "Amen." Our grief was cumulative.

Jerry, the patient who wanted to lose his virginity, died at home on Christmas Day. I was one of the family and neighbors gathered around his bed telling stories, sipping brandy, and sharing tissues, the lights on the tree blinking on and off while we waited for the undertaker's arrival. Death, the ominous shadowy figure who had haunted me for so long, was among us.

At the Center, it was the teachers in our hospital school, the psychologists, and the child psychiatrists who taught me about childhood in ways I hadn't learned in medical school. I learned about obligatory egocentrism—the three-year-old really believes the sun comes up when he wakes up and the sun goes down at night because it's his bedtime. About being five and struggling with what is "right" and "wrong." Experimenting a lot with telling lies and partial truths and experiencing a wide range of consequences before conscience gets internalized by six and becomes relatively constant. Understanding later that people make the rules.

After Alan's death, the Mill became my own personal laboratory to observe how children understood death. We all struggled to find a way to move on. Kaki had Copy Cat. I had my talk sessions with

Dr. Josephthal. Dylan played Monopoly and chess in his sessions with child psychologist Jerry Saffer. Beverley had Chivas Regal, and Yvonne had her conversations with Alan in heaven.

When Dr. Elisabeth Kübler-Ross presented medical grand rounds, people from every imaginable discipline crowded the aisles of the auditorium. Teams at the Center ventured into structured conversations about patient and family decision-making around death—whose perspective to consider, who was allowed to initiate, and who should be included. Planning was challenging at first and filled with conflict. We forgot the importance of clarifying values. We were surprised when our belief systems were in conflict. But the work started.

When death occurred among my colleagues, I was often the one at their back door with a warm loaf of pumpkin bread, baked by Yvonne of course, or sitting at the kitchen table planning a funeral. My actions were not deliberate, but I knew how it felt to be the mourner, alone and terrified. I was comfortable knocking on the door, inviting myself in, and listening.

And then, I was a thirty-seven-year-old widow. Death spilled out in stories I told on the couch. About Alan. About my patients. And about my childhood.

So, yes, I accepted the invitation to give a keynote speech in Rochester without hesitation.

My assignment was to lay out the development of the child's concept of death. I projected two carousels of sixty slides each, using a machine that allowed me to dissolve one image into the next, which I timed from the podium to synch with my verbal presentation. I knew the process was like black magic for academic audiences. In 1977, before computers, before thumb drives, and before embedded videos. The audience listened intently.

I concluded: "The kingdom where nobody dies is and always has been a fantasy. Death can occur to a child's pet, relatives, friends, parents, siblings, or he, himself may die. The child's struggle to understand and to grieve such losses should not distress adults, parents, and professionals."

When I finished, I stayed at the podium. The last slide remained projected behind me. I looked out at the amphitheater, rows of people, probably five hundred or so, sitting in silence. By then in my career, I had learned to stand quietly and wait, but it was never easy. The first person who started to clap did so tentatively. Others followed, then everyone was on their feet, applauding. I had set the stage intellectually and emotionally for the next two days. I thought my work was done.

Instead, my own work had just begun. The conference was a dramatic demonstration of the professional coterie formed around death across different disciplines, conceptual frames, and childhood diseases. The speakers were distinguished professors from across the country. The academics were pediatricians, psychiatrists, pediatric hematologists, internists, and geneticists, but there were also nurses, social workers, teachers, students, nuns, and funeral directors.

I listened as they described conflicting perspectives on family dynamics; the wide range of trust and collegial support across disciplines, rank, and hospital boundaries; and the expansive nature of teams that included religious representatives, community groups, and even funeral home directors. I focused on how to bring some of the models presented at the conference back to UVA.

By the end of the first day, I was exhausted. I resisted the faculty dinner debrief, but protocol prevailed. After dinner, Dr. Sahler introduced the conference speakers and distinguished members of the University of Rochester faculty. Among them were the psychiatry professors who first described the "anniversary phenomenon" in the scientific literature. The next morning, I received signed copies of their articles. How could I not have known that there was not only a community of death scholars but that they had developed a formal literature?

By the time I left Rochester, I had learned different schema for understanding death and dying, unique ways to support children and families nonmedically, and how varied healthcare teams could be in form and function. There was a national network of professional death scholars, and I was now one of them. I received many invitations from other presenters to be a visiting professor or give grand rounds, and the chair of Pediatrics offered me a faculty position at the University of Rochester.

Dr. Blizzard was surprised when I let him know that I was being recruited to the University of Rochester and was making an official candidate visit. I smiled when he reminded me that I had tenure at UVA. I spent a heady three days at Rochester presenting grand rounds, making teaching rounds, and meeting with the dean. On the drive to the airport, the chair predicted an invitation to join the faculty would be in the mail.

But by the time my flight landed, I understood Charlottesville had become our home. I had plenty of work to do at the University of Virginia.

· 26 ·

The Year of Drying Out

1978

The seemingly spontaneous safety net that saved me after Alan died was stitched solely of women's friendships. AV came through the kitchen door of the Mill the night of the crash with a tenderloin of roast beef, Erla with the basket of still-warm bread. Patty arrived the next noon from Philadelphia to take over the house through the funeral. Ruth appeared at the supper table to assure me that seeing Alan in the kitchen rocking chair was perfectly normal, if not expected. Jan brought art projects for Kaki and Dylan. Clariece, Beth, and Helen from C&Y. Nancy, Peppy, and Jean from the Center. The docs—Carolyn, Margaret, Ann, and Ruth. And always, Beverley and Yvonne.

Beverley was my first and best friend. The women at the Center sanded my rough edges and softened my "command and control" leadership behavior. I survived and started to thrive. After Alan's death, Yvonne and Beverley coalesced around Kaki, Dylan, and me. Beverley provided the unconditional love I had never received as a child, the unconditional love I had received from Alan and learned to trust for twelve years. Then abruptly lost. Beverley still supported and sustained us. How could we lose her?

Beverley's drinking had gotten out of control. In the early days at Beau Pré, I'd believed her cockamamie tale that an errant Black Angus had forced her Alfa off the road and into the woods. After one disastrous drunk, Alan and I were so distraught we dumped out all the liquor. Yet, a few weeks later we were sipping cocktails together, and so it went.

After Beverley fell down the circular staircase at the Mill and broke her leg, she had acquiesced to seeking help and consulted Dr. Respess, an internist respected for his skill in managing UVA's academic alcoholics.

Beverley took the prescribed Antabuse for a month or two and complained vociferously about the garlic taste in her mouth. She calculated exactly how many days she had to stop taking it before she could reliably take a drink without retching out her insides. She discovered that it required one full week, precisely as the label indicated. That abstinence trial was short-lived.

We argued about her drinking, each time ending with screams and ultimatums. The kids still talked about the hike up Old Rag when Beverley left the trail to circle back to the six-pack of Heineken she'd stashed in the creek.

Over the past year, I hadn't trusted Beverley to drive the kids anymore, but I couldn't stop her from driving altogether. When I demanded that she stop drinking *or else,* Beverley moved out of the Mill and settled back in her apartment at Mrs. Baker's in Ivy. We rattled around the Mill without her. The kids were worried and angry with me. Yvonne "tsk-tsked" under her breath. The Danes moped around the kitchen.

After a time, Beverley finally acknowledged the drinking was a significant problem and agreed to consult with our colleague, the psychiatrist Dr. Ruth Weeks, who had left UVA for private practice. Beverley's friends naively believed—or maybe just I believed—that after a few talk sessions, Ruth would conjure up a miracle—a miracle to enable Beverley to drink socially, never to excess.

None of us had a grasp on alcoholism and its treatment or insight into our own drinking patterns. The structure of my on-call schedule protected me. I couldn't drink if I had to go back into the hospital. But we were Beverley's drinking partners. Later, I would understand the more accurate descriptor: We were Beverley's enablers.

The spring of 1978 marked the official beginning of the end, characterized by early-morning phone calls of distress.

"Oh, my God, Sharon. I have some neurological disease. My legs are too heavy to lift. Maybe it's cerebral palsy—"

"Cerebral palsy is congenital," I said. "You don't just catch it."

"Maybe, its Guillain-Barré. I can't pick my feet up off the floor and my toes are all tingly. No way I can work." She'd pause. "Maybe this afternoon."

The first time or two, I drove out to Ivy at noontime to make sure she wasn't seriously ill. The day I found her sipping a cold beer "to clear my head," I lost it. After another bout of empty threats, I vowed to keep my distance. No more rescues.

Beverley was respected and beloved by the tolerant staff at the Center, but they started to worry. Whispers began. Much later, I would learn that Peppy, the adolescent program coordinator who reported to Beverley, had consulted Alcoholics Anonymous on her own. She confronted Beverley about her drinking and specifically suggested that Beverley was alcoholic. "It didn't go well," Peppy reported.

Eventually, staff filed complaints. They documented when Beverley had alcohol on her breath at morning meeting or forgot a meeting or missed a report deadline. Everyone knew that Beverley was my friend, but still they looked to me to intervene, take charge, do something. I was the leader. I had to act before rumors got to Dr. Blizzard. It wouldn't take much for him to react. He and his wife were still perplexed by the enormous banana tree topped with a red satin bow Beverley had delivered at Christmas. He would have no sympathy.

Ultimately, I acted. In mid-July, I placed Beverley on medical leave with pay and directed her not to return to the Center.

The very next day, Beverley invited the nursing director for a round of golf at Birdwood and pulled out a bottle of gin from her golf bag on the first green. Jan reported that Beverley had accessed the liquor closet of Mrs. Baker, her eighty-two-year-old landlady, when her supply of Scotch was depleted.

I threatened to change Beverley's status to medical leave without pay. Ruth discouraged me. "Beverley will need access to every penny of her medical insurance."

Beverley complied with one thing—she continued to show up for appointments with Ruth. When Ruth confiscated her car keys, a former drinking buddy chauffeured her to her appointments.

I was afraid that Dr. Blizzard would fire her, that she would hurt herself or someone else, and the kids and I would lose her forever. By early September, Ruth assured me that a solution was in the wings.

Beverley's trajectory differed from that of my parents. Hop and Nellie had always slept off the big drunk, missed work, and found another job when they were fired. After Hop died, Nellie was drunk and smoking in bed when she passed out and set the bedcovers on fire. Disgusted at thirteen, I rolled her onto the floor and shoved the smoldering mattress out of the window into the backyard. Nellie lost one job after another, but she always found the next one—hostess, waitress, short order cook. Over the years, some of the guys Hop hung out with took "the pledge." Not Nellie. She had no desire to give up her Pall Malls, her sleazebag buddies, or her booze.

On Thursday after Labor Day, Ruth called me to share the news. Beverley and she had found an inpatient alcohol treatment center in Florida near Bradenton, where Beverley's brothers, Allen and Tom, lived. Beverley agreed to be admitted.

Beverley's brother Allen would meet her flight and deliver her to the treatment facility. My assignment: get Beverley packed, reserve a seat on a nonstop flight, and drive her to the airport. At the time, it sounded perfectly doable.

The next day I asked Yvonne to stay late with the kids, and I left work at noon for the drive to National Airport.

When I pulled up at Mrs. Baker's house, Beverley was not in the driveway as instructed. I stormed inside.

"I need to borrow another suitcase from you, Sharon," she said with a smile and a nonchalant shrug. "I'll never get all this stuff in one suitcase."

I stared at the pile of gear. "You're not jetting off to the Caribbean on vacation, you're being admitted to a damn hospital."

"Now that's where you are wrong, dead wrong, Sharon Lee Hostler." She pulled herself upright for a beat or two and glared at me. "No hospital is involved. I am traveling to join a therapeutic community in Florida."

It took a lot longer than it should have, but I finally understood. We were not going anywhere, at least that day.

I canceled her flight reservations, apologized to the airline, and upgraded her seat to first class for a few days later. Round one for Beverley.

"I'm not surprised," Ruth said when I reported the packing fiasco. "She sees the end game, but that doesn't mean she will go quietly."

"She was drunk as a skunk, Ruth."

"First class was a good idea. Not because of the luggage, but they'll keep the booze flowing. Withdrawal is the last thing Beverley needs to endure at this point."

My mind flashed back to my patient with the DTs, delirium tremens. It was the beginning of my third year of medical school on the surgery rotation. I sat with the forty-year-old guy for three days. His family refused to come to bedside, and my attending refused to sedate him as some kind of punishment. "Let him dry out enough to understand the terrible damage he's done to himself and his family," he'd said on rounds.

My patient was hallucinating, hollering to hell and back about the demons pinching his flesh, the ogres on the ceiling, and the devil himself carving out his soul. It was the first time I'd ever seen delirium tremens from alcohol withdrawal. I was terrified. He sobbed for his mother between screams. He had cirrhosis of the liver, bleeding esophageal varices, and died of liver failure.

So, no, we wouldn't let Beverley dry out on her way to the treatment center. I needed assistance, so I recruited Jan to the mission even though her baby had a fever that day. We failed again.

The third attempt looked like a go. I had Beverley's golf clubs, one packed suitcase, and her tennis racquet in the trunk of my car. In my hand was a list of athletic equipment to ship to the treatment center as soon as I had a mailing address.

We were almost driving out of Charlottesville—so close—but Beverley insisted on stopping at the Wayside Deli for a hoagie.

Jan glared at me in frustration. I shrugged. If we could keep Beverley safely in the car, titrate her alcohol intake to some magical point between upright equilibrium and withdrawal, and manage to drive safely to National Airport—if and if—we might succeed.

It had been a week since my first attempt. Beverley's flight to Florida departed at 7:40 p.m. I didn't know whether I was most worried about keeping Beverley in the car, not missing my exit on the Beltway, or getting her physically on board the plane. The beers and napkins and hoagies were minor annoyances.

It was nearly dark by the time we exited the Beltway into National Airport. I unloaded Jan, Beverley, and the luggage—with firm instructions to stay in place as I parked.

Beverley sent Jan for more cigarettes and easily found her way to the bar.

"Chug it down," I said to Beverley. "It's time to board." One on either side, Jan and I handed a wobbly Beverley over to the stewardess. "Double Chivas on the rocks," we heard Beverley order as we left.

I called her brother Allen to report that Beverley was on board, and she was still drinking. I advised him to have a six-pack ready for the drive to the treatment center.

"I thought she wanted to stop drinking," he said.

It was pitch-black outside and inside as Jan and I drove down Interstate 66 in silence. Our minds were reeling. I missed the exit to 29 South and headed off toward Front Royal for a good fifteen miles before I realized my mistake. Jan hated driving, especially in the dark, but she drove the rest of the way home.

By Warrenton, nearly halfway home, we started whispering little stories about Beverley, trying to comfort ourselves, trying to make some kind of sense of what we believed was our betrayal. Before long, we were both sobbing. It was like a wake without a body. Again. Just like Alan's. No other mourners were in the car or along the highway. No one was present to bear witness to Beverley's death. Together, Jan and I had dropped her off, pushed her off the edge of the earth, and abandoned her.

We never expected to see Beverley again. We didn't talk about it out loud, but I don't think either of us could visualize a circumstance where Beverley would return to the social shame and academic embarrassment of the previous year. We had no experience with Alcoholics Anonymous. Beverley's abstinence from alcohol seemed impossible.

Primum non nocere. I understood that I didn't have a choice. I believed that I had done Beverley significant harm by putting her on that plane. I wasn't wise enough then to recognize that sometimes doing harm to someone you love may be necessary to save that someone.

The next morning at breakfast, I explained to Kaki and Dylan where Beverley was and why. I tried to reassure them when I was the one who most needed reassurance.

Dylan slid down from the table and brought me the phone. "Call her, Mommy. I bet Beverley is afraid. She's all alone and far away from home."

"It's a hospital, Dylan. They won't let us talk to her."

On top of Friday evenings without Alan at the Mill, that first Friday evening without Beverley was even worse. We heard not a word from Florida.

Jan started to question whether we'd done the right thing. The staff at the Center looked to us for news, for reassurance. We had none. Ruth assured me that we wouldn't hear anything from Beverley or from the treatment center staff.

After a few days, Beverley finally called—collect. In a tiny voice so shaky and wobbly that I hardly recognized her, she said, "It's beyond awful. We need a ping pong table, paddles, and lots of balls. And good coffee, we—"

The call was disconnected.

Ruth advised against sending the ping pong table. At supper each night, the kids looked to me for news, but there was none.

Finally, I got a letter in feathery script that was barely readable, a generic apology. The handwriting looked as if a frail old lady had written it, someone close to death. An apology made no sense. We should be apologizing to Beverley for sending her away. That was the moment we knew Beverley was never coming home. We mourned out loud. Dylan most of all.

"Beverley was always kind to me," he said. "She always listened. She threw the ball when I asked. Beverley loved us. She never hurt me, she never made me cry, ever."

"Miz Butler, she did drink too much of that damnation Scotch, no doubt about it. Like Spencer, she got the thirst, that thirst what can't be stopped," she said. She sniffed a little, pulled out her handkerchief, and started the chest-shaking sobs.

She hefted Dylan up, laid him over her shoulder, and rocked him. He was almost nine by then, growing long. "But Miz Butler, she's a child of God, loving and good. She be back, Dee. She love you. She be back. Just you wait."

"Mommy, what do you think?" asked Kaki. For a minute, I thought that she might crawl up into my lap, but instead she settled herself in the rocker opposite me and glared. "I mean *really* think?"

"I don't know," I said. "I just don't know."

Nearly two months later, Ruth called me to let me know Beverley was being discharged and asked me to drive her car out to the airport. No welcoming committee. No announcements. No children.

On the drive into town, Beverley was quiet, subdued, withdrawn.

"How was it?"

"A lot of meetings," she said, "Group meetings we had to go to. All day long."

"And—?"

"We ate a lot of prunes and drank really bad coffee."

"Prunes?" I asked.

"Constipation was almost worse than the shakes."

She made a few passing comments about the white chip for twenty-four hours of sobriety, the red chip for thirty days, and how the AA meetings worked.

"I need to attend a daily meeting now that I am back. Probably St. Paul's over on the Corner after work." I was speechless. *Beverley was coming back to work?* Did she not remember the mess she'd left?

Mrs. Baker did not allow Beverley to return to her place in Ivy. Instead, she stayed in Miriam Birdwhistle's empty condo until AV's friend Caroline found Beverley a little house on Rugby Avenue. It felt awful for the kids and Yvonne and me that she didn't come to the Mill. The past year had been crazy and chaotic and conflicted for all of us.

The kids and I rarely saw Beverley. When we did, she was silent, preoccupied, lifeless. At work, she remained sequestered in her office with the built-in shelves and desk Alan had crafted for her. She kept the door completely closed. The staff tiptoed by the office and left her alone. Eventually, Beverley started seeing patients in clinic and supervised her staff. Very quietly. I wasn't aware at that time, but Beverley was making her personal amends to the Center staff, one by one.

At home on Rugby, Beverley locked her doors, pulled down the shades, and didn't answer the doorbell or the phone. Kaki folded origami swans, created get-well cards with horse scenes, and wrote poems that she taped to the kitchen door. Dylan asked over and over, "Why, Mommy? What did we do wrong?"

After a while, things started to change. A different Beverley showed up. It was more than just the fact that she wasn't drinking. She was flat, lost inside herself, barely responsive to the world around her. There was no light in her eyes, no spring in her step. She seldom smiled. We tried to reassure ourselves that her energy was directed toward the daily AA meetings at St. Paul's.

We couldn't fathom why she wouldn't answer the door, not even on Thanksgiving morning. At Christmas, we left homemade cookies, casseroles, and fancily wrapped presents at her door. Untouched, days later. Yvonne, the kids, and I reluctantly began to learn the lessons of depression.

Later, Ruth explained that Beverley's drinking was an attempt to self-medicate the symptoms of serious mental illness. That Beverley's diagnosis was bipolar disease, a manic-depressive disorder that could be managed—but not easily—with drugs like lithium. And that AA was for—forever.

Years later, Beverley and I would reconstruct the timetable of her manic periods. They were times I remembered with great glee because they were so outrageous—Alan and Beverley bringing home two Great Danes to the Mill, the two of us taking our mothers to Jamaica for Christmas, and her convincing me I deserved a Mercedes.

During the first months, none of us grasped how important the daily AA meetings were for Beverley's recovery or how the meetings worked. Gradually, Beverley shared the structure, the ritual opening: "*I am an alcoholic. I am powerless over alcohol. My life is unmanageable.*" The importance of the chips: green for four months without a drink, deep blue for six months. A medallion for a year. Working the twelve steps.

Something critical happened between her ignoring the cookies and her sharing details of the meeting ritual—her absolute commitment to sobriety.

I continued seeing the shrink three times a week. He listened and nodded as I lay on the couch trying to make sense of what was happening.

Yvonne continued to profess that God would take care of everything for Beverley, just "maybe not in this lifetime." Her husband, Spencer, had uncontrolled insulin-dependent diabetes. Blind and with double above-knee amputations, Spencer sometimes sat in Yvonne's car outside the Mill sipping on his bottle of generic booze. When Dylan and his buddies tiptoed around the car, Spencer would scream out strings of colorful curses. The kids ran away, excited. Yvonne shrugged.

On Beverley's first-year anniversary of sobriety, Jan, Kaki, Dylan, and I went with Beverley to the open AA meeting at St. Paul's Church and watched her receive the one-year medallion. Peppy attended too, but she remained in the back of the room. That original medallion remains on Beverley's keychain.

A more familiar version of Beverley gradually emerged. One day she showed up unannounced at the Mill to "check in on Mattie" and stayed for supper. A week later she surprised Dylan at a Little League game. The next day, she appeared at the Keswick Horse Show in time for Kaki and Copy Cat's round over the fences.

Looking back later, Beverley dated her emergence as "human" to a Florida visit with her brother in Bradenton for her thirty-eighth birthday in May 1979—eight months after the intervention.

My personal benchmark was in September 1979, almost exactly a year after the National Airport run. Beverley showed up unannounced in my kitchen, greeted me with a hug, and asked what time we were leaving for the evening wedding of Caroline's daughter. And what did I think she should wear?

For Jan, it was when the three of us went out for our first post-recovery supper at Lena's Dance, the Mexican restaurant on Elliewood Avenue where, for years, we had regularly met on Wednesdays for chalupas.

"I'll have sparkling water on the rocks with a twist," Beverley directed the waitress. "Chardonnay for them."

Eventually, Beverley invited Kaki and Dylan, one by one, to spend the night at Rugby.

On the second Thanksgiving, we created a version of a rotational dinner. After the Blessing of the Hounds, the first stop was Rugby Avenue. Beverley served scalloped oysters she'd prepared from the Bradenton cookbook. Peter agreed to skip the traditional Bloody Marys.

Jan set her fancy table for an elaborate turkey spread. I served the traditional pear, pomegranate, and spinach salad course at my table, followed by a long, circuitous walk. It was long after dark when the self-appointed pie maven Peter proclaimed this year's pumpkin and pecan pies as "the ultimate holiday dessert."

Champagne for toasting, sparkling water for the kids and Beverley. It had been a very long two years.

Beverley ended up embracing sobriety. It's been forty-seven years and counting. Some of that initial network of women friends who stepped up and rescued me after Alan's death are still around and remain tightly connected. Some friends have died. Somehow, new friends got folded in along the way.

Beverley remained my very best friend and the fairy godmother for Kaki and Dylan.

· 27 ·

Leaving and Losing

Summer 1979

For the first time, I was uneasy about living at the Mill alone. One night, a motorcycle crashed through our fence and ended up on the porch. The Mill sat right next to the road, tucked into a sharp curve approaching the bridge. I installed new locks and exterior lights.

Then the Great Danes got out of their pen and ended up in the cow pasture across the creek. I received a call at work: "Listen lady, the next time I'll shoot the damn dogs."

The twelve-mile commute to town from the Mill was getting complicated. It was twelve miles to town and back for work, twenty-five miles to Darby's Folly and back for Kaki to ride Copy Cat, twenty-two miles to Darden Towe Park for Pop Warner football, twenty miles to Preston Avenue for Little League baseball.

Beverley was no longer part of our shuttle system. After she'd found another home for Mattie, Beverley visited the Mill less and less. Yvonne couldn't manage the trips to town alone. Spencer was always in her car, sipping booze and cursing at the kids while she worked. That wasn't such a problem out in North Garden, but the in-town drop-offs were a challenge. Kaki was embarrassed by Spencer hollering at the barn. Dylan felt the same at the playing fields.

My days at the hospital became more scheduled, with less opportunity to disappear for a midafternoon trip to run out to Darby's Folly. And it was not only inappropriate but illegal to ask my secretary to make the emergency runs. But sometimes I had to.

The cost for one month of paying a UVA student driver by the mile was $1,285. It was not feasible! We couldn't afford an annual expense of over $20,000 for after-school chauffeuring.

There was a lot of weeping about leaving the Mill. Not so much about leaving Red Hill School or North Garden. I would hear much later that Kaki's fifth-grade teacher pinched her upper arm until it was black-and-blue and complained about how "hoity-toity" I was when I took them out of school for travel. The mother of her classmate Virginia Ann ended up reporting the abuse, and she lost her teaching license the next year. Much later, Dylan would describe how lonely he was without the Page boys from North Garden, how hard it was to move into a new neighborhood and to attend a new school without friends.

But, at that point, my focus was on one question: Where would we live? I was rescued by Caroline, AV's friend who had become my good mother surrogate.

In early August, I headed, with a group of women, to the Kennedy Center to see *Getting My Act Together and Taking It on the Road.* I was surprised and delighted that Beverley wanted to join us.

The five of us were ready when the defiant redhead strutted across the stage and belted out: "I'm doing my strong woman number. I know I've got such self-esteem. I can handle any crisis. I'm so capable I could scream."

We knew the words and sang along. We clapped, pinged our glasses, and pounded our feet.

Caroline was a diva in her fifties, the mother of five daughters. Peppy was childless in her late twenties. Both were recently divorced from men of self-appointed importance. AV was suspicious that it wasn't just poker and bourbon keeping her husband out until dawn. Beverley was about to start her second year of collecting AA chips. And I was the not-so-merry-widow about to turn forty.

All of us were damned tired of being capable, strong women. Done with smiling for Daddy at home, at work, wherever. We were all wondering about our next acts.

I rode in Caroline's car when we drove back to Charlottesville in August 1979. I had a decision to make about my moving on. We'd narrowed the decision down to a house perched up on a ledge in Flordon, right around the corner from Kaki's friend Kate, and a Cape Cod set back in Canterbury Hills. Flordon was by far the higher-end neighborhood, but the driveway was steep, and the first-floor layout was strange.

The negative about the Cape Cod was that the seller was a faculty colleague. He was moving his family to a house in the same price range in a neighborhood just across Barracks Road. "For a larger screened porch," he explained. It didn't make sense to me. I was suspicious, but I didn't pursue my concern. That would turn out to be a mistake.

Finally, Caroline gave up on Flordon. I think even she thought the floor plan truly weird. Caroline went on and on about the convenience and charm of Canterbury Hills. We put in a bid below the asking price, and it was accepted. That should have been a red flag.

I just wanted to find a place that was NOT the Mill. Maybe I could get free of Alan's implicit expectations of who I should be. Who we should be as a family. How we should be living in the world.

In contrast to the chaos at home, work was great. A formal fellowship program in developmental pediatrics had been approved for two positions, each two years long with funding from the Department. I'd recruited faculty member Dr. Peter Blasco from Hopkins. He'd finished his training at the Kennedy Center, and he'd start attending on the wards in September. Peppy recruited UVA undergraduates as summer interns and set up an apartment, kind of a teenage clubhouse, for our inpatients in an abandoned motel across the lawn from the Center.

An ethics conference for a national audience was funded and scheduled for fall. UVA students would perform *A Day in the Death of Joe Egg,* a play by Brit Peter Nichols about a family in crisis around their severely disabled child. And listen as two famous ethicists discussed opposing perspectives: Joseph Fletcher, *Situation Ethics* author, UVA professor of medical ethics, and my hero from the 1972 abortion roundtable; and Edmund Pellegrino, professor of medicine and medical ethics at Georgetown University.

It took a week at the end of August to move from the Mill into town with all hands on deck. No creek to rise. No gun-toting neighbors to shoot at Max. No snakes in Canterbury Hills. No rats were immediately evident, but the next-door neighbor, the one whose wife had just left him and with whom I shared side-by-side driveways, was nowhere to be seen while we were doing the heavy lifting.

The neighbors watched the proceedings with interest. Some wandered over and introduced themselves. It was great entertainment for the neighborhood kids. The Center staff pitched in after work, loading and unloading my rental truck, and making the run from North Garden. AV set up the kitchen cabinets. Even Peter Blasco unpacked boxes of my books and stacked the shelves as we discussed the role of the ward attending.

Max ran from room to room, leaping up and down the stairs, jumping up at the windows in the living room and the dining room to bark at the parade of cats and small dogs along Smithfield Road. I was startled by how massive he seemed in the little rooms. But eventually Max calmed and lay across my feet on the screened-in porch while I sipped a glass of chardonnay and gazed out over the backyard. It was dusk, but I could still make out the mounds of overturned dirt where the azalea bushes had been.

I hadn't really thought through how we would live in this house. It was like a fragile doll house compared with the Mill's massive chestnut beams and thick walls. I still had to figure out a pen for Max. The only way I could manage him on a leash if he was uncooperative was to sit on the ground until he tired of pulling me along.

While I went to play tennis Sunday morning, I put Max downstairs in the family room and closed the door into the kitchen. I pulled into the driveway two hours later. I could see him from the car, standing up on his hind legs leaning against the dining room window. Barking!

The guy next door already had beer in his hand and hollered, "You better muzzle that big guy. Danes are a dangerous breed. We've got little kids around here."

I slammed into the kitchen and ignored the end of the diatribe. Max wagged his tail and stood up to greet me, lapping away, delighted for my return. I could see the plank door was shredded where he burst through from downstairs. The drapes next to the dining room windows were ripped, and the windowpanes had claw scratches.

I should have known. How could I have been so stupid?

I gathered up Max's bowls and his brushes. I snapped the leash on his collar, and we got back in the car. I didn't even look at the other driveway. I continued to bawl all the way out and back to the SPCA. Max keened along. Alan would never forgive me.

I wandered from room to room, moving things around, straightening and adjusting. I tried to read the *New York Times,* but I couldn't concentrate. What had I done?

The ringing phone startled me. It was Berta from Beau Pré. Berta with the Swiss accent. I was confused.

"Sharon, I just met your beautiful Max. The SPCA called me right away when you dropped him off."

"Berta? You're with Max?" It didn't make sense. "My Max? Really?"

"Yes, Max is right here, but I want to make sure that you approve of Max to coming to live at Beau Pré. He's magnificent."

I started to cry again. "Oh, yes, of course," I said. "Berta, may the kids and I come to call, every now and then?"

"Of course."

On Wednesday, I drove to Camp Strawderman, watched as Kaki loaded Copy Cat into the horse trailer, and prepared to tell her about Max on the way home. "You did what?" she said. After some quiet tears, she glared at me and said I had never really trained Max or Mattie. "You do know, Mommy, that it wasn't Max's fault."

On Thursday, Kaki and I shared a quiet drive to North Carolina. On Friday's drive home, Dylan cried most of the way. "Losing Mattie was bad enough, but Max took care of us after Daddy died." Kaki did her best to soothe him as I drove home. We ate the fried chicken Yvonne had left on the stove in silence. We unpacked, and I called Berta. No one paid the slightest attention to the new house.

First thing the next morning, we went out to visit Max at Beau Pré. Berta had assigned him to the butler's pantry off the kitchen and covered it in mattresses.

Dylan lay on the ground next to Max and they embraced, full body. Dylan cried. Max groaned. Kaki squatted and patted his head, "Good Max. You did your best."

On Sunday morning, the kids were still asleep when Yvonne slammed the door and stormed into the kitchen. "Come on, Doc. Get your bag. Now." I recognized the look on her face, wrote a note for the kids, and got my bag.

Spencer had died sometime during the night at the hospital. The nursing staff called to let her know.

"We've got to visit Spencer," she said and grabbed my arm. "To say goodbye."

I tried to explain he was already tucked away in the morgue, and she wasn't allowed there. Besides, it was Sunday. No one would be there.

"I know, Doc. They told me that on the phone. He's in a drawer. In a refrigerator."

I continued to protest as Yvonne dragged me to the car. "We can't visit Spencer. He's dead, Yvonne."

"I need to know for sure. Besides, I've got a few things to say to him. And that's not all."

"But—"

"Aren't you Doc Hostler, the professor with tenure, the high and mighty director of the Children's Rehabilitation Center? Isn't that you?" She paused and thought. "Yep, sure is you. We be paying our respects to Spencer. You and me, now."

So it was that an hour later, Yvonne and I were in the empty Medical School Auditorium between the raised podium in the front and two hundred fixed seats sharply slanted up to the rear. Yvonne, the administrator-on-call, and me—we stood around Spencer's body laid out on a gurney from the morgue, a white sheet covering him from head to toe. Yvonne and I were on opposite sides of the gurney. The frantic MPA graduate student, who unluckily for him just happened to be on weekend call, stood next to Yvonne. He was poised to roll that steel gurney back to the morgue in a skinny minute.

"Are you ready?" I asked.

Yvonne nodded. I slowly pulled the sheet off Spencer's face and folded it onto his chest. We stood in that huge auditorium just staring at him. For a moment, it was deadly quiet.

Then, Yvonne shouted, "Look at you, you beautiful Black bastard! How I loved you. You were the best dancer ever!" The student administrator stared at me, terror on his face. First, I worried about him fainting, then that someone in the corridor might have heard Yvonne.

Yvonne bent down and lifted Spencer's head, stiff as it was, to her face, kissed him and hugged him. Still cradling him in her arms as best she could, she looked at us, grinning. "He's still a right fine-looking bastard, isn't he? And what he could do with his hips. Oh my."

The administrator paled. I worried he might vomit or pass out.

She lay Spencer back down on the gurney and slowly pulled up the sheet, all the time stroking his cheek. Then suddenly, she was trying to pry open his jaw. It was difficult. Rigor mortis had well set in.

"What the hell are you doing?"

Yvonne giggled like a giddy school kid. "Checking to see that my gold crowns are still there. Cost me a small fortune."

"Yvonne, if you want the crowns, we can request them. From the funeral home."

"Bell's over on Sixth Street," she interrupted. "No, I hear stories about the University stripping out the gold from the colored folk." Yvonne grinned and reached over the gurney to poke me. "Just checking up on your people, Doc."

Much later, I stood on Yvonne's doorstep with a bottle of Glenlivet in my hand. I had never been to her place in Palmyra, not once in ten years, but soon, Yvonne and I were settled in at her kitchen table with the open bottle of Glenlivet between us. Her kinfolk, all women, whispered and worked around us. When they tried to engage her, Yvonne waved them away. It was way after midnight when she finally let me go. She wasn't pleased that I wouldn't be at the funeral, but I had to present grand rounds at the Children's Hospital in Washington, DC.

It was Beverley who showed up at the Baptist Church in Palmyra with Kaki and Dylan in tow. And as Yvonne instructed, for the open casket viewing, the funeral service, and the graveside service in the family cemetery at her homeplace.

"Front row. Right next to Yvonne in the front row with the kids' shining white sneakers almost glowing in the dark," Beverley reported that evening. The stories from Kaki and Dylan were more detailed. How they had knelt with Yvonne next to the bier and she showed them how to cross themselves and how to say the prayers after her. How Spencer was laid out in his black suit, a tie, all fancy in the casket.

Dylan said, "You couldn't tell that he was blind and didn't have any legs." They didn't mention Alan, but I think we were all remembering that when Alan died, we didn't have a body, just ashes.

Whenever I came home from work that fall, the divorced neighbor next door was tossing the baseball with his catcher-son, Tony, or sitting in the driveway with a beer. One evening he referred me to the covenants of the Canterbury Hills Neighborhood Association, read aloud the exact height at which lawns were to be maintained, and pointed out just how tall my grass had gotten.

"Maybe I'll let my yard go to seed," I said and slammed my kitchen door.

The next week, the lady bus driver reported that on Monday morning Kaki had kickboxed Tony on the school bus because Tony had been harassing Dylan. "Laid him out cold in the aisle," the driver reported proudly. "The kids cheered as Kaki took her seat. My bus kept moving. No reports were filed."

From then on, Kaki was the neighborhood hero.

"Great legs from riding," Kaki explained.

Many years later I learned that my colleague's family moved out of 2501 Smithfield Road not for a larger screened-in porch but because the neighbor ballplayer had bullied their son.

No rats. No snakes. No twelve-mile commute.

Just the blond-headed bully next door.

· 28 ·

The Birthday Party

Fall 1979

I learned about the party when an elaborate parchment scroll was delivered to my office. The scroll was wrapped in blue satin ribbon with purple asters and signed by Beverley, AV, Jan, Caroline, Ina, Peppy, and Ann. The calligraphed instructions indicated time, place, and suggested attire. On October 24, 1979, I had to wear a long dress to celebrate my fortieth birthday.

Any event at Ann's home was special. A red wooden bridge led to her elegant house, furnished in stylish Scandinavian décor.

I circled the table and scanned the name cards, self-conscious in my ankle-length chiffon. There was no place set for psychiatrist Ruth Weeks. In theory, she should have been here, but her patient list included both Beverley and Jan. From the head of the table, Ann offered a champagne toast to friendship, the champagne provided by Beverley, the one-year-chip-carrying AA member.

In the background, the music from "I'm Getting My Act Together and Taking It on the Road" played softly, cued up by AV.

The first course was snails, prepared by our hostess. We were clumsy, quiet, and generally unenthusiastic.

Caroline presented the molded lobster and shrimp aspic. I loved lobster from summers on Cape Cod, and Caroline knew it.

As the next course was served, an elegant veal Marengo, Peppy reported its preparation in detail. The veal was purchased at the farm stand, cooked in several stages, and finished with an elaborate sauce. Which spilled on the car floor on her way to Ann's house.

When we were done laughing, we sang along with the Miss America song. When the vocalist reached the line about "taking her trophy and smashing the television set," I thought about Nellie, but only briefly.

I loved presents. I loved attention. And I loved dress-up parties. As I unwrapped the presents after dinner, I noticed the background music, which had moved on to "Now I'm doing my strong woman act."

AV stood up, glass in hand. She was the oldest of our group and the wisest by self-report, as well as the worst, but most enthusiastic, dirty joke teller. Clinking her glass for attention, she announced, "It's official. I decree that tonight is the absolute end of the mourning period for Alan Dimock. May he rest in peace!"

"Hear! Hear!" the others answered, raising their glasses.

"Even for a saint, and we all know Alan was beloved, but no damn saint, five years of mourning is enough!" She paused, waiting for the chatter to quiet. "Tonight, it must end!"

"Hear! Hear!"

Beverley lifted her champagne glass filled with seltzer water, "To Sharon. Make forty the beginning of the rest of your life."

I was wrong to think the party was winding down. It took me a while to understand that AV's declaration of mourning's end was just the beginning of the evening's official program.

A stack of envelopes appeared. One by one, I opened the gift certificates, each one of them focused on self-improvement. *My* self-improvement.

First, a session to learn my colors. *Was I a spring, a summer, an autumn, or a winter?* I would learn how my skin tone, hair shades, and eye color determined my season and what was the preferred palette of clothing, cosmetics, and accessories. Second, a consultation with a hair stylist. Third, a makeover with a cosmetologist. Ina Levy was Bob's second wife. Her envelope contained an offer to assist me build a basic wardrobe consistent with my professional status and my soon to be very busy social calendar. I laughed. They were so earnest.

AV poured more champagne. I was relieved by the break. I wondered how they thought I'd work these beauty routines into morning rounds, the kids' after-school schedules, and grocery shopping. Of all this group, only Ann understood the academic demands.

I doubted Ann had any interest in what season she was. On the other hand, her home was beautifully decorated, and she did wear an embroidered Loden jacket with a long black skirt that didn't come from Levy's. Beverley's Lacoste dresses came in different colors, but one shirtwaist style. AV had a consistent preppy look, khaki skirts, navy jacket with Kelly green or hot-pink piping. My work uniform included Birkenstocks, something long under my white lab coat, and a stethoscope. My only point of style was the collection of funky pins I wore on my lab coat to divert my young patients.

The next section of the program focused on topics currently recognized as self-care. It was as foreign to me as knowing what season I was. Jan presented a tutorial on skin care, emphasizing the urgency now I was forty. With much fanfare, she presented me a gift certificate for a year of monthly facials, manicures, and pedicures.

"I booked you on the first Saturday of November and December to get you started!" And if that wasn't enough crossing of personal boundaries, Beverley gave me a year's worth of massages scheduled for Fridays at four thirty. A theme was emerging, one that even I recognized.

I thought yoga sessions were over the top until AV introduced tennis as the path to meeting new people, learning to leave the hospital at a reasonable hour to join her foursome on Wednesdays, and, incidentally, to improving my physical fitness. Ann gave me six tennis lessons on Saturday mornings at nine o'clock. Jan quietly mentioned that we, the two of us, were signed up for the UVA's new Nutrition Clinic.

Mercifully, AV distracted us by pouring more champagne. I hoped the evening was winding down. It was increasingly difficult to nod and smile as the fortieth birthday self-improvement course unfolded. Maybe, I mused, my loving, kind friends would offer weekly grocery shopping, dry cleaning pickup, or a landscaping service so the height of my grass wouldn't exceed the neighborhood association's standards.

I sipped my champagne, but I was starting to feel something more than just being celebrated and loved. After all, I was still standing upright after five years. With a little help, I had gotten promoted and tenured. I'd had my tubes tied despite the indignity of appearing before a hospital committee to get permission, since my husband wasn't alive to approve the decision. My son was only ten at the time. I thought I was doing more than enough. My friends had other ideas.

I don't remember who introduced the last topic for discussion, but everyone joined the melee. First, Jan read a list of recently divorced faculty members from the School of Medicine. Ann suggested some unwed colleagues at Hopkins. Caroline volunteered to get me into the Farmington Country Club or the Keswick Club to access a richer pool of eligible bachelors, but AV thought the round robins at the Boars Head would be a better place to meet men, especially athletic men. But first, my tennis game had to improve.

What about Parents Without Partners? Was I attending my Middlebury reunions? What about the guys I used to date before Alan? How were their marriages going?

I was overwhelmed by the dinner and festivities, the generosity, the concern, the love. But I was stunned that anyone, especially this group of savvy women who purported to be my close friends, thought I should get over Alan.

A year later, in the fall of 1980, Kaki and Dylan were both at Jack Jouett Middle School. Beverley was still picking up her chips at AA meetings. There were recent reports about Beverley laughing a lot with a new female friend over ice cream cones. We'd learned that adjourning to the closest ice cream parlor after AA meetings was standard practice.

I had worked through the stack of fortieth birthday gift certificates. I had struggled at first, but eventually I learned to establish some work boundaries. I maintained a routine of weekly massages and monthly spa visits. Jan and I counted calories, walked in the neighborhood before dawn, and slowly shaped up. My dress size went down, my skin glowed, and my tennis serve snapped.

I regularly showed up at social occasions around the University with an escort. But I was no closer to identifying a suitor.

I didn't meet any eligible men on the tennis court, but I did make new friends at the tennis lottery, shared beers with the guys who played next to us, and subbed in other games. Then I met Betta at the Boars Head Sports Club. Betta had just moved to town with her husband, set up a travel agency, and she was looking for a tennis partner. Betta was a strong player, way better than I was, but she hated playing the net and I loved it. We remained doubles partners for over twenty years.

Another year passed. In the fall of 1981, I was still on the couch with the shrink at exactly 10:00 a.m., three times a week. We had talked and talked about Alan. We'd talked about the children. We'd talked about Nellie, Hop, and Pa Hostler. We'd talked about the times after Hop's death when Nellie went totally off the rails and her evil stepfather lurked around 15 Vernon Street.

We'd talked about the competition in academic pediatrics, the upcoming promotion to full professor, and the relentless sexism throughout the University, but especially in medicine. We explored how I could modify some of my self-defeating behaviors. How could I tackle the rampant sexism in the Department and the School without derailing my own career?

We talked about the family crises—that Copy Cat had developed a malignant hemangioma and would have to be euthanized; Dylan was selling candy at school, which he charged to my account at Foods of All Nations after biking there on the 250 Bypass at recess; and that Nellie's repeated hospital admissions in Vermont with elevated blood alcohol were getting more frequent.

Two years after the fortieth birthday party and five years of being on the couch, I was unprepared when even Dr. Josephthal suggested it was time to focus on finding a man. I had described the local dating scene—the crazies, the drunks, and the social misfits. We finally agreed that maybe there were no eligible men in Charlottesville—or at least no one ready to take on a widow with adolescent kids and stepchildren; an academic pediatrician who liked taking care of sick kids, teaching medical students, and taking night call. One quite comfortable as head of household. Yvonne didn't see a need for a man in the house, either. We were both widows.

And then, in a startling demonstration of nonstandard practice, or maybe loving desperation, the shrink proposed that I consider Club Med for a practice run out of my milieu, without the children. An experiment was how he framed it. Married friends of his had recommended the one in Martinique.

I signed up for one week at the Club Med in Martinique in February 1982. Betta, travel agent and tennis partner, assured me that I would have a single room, the Club had a white sand beach and tennis courts, and the guests would include French-speakers from the Continent and the Caribbean, and public-school teachers on holiday.

Martinique seemed very far away when the time came to euthanize Copy Cat. Muffin, Kaki's trainer, arrived to take her to the barn. It was the Saturday before Christmas. Kaki was there when the backhoe dug a ditch in the field. She held Copy Cat's massive head as the vet gave the injection and helped shovel the dirt over him after he fell into the ditch. Still grieving, Kaki was excused from the run up to Vermont to retrieve Nellie on the day after Christmas.

Early that morning, Yvonne, twelve-year-old Dylan, and I left for the twelve-hour drive to Burlington to move Nellie to Charlottesville. Dylan would stay overnight with Nellie, the boxes, and her two Siamese cats. It was nine o'clock when Yvonne and I got to the hotel. While I checked us in, Yvonne went to the restaurant to order supper before the kitchen closed. I took the bags up to our room and joined Yvonne.

"Wouldn't take my order, sorry, Doc," she said.

I waved to a waiter. "What's going on? We don't want to miss supper."

"That one," he tipped his head toward Yvonne and glared at me, "She ordered champagne and lobster." He shrugged.

"I hope you got our order in on time. We drove twelve hours from Virginia."

"That champagne better be cold," Yvonne said. "We earned it!"

That night, we shared a king-sized bed with an eight-by-twelve-inch, framed photograph of Spencer propped on a pillow between our two heads. "Can't sleep without him," Yvonne said and turned out the light. "Nitey-nite, Doc."

In the morning, Yvonne drove the U-Haul truck with Dylan. I had Nellie in the front seat of the car, her indoor plants, and the howling Siamese cats in the back. I lost sight of the truck at the rotary in Glen Falls, New York, but kept driving, convinced they were ahead of me on the interstate.

After an hour driving with no sight of the U-Haul, I stopped at a New York State Trooper Station and described my dilemma. As I spoke to one officer, I could hear Dylan over the speaker at the next window, "We've lost my mother. She's driving a yellow Mercedes with Virginia tags."

Yvonne had been afraid to stop, worried that the troopers would think she, a Black woman, had kidnapped the blond, blue-eyed Dylan. That was long before cell phones.

After two days of snow, rest stops for the cats and Nellie, and repeatedly being separated, we arrived back in Charlottesville.

Beverley and Jan unpacked the truck. AV and I set up Nellie's apartment, made the beds, and put away the kitchen stuff.

Yvonne was slamming pots around when I got home that night. "Thought you said it was different in the North, Doc."

It didn't take long for Nellie to include Kaki in her baking activities nor to con Kaki into buying cigarettes and scratch cards at the nearby 7-Eleven. And invite Kaki to take a puff. I'd learn later that Nellie arranged for a taxi driver to pick up her weekly liquor at the ABC store and deliver it. Yvonne answered the crisis calls. I did the weekly grocery shopping and paid the bills. When I would be at Club Med in late February, Kaki and Dylan were scheduled to visit Nellie after school and be picked up for supper by Yvonne or Beverley.

Martinique was magical. The air smelled of bougainvillea and the sea. Misted mountains framed long white beaches. The cemeteries had aboveground graves decorated with photographs, crucifixes, and sometimes, fresh flowers. Club Med was a camp for grown-ups, complete with competitions around sports, drinking, and sexual scoring.

On the other hand, I loved attending yoga at sunrise, swimming in the turquoise water off the coast, and reading my book on the beach. Some of the other guests were as advertised—the topless French, the ones still clothed seeking the nude beach, and the young studs perennially in the heat of a basketball game or on the make. Mealtimes, I elected to sit with the teachers who were delighted to be on vacation from public school. They were curious about my being alone and often offered tips about activities to try.

Which is how I ended up in line for water-skiing. I was a good snow skier, but I had never tried to water-ski. I observed and quickly understood that the challenge was getting up on the skis. There was a lot of screaming and splashing as people fell into the water right at the start. And they were young, not like this widow in her forties.

When it was my turn, I bent my knees, kept my arms straight, and, as instructed, let the boat pull me up. I got up on my first try! I was stunned by the cheering as I took off from the dock. I sailed around that bay like it was an early-morning run downhill at the Middlebury Snow Bowl. It was glorious. I skied between the ocean and the clouds, the wind soft on my face, and with just a little bend in my knees. I didn't want to ever get off those skis, but the guy in the motorboat pointed to the line waiting on the shore and shrugged. There was more cheering when he dropped me at the pier. I got right back in line.

At the tennis courts, I was toweling off when an older player approached me. He was fit, tanned, and had just whipped one of the arrogant young studs, 6–0, 6–0. "If you're willing to work on that backhand, we could take the mixed doubles tournament," he said to me.

For the rest of the week, I met Joe Boardman every morning at the courts. We won the mixed doubles tournament hands down.

At the awards ceremony, Joe and I were recognized for our tennis victory, as expected. But unexpectedly, I received a huge blue-ribbon rosette for expertise in water-skiing. I was giddy.

Joe was fifty-nine, sixteen years older than me, and as different from me as could be. Joe was the founding cantor at Westchester Reform Temple in Mamaroneck, New York. He had entertained the US troops in Burma during World War II, sung opera for ten years in Germany as a Fulbright scholar, and been a tennis pro in the Catskills. Although we went dancing after the awards ceremony, I never expected to see him or anyone from Club Med again.

I flew directly from Martinique to Florida for a four-day conference about hospital finance designed for physicians. In Florida, I rejoined a doubles game from our previous training session six months earlier—an endocrinologist from St. Louis, a psychiatrist from Boston, and an internist from Norfolk. All men, all terrific, and all happily married. They remarked on how much my game had improved.

The last night in Florida, Beverley called to report that Nellie had broken her femur on the day I flew to Martinique. The kids found her on the floor and called 911. Nellie was stable on the orthopedic ward at UVA, but the team delayed her transfer to an alcohol rehab center until my return.

And she told me that a bouquet of roses had been delivered for me that afternoon. "I am guessing you've had a better two weeks than we have had here," she said.

It was a complicated courtship. When Joe and I announced we were spending a sabbatical year in Israel, Nellie worried aloud about "all the Jews."

In 1983–84, I sublet the house in Canterbury Hills, found a sabbatical position, and moved to Jerusalem. Kaki commuted in a *sherut* to the

International School outside Tel Aviv. Dylan stayed behind at Cardigan Mountain School in New Hampshire. At Christmas break, Dylan carried ten thousand dollars in his socks when he came to visit with Beverley and Peter. We lived in a cash economy; inflation in Israel was out of hand. Yvonne and Nellie not only visited Israel, but Joe managed to get them to the top of Masada and the Galilee. Later, Dr. Blizzard's secretary reported how much he looked forward to the interim reports I sent summarizing my activities. No other faculty member on sabbatical had done that.

I was based at the Hadassah Hospital in Jerusalem but not welcomed. The chair of Pediatrics assigned me a study carrel in the library and the middle drawer in his secretary's desk to store my purse. Inpatient rounds were in Hebrew. I struggled to find something wise to add when the chair nodded in my direction. I ended up commuting through Bethlehem and the West Bank to Beersheba, the gateway to the Negev Desert. I worked with Dr. Mickey Karplus, chief of Neonatology at Ben Gurion Hospital, to create a follow-up clinic for their premature babies. Each Thursday, I sat on the ground in a tent with Bedouin mothers and babies, answering questions about their babies, translated from Arabic to English and back again by Zippy, the neonatologist's wife. The men, away from the village herding goats, would not have approved.

Midway through that year, I was awakened in the middle of the night by the chief of Surgery at Hadassah—they needed an emergency consult for a two-year-old with liver failure. A hospital in England had a genetically matched donor organ, but they required that the recipient have normal development documented. The military jet waited at the nearby base, and the surgical team formed a circle around the crib as I shook rattles, stacked building blocks, and babbled with my patient. It was 3:00 a.m. when I signed the consult form, attesting normal cognitive and fine motor development, but gross motor delays secondary to his huge liver and prolonged confinement in the hospital crib.

In the summer of 1984, we returned to the States and continued parallel lives. Joe arranged a New Year's Eve celebration—black tie, champagne, a performance of *Les Misérables,* dinner after theater, the ball falling in Times Square, dancing in Peacock Alley at the Waldorf, and breakfast at P. J. Clarke's in Lincoln Square. Although I interviewed for faculty positions in New York City and we looked at apartments, it became clear that my moving to New York was not going to work. Geography wasn't the only conflict, but it became the designated conflict for discussion.

My friends in Charlottesville worried that I would be a widow again were I to marry someone so much older. Dylan had become a model citizen at Woodberry Forest School while Kaki was raising hell at Foxcroft, a boarding school for girls and their horses. She refused to dress for morning report, smoked in the dorm attic, and sold minutes on my AT&T card for cash. Dylan was All Prep in wrestling, varsity in football and lacrosse. Kaki took her chestnut Country Fiddler to the International Horse Show and won blue ribbons. Gioia, by then an international photojournalist working out of Washington, DC, spent an exciting but dangerous year with Stevie in Palau.

By the fall of 1986, I petitioned Dr. Blizzard for promotion to full professor. It had been ten years as an associate professor, well beyond the period for my male peers. He was not enthusiastic, but I persisted, asking for the rules. I was told there were only two copies of the Promotion & Tenure Policy manual for the School of Medicine. One resided with the School of Medicine Promotion & Tenure Committee and the other in the second drawer of the dean's desk. I arranged with Linda, the dean's secretary, to read the manual when the dean was out of the office. I developed my portfolio, listed names of external referees to write letters in support of my work in patient care and medical education and my national reputation. Dr. Blizzard supported the promotion.

At Thanksgiving dinner in 1986, Joe asked Kaki, Dylan, Gioia, Stevie, Dorothy, Beverley, Yvonne, and Peter for my hand. He presented his bed pillow from New York and asked their permission to put it on the bed next to mine. And gave me a tiny bag of loose diamonds and sapphires for an engagement ring. There was much laughter and cheering that weekend. I completed my study with the local rabbi, petitioned the Beit Din (rabbinical court), and visited the *mikveh* to complete my conversion to Judaism. I found that Reform Judaism was not significantly different from Unitarianism. We shopped for a house in Charlottesville. Kaki and Dylan lobbied to return to the Mill. Joe vetoed that suggestion. He was not living in "Alan Dimock's mausoleum."

Joe and I were married in May 1987 by Rabbi Dan Alexander from Charlottesville's Congregation Beth Israel with the assistance of Joe's colleagues from Westchester Reform Temple, Rabbi Jack Stern, and Rabbi Debby Zucker. Debby served as the cantor under a *chuppah* at Alumni Hall. Dylan gave me away, and Kaki served as maid of honor. Gioia and Dorothy joined Joe's niece, Shira, as bridesmaids. Groomsmen included Stevie, Joe's nephew Joel, AV's sons, Mike and VG, and Jan's sons, Tim and Ben. The festivities had started Friday night with the congregation at Westchester Reform Temple in New York City and continued on to Charlottesville with a dinner party Saturday, a brunch with bluegrass music before the garden wedding that afternoon, and brunch the following Monday for the 125-plus out-of-towners in the backyard of our new home in West Leigh.

We all had significant changes to make. I had never lived with a man under the same roof. The longest Alan and I had ever spent together was the week after Kaki had been born. Joe never had children and was accustomed to giving his bar mitzvah kids orders at the temple. That did not work with Kaki or Dylan. Joe introduced all of us to international travel starting in the Middle East. He taught the kids currency, public transportation systems, and a little language, then turned them loose. We all traveled with tennis racquets and extra cans of balls. Most family battles took place on the tennis court or in some distant piazza.

When AV or Ann called Joe at the last minute to substitute in women's doubles, he showed up. When Joe's Italian teacher's child had an ear infection, Joe called me. Joe quickly learned to add an additional hour to any time I said I would be home from the hospital.

Joe and I struggled over little things like my insistence that the UVA uniform for men was a navy blazer and khakis or what hour I would really be home for supper. We struggled over big things like money and who made what decisions, when, and why. We had screaming fits and long no-talking spells. Sometimes for weeks. I went back to the couch then.

We argued about Kaki and Dylan, their decision-making, their choices. Yvonne and her tone of voice when she called him "Mister Boardman, sir!" And when was I going to learn to get my backhand back early, *before* my opponent's racket hit the ball? But when Yvonne and Linwood decided to get married, it was Joe who made the food (ham biscuits and chicken livers), and I arranged Yvonne's dress and bouquet for the wedding in her front yard.

Joe and I danced in the kitchen. Eventually, I stopped trying to make our bed when Joe was still asleep. He always took me to the airport and picked me up, no matter the hour or the weather.

And for so many years when I was invariably late for events at the Rotunda or Carr's Hill, I knew Joe would stand up immediately when I entered the room and bow slowly. Then, I knew exactly where I was headed.

· 29 ·

Yankee Woman in the Birdsong Chair

March 1991

It was March 1991. Dressed in formal attire, I arrived for dinner in the Dome Room of the Rotunda to receive an endowed chair, one of the most prestigious honors bestowed by the University of Virginia on a faculty member. I was being recognized by President John T. Casteen as the McLemore Birdsong Chair of Pediatrics—an honorific title that came with enhanced academic rank, a salary subsidy, and a traditional captain's chair with a bronze plaque.

The glorious spring evening and the accolades were shared with Dean Bob Carey, who had nominated me, esteemed colleagues from across Grounds, and my husband, Joe Boardman. Yvonne said that the neckline of my dress was too low, Nellie ignored the event as it wasn't important enough to be televised, and both kids were away at college. I wished that Dr. Mac had been alive for the endowed chair ceremony. And that Dr. Smith, Dr. Ryan, Dr. Lucey, and Dr. Thurman could have been present at our table in Mr. Jefferson's Rotunda. I wondered what Alan would have thought about my staying in one place for twenty-six years.

At the end of the evening, the awardees stood up to toast Mr. Jefferson. By then Joe was accustomed to toasting Mr. Jefferson, as well as having Beverley drop by for supper.

Joe continued to play tennis nearly every day, take Italian classes at UVA, and fix dinner every night. Once he'd enrolled in the associate chef course at Piedmont Virginia Community College, the level of cuisine at home changed significantly. Joe convinced me to bankroll my vacation days so that each May we could set up housekeeping in a different Italian village, from Sicily to Cinque Terra, Siena to Ravello.

By 1991, Beverley was director of social work for the UVA Hospital, still collecting her chips, and breaking ground for a post-and-beam house on fifty-five acres in Schuyler, where she would live with her partner, Nathou. Peter dutifully came from Nashville for birthdays, graduations, and Thanksgiving. At home, Yvonne was still negotiating with Joe about most everything but especially whose domain was the kitchen.

Kaki would graduate from Vassar in May. She was still trying to decide between a career as an equine vet or a social worker. I had refused to send her horse to college. Kaki worked at a residence for burnt-out alcoholics in Charlottesville and at a shelter for abused women at college, but her plan for the coming year was to intern with a vet in Vermont who specialized in equine athletes. It wasn't clear to me what became of her beau, the captain of the rugby team. But, after one year in Vermont, Kaki returned to Columbia University for graduate school and received her MSW, then headed cross-country with her girlfriend. She readily landed a position with the King's County district attorney to reform Seattle's juvenile court system. Joe and I kept their cats.

Dylan was a rising senior at Middlebury College, writing his thesis on General Stonewall Jackson and taking courses in feminist literature. Dylan played offensive tackle on the football team, volunteered with the Middlebury Fire Department, and commuted to North Carolina for his girlfriend Julie's debutante season. Dylan had taught Julie to sail at Camp Morehead when they were thirteen. Both stayed on as counselors during college. Joe helped him buy a tux, but I refused to pay for the plane tickets.

The years leading up to that March night at the Rotunda had seen changes at the Center as well. We had recruited outstanding faculty and developed model clinical programs, training programs that brought graduate students to the Center from throughout the mid-Atlantic region. By 1991, the Center faculty and staff were presenting at national academic meetings, publishing peer-reviewed research papers, and winning competitive research awards. The Center had been renamed the Kluge Children's Rehabilitation Center (KCRC). We'd received a significant donation from billionaire John W. Kluge to build a new outpatient wing and to fund research projects.

As planning began for the construction, I gathered a group of parents in the conference room at KCRC and asked what they would like to have in the new building. I expected suggestions about parking and maybe a parent lounge or library. We were worrying about children who needed ventilators having to live their lives in the hospital intensive care unit. About the adolescent boys with muscular dystrophy and what they needed to know. We weren't focused at all on the families and what their questions were. We were, in fact, disinterested and arrogant.

"Respect," one mother said. "We want to participate in the team meetings when you professionals make decisions about our kids," a second added. "We know more about what our kids need than you do, and you never even ask." It got more and more heated. "We want to read the medical chart." "We want to be able to disagree with you and not lose medical care for our kids."

We were one of several groups across the country grappling with the role of families that eventually mobilized around the concept of family-centered care, or FCC, as parents became significant advocates for their children and their rights as parents to participate in decision-making and be present at bedside and during treatment. Parents told us that we organized hospitals with the staff and the staff's convenience at the center of our universe when we should have organized our care around the patient. At that time in history, those ideas were revolutionary. Today those words sound like marketing phrases, but at that time, FCC was a revolution in how children and eventually adults were cared for.

I continued my advocacy work in another area even closer to home. Dr. Carolyn M. Brunner, my colleague in Internal Medicine from my internship years, and I had begun an effort several years earlier to seek gender equality for women in academic medicine. When we had visited the offices of the Association of American Medical Schools (AAMC) in the early 1980s, we were listened to politely but informed that until we had hard data, our anecdotal observations had no meaning. So, when Dr. Robert M. Carey was named the new dean of the School of Medicine in 1986, we immediately petitioned him to create a Committee on Women, and he did, naming senior women and men from both the basic science and the clinical departments.

We consulted peers and the medical literature, sought advice from experts, and developed questions about the student, house staff, and faculty experience at UVA School of Medicine. We collected and analyzed data from UVA School of Medicine, an identified peer group of medical schools, and the published literature. Later, we realized that our design had omitted three important groups—the experiences of nursing students and faculty, Persons of Color, and our gay and lesbian colleagues.

In 1989, the group had completed a five-hundred-page report to submit to Dean Carey, who immediately requested we present the findings to his council of department chairs. Although we had anticipated that salary inequity would be the first and easiest intervention, the School of Medicine leadership instead committed to revise the School of Medicine promotion and tenure guidelines to avoid the conflict between the tenure and the biological clocks, to redefine scholarship, and to define and value excellence in medical teaching and clinical work. It was a heady period as UVA's report was used as a model to examine gender fairness in other schools of medicine. The AAMC was ready to develop national leadership programs for women in academic medicine, starting with midcareer women from the 135 medical schools in North America. Alec Horniman, Darden School of Business professor, stood with our team when the UVA School of Medicine received the annual AAMC Award for Excellence in Leadership.

In the days following the endowed chair ceremony in March 1991 at the Rotunda, the congratulations continued. My women friends were not included in the Rotunda celebration. Not to be upstaged, they threw a party for me in the garden of Pavilion I with champagne, little cakes, and fancy dresses. And speeches.

"Had we known the importance of the chair," they said, "we would have done this years ago."

Then they, too, gave me a chair. But this one was a polished mahogany commode with a white porcelain pot and a rush weave lid.

Many of my colleagues across Grounds congratulated me as well. More than a few chuckled and commented, "I suspect that Dr. Mac is turning over in his grave. A woman as the McLemore Birdsong Professor of Pediatrics? Hell, no!"

"Maybe, but I'm not so sure about that." I smiled and shook my head. "If Dr. Mac turns over in his grave, it's because a Yankee is in the McLemore Birdsong Chair. Not a woman."

Epilogue

1990–2025

I was seventy-six years old when I retired from the University of Virginia in 2016—fifty-one years after the first day of internship in 1965. Caring for my patients was how I established my identity, my meaning, my path in life. And it has been through remembering and retelling their stories and my stories that I've made sense of my life.

After President John T. Casteen named me to the McLemore Birdsong Professor of Pediatrics Chair in 1990, the Center flourished, and another important chapter of my academic life began. I was invited to participate in restructuring the policies for academic advancement within the School of Medicine.

At the national level, the Association of American Medical Colleges (AAMC), under the leadership of Dr. Jordan Cohen, initiated the Women in Medicine program (WIM), with its focus the development of midcareer women faculty as medical school leaders. For more than a decade, as a member of the WIM faculty, I collaborated with outstanding senior women leaders from across the country in the basic science and clinical disciplines to develop leadership seminars for women. I convinced Dean Robert M. Carey that our medical school should replicate these ideas. When our program at UVA received national recognition, I was invited to present our findings to the AAMC Council of Deans, which included the leaders from all 135 medical schools in North America.

Although I was still taking inpatient call during the 1990s, my home life was relatively calm and orderly. Kaki and Dylan were at college. Gioia had returned to Cape Cod. My husband, Joe Boardman, had retired and relocated to Charlottesville from New York City. Not only did Joe concoct increasingly complicated menus for supper each evening, but he also organized our tennis games and planned our yearly excursions to Italy.

Kaki graduated from Vassar College and Columbia University's School of Social Work, migrated to Seattle to work for the district attorney of Kings County, and soon found her wife, Deborah. We celebrated a series of nuptial events, first in Seattle in 1999, and then in Vermont and New York City. Their marriage finally became official with the Supreme Court's 2015 landmark decision in *Obergefell v. Hodges.*

After Dylan graduated from Middlebury College, he coached football at Delaware Valley College, Princeton University—with one year in Bergamo, Italy—and the College of William & Mary. After a year of the traditional prenuptial festivities and parties, Dylan and Julie married in 1998. They settled in the beach community of Wilmington, North Carolina. Dylan coached high school football and taught American history as Julie established her pediatric dentistry practice.

Along with the many celebrations, we endured a season of losses. Nellie died at age ninety. My stepdaughter Dorothy's eleven-year-old, Becca, died in a horseback riding accident. Peter Kaplan suffered a painful death from a neurological condition. Yvonne lost her only daughter, Frederika, and her second husband. It seemed I had returned to my death maven days. The final blow was when Dr. Blizzard, my former nemesis, named me as his medical executor.

Joe increasingly agitated for me to retire, admonishing me that I was wasting years of good health and deferring international travel. And with the hospital administrator's announcement in 2002 that we would not build a freestanding children's hospital at the Center site, I scheduled an appointment with the newly appointed dean, Dr. Tim Garson.

Instead of accepting my resignation, Dean Garson recruited me to his office as senior associate dean for faculty. Here was a new challenge and opportunity—to oversee the promotion and tenure process and to develop outstanding faculty, *men and women,* into leadership roles as chairs and deans. In January 2003, after one last month on inpatient call, I retired, properly celebrated, from the Department of Pediatrics and moved to the Dean's Office in McKim Hall on Hospital Drive.

For the first time in my career, I negotiated for major resources, administrative support, and a 90 percent time commitment. By this period, I was anticipating grandmother responsibilities. And in September 2003, I walked out of the Dean's Office midafternoon, en route to Wilmington, North Carolina, where Julie was in active labor. As the designated neonatal nanny, I bonded with the young Alan Dimock, early and tightly. I was delighted to reprise my nanny assignment with Lucy Nell two years later.

I loved every aspect of my role, from playing the utility infielder on the dean's team to rounding regularly with the clinical and basic science department chairs. The Leadership in Academic Medicine program soon became a major success with more chair recommendations than we had positions. The only complaint was from Joe—he expected me home for his increasingly complex dinners by 6:30 p.m. instead of my usual 7:30 p.m. Yet Joe was always ready, when called upon, to don his black tie, save me a seat, and raise a glass to toast Mr. Jefferson.

In May 2007, President Casteen appointed Dean Garson as vice president and provost of the University and me as the interim dean and vice president of the Medical School. When I approached the podium at my first State of the School address, I was stunned when the faculty stood and clapped. Joe cheered as I regaled him with all the details at dinner that evening.

I lost my most ardent supporter when Joe was diagnosed with lung cancer that summer. Joe died in early January 2008, taking to his bed only after one last tennis game, a final Beefeater martini, and a trek to visit the grandchildren on Christmas Day. Following the public and private death rituals in New York City and Charlottesville, my family and friends gradually returned to their homes. Beverley and Kaki were the last ones to leave. Joe's Maine Coon cat, Florrie, and I rattled around the empty house. It was then Yvonne announced, "Enough dying" and, after thirty-eight years, she left. I'd mastered the role of death maven and dean, but I had to relearn how to be a widow and how to live alone.

It was a relief to return to the demanding academic schedule and the support of friends and colleagues in the Dean's Office. By late 2008, I resumed my role as senior associate dean and added a new one as vice provost for faculty development. Provost Garson charged me with extending the Leadership in Academic Medicine program across Grounds. It was an exciting time of learning and personal development. My women friends once again created a safety net for me.

President Casteen, amid much controversy in the Faculty Senate, had recruited the Semester at Sea program to the University in 2006. The old dreams of sailing the world with Alan Dimock resurfaced. I became determined to sail as academic dean and circumnavigate the world.

"No way, Sharon," is what President Casteen said. "We need a dean from the College of Arts and Sciences. Forget about it."

But I persisted.

I was only an observer on the Maymester Voyage for Engineering Students in 2011, but I was the academic dean for the spring semester of 2013. It was a new and exciting challenge for this pediatrician. In January 2013, the MV *Explorer* departed San Diego Harbor for Japan with 722 students, 300 crew, 35 faculty, and Visiting Scholar Archbishop Desmond Tutu. Our days at sea were marked by a major storm in the Pacific, a faculty death in Shanghai, and one honor trial. After 110 days at sea, we proctored semester exams, donned academic robes for commencement, and disembarked in Barcelona.

Exciting days on Grounds included faculty programs, officiating at the opening of the Sharon L. Hostler Child Care Center for the children of medical residents, and traveling to sports competitions in North Carolina for Alan and Lucy. I was determined to cheer for the entire competition, not just a frantic round or inning as I had done with Kaki and Dylan. I sailed again as academic dean for the fall 2015 Semester at Sea.

I retired from UVA in 2016, and I relinquished my medical license in 2020 at age eighty. Inspired by both husbands and emboldened by my experiences at sea, I keep traveling and exploring the world with friends and family. Adventures with Alan or Lucy remain the most fun.

The practice of medicine today bears no resemblance to that of the summer of 1948, when Dr. Smith delivered babies at home and accepted chicken, eggs, and fresh tomatoes in barter for payment. Instead of barter, we have Medicaid, Medicare, and private health insurance programs.

So much change. Today, 85 percent of children diagnosed with acute lymphocytic leukemia have normal life expectancy. Cystic fibrosis is treated by designer drugs that extend patients' lives by up to forty-five years but cost three hundred thousand dollars a year. Gene engineering techniques show promise for the treatment of many diseases, such as sickle cell disease, beta thalassemia, and congenital deafness. Public health initiatives in vaccine development, accident prevention, and no-smoking laws have shaped healthier childhoods. Gunshot wounds have become the most common cause of death in childhood.

Today, medical residents have limited duty hours, competency standards to demonstrate, and networks of social support including parental leave and their own daycare center. We recently had a class of medical students in which the women outnumbered the men. Women and Persons of Color are included in drug studies and clinical trials. Telehealth networks reach out to isolated, rural families. Rescue squads intervene with suspected stroke patients before reaching the emergency room. The UVA Hospital is no longer a single building but a complex system with an extensive network on Grounds and across the Commonwealth and telemedicine around the world.

I still remember being trusted by Dr. Smith alone in his office when I was ten. I'll never forget Dr. Ryan picking me up from school two years later to explain that Hop would soon die from Hodgkin's disease. And the excitement and terror of that first day of July 1965 when I entered the hospital at Mr. Jefferson's University is still fresh. The hospital was yet to be integrated, and there were few women in training. The University did not admit women to the College of Arts and Sciences until the 1970s.

In 2010, UVA appointed its first woman president, Terry Sullivan. In 2019, UVA appointed its first woman provost, Liz Magill. In the summer of 2025, women are deans not only of the School of Medicine and the School of Nursing but also of the College of Arts and Sciences, the Law School, the Engineering and Applied Sciences School, the McIntire School of Commerce, and the School of Education and

Human Development. The dean of the School of Architecture is Black. And the rector and vice rector of UVA's governing Board of Visitors are women.

I hope that Mr. Jefferson and Dr. Birdsong are cheering.

I am.

ACKNOWLEDGMENTS

I have been writing this book in my head and on sundry pads of yellow legal paper from the day I met my first pediatric patient. It was the fall of 1962 in Burlington, Vermont. I was a second-year medical student in the hospital morgue. My patient was eight years old and she had died of a disease I'd never even heard of: cystic fibrosis. My patients and their families became my teachers, their stories part of my story. I was always writing medical chart notes, journal entries, and, sometimes, sympathy notes.

I had developed a strong writing habit long before medical school. My English teacher at Rutland (Vermont) High School, Mabel Morrill, was to blame. She required that we maintain daily reading diaries and submit them weekly. That she regularly made notes in my diary was reinforcing and magical. Arthur "Beowulf" Brown, my freshman English professor at Middlebury College, demanded student journaling, and I never stopped squirreling away my wonders and my rages.

The practice of medicine was one series of storytelling sessions from morning work rounds to attending teaching rounds to weekly grand rounds. That is, to be quite clear, before the introduction of the electronic medical record in the 1990s. I always used patient storytelling to ground my academic presentations and scholarly writing. I was envious when I discovered a colleague—poet and doctor—completing an MFA during his tenure year instead of doing research in a basic science lab.

The doctor poet, Dr. Danny Becker, and the University Professor, writer David Morris, graciously invited me to co-teach a series of writing seminars for faculty physicians. I understood I was a student. In 2003, I stopped taking night call and signed up for a writing class at the Charlottesville Writing Center taught by Lauren F. Winner, celebrated author of *Girl Meets God.* We learned the etiquette of workshopping, wrote to weekly deadlines, and received footnoted comments on our submissions. A humorous essay about my early morning gym experiences was accepted by *Pharos,* the academic journal of Alpha Omega Alpha, the medical honor society. I was hooked.

When Winner's course ended, a group of students continued as the Ivy writing group, recruited others, and went on to meet monthly through to the present. I am grateful to those gentle critics who read endless iterations of my doctoring stories—Susan Guerrant, Gerry Kruger, Sharon Davie, Muriel Humphry, Margaret Browne, Marti Snell, Bruce Hillman (deceased), James Plews-Ogan (deceased), Madaline Harrison, and Leigh Grossman. And every year or so, I celebrated a piece published.

As the Academic Dean on the 2013 and 2015 circumnavigations of Semester-at-Sea, I audited writing courses with the undergraduates and contributed to the *Squid,* the online student newspaper. Teachers John Miller, Paul Shepherd, and my fellow students were tougher critics. I thank them for the tough feedback and fearless prodding as I explored themes of loss from my personal life.

Late in 2019, the Writers House in Charlottesville listed a Memoir-in-a-Year class taught by the memoirist and novelist Sharon Harrigan. In January 2020, the first case of COVID-19 was reported in the United States. On March 18, 2020, I was one of the eight members of the memoir class gathered in a conference room at Writers House. It was our first and last in-person meeting. The next day UVA President Jim Ryan announced all classes would move online. Every Monday at 9 a.m., our class met with our teacher, Sharon Harrigan, for three hours by Zoom. For each of us, it became a focus and a strategy to survive the pandemic. In March 2021, the Memoir-in-a-Year class morphed to a second full year.

These students were serious, accomplished, and published writers of various ages and stages. My memoir initially focused on my years in pediatric training at UVA during the civil rights era. They had little or no patience with my endless patient histories, detailed physical exams, and laboratory data. It was a slow and painful experience, but their relentless questioning about "where I was in my own story" was effective. It was in 2022 at our last scheduled class when I acquiesced to writing about growing up with Nellie and Hop in Rutland, Vermont—now the first two chapters of *Making Rounds.*

The COVID memoir class under the mentorship of Sharon Harrigan became not only an intense learning experience but a trusting support group. Without the support and challenges of my respected and respectful classmates Linda Hewitt, Erin James, Jessica Lowe, Sue Murdock, Fran Slayton, Stan Trent, and Rowena Zimmerman, there would have been no *Making Rounds.* I recognize and honor each of you.

I am grateful to editor Kimberlee Walker's insightful review of the manuscript. She identified examples of my white assumption, pointing out stereotypes of the Sapphire Caricature, and educating me that what happened to the Tuskegee airmen was far beyond my naïve description as a disaster. The African American Heritage Center was a useful resource for my understanding of the urban renewal movement that resulted in the destruction of the Vinegar Hill neighborhood in Charlottesville.

Manuscript reviewers selected by the press and initially blinded to me were Dominique Tobbell, a scholar of twentieth-century US healthcare in the post–World War II period, and John T. Casteen III, a medieval scholar and former University of Virginia president. I am grateful to both for the time and attention devoted to the review process and the importance of their detailed and supportive feedback. Tobbell pointed out my misogyny, especially how I overlooked the critical mentorship and advocacy I received in my training from the nurses at UVA Hospital. Casteen commented on the importance of the sharing of my "open-faced maturation as a woman, wife, and mother, a practitioner and a teacher."

My guide at UVA Press has been Mark Mones since I submitted the manuscript in September of 2023. He has been a patient mentor and shepherd to the complex processes of taking the manuscript to its final form as a book in the hands of a reader. His helpful colleagues include EDP director Ellen Satrom, art director Cecilia Sorochin, marketing director Jason Coleman, publicist Mary Kate Maco, and press director Eric Brandt. I have learned important lessons from all of them. I still think "badass" is a better descriptor than "indomitable" in the book's subtitle, but marketing knows best. *Making Rounds* is a far better book because of them. Thank you, each and every one.

Thanks to Dan Grogan, my friend and KCRC colleague, the photographer for the cover of *Making Rounds.* Dan patiently clicked away as Daphne, her parents Skyla and Trey Beverly, and I played doctor in Michael Bailey's studio. Daphne is three years old, Gioia's great-granddaughter and Stevie's granddaughter.

I take full responsibility for the content of this book. The names of my patients and their families have been changed. I have described people, situations, and conversations to the best of my memory. However, it is my description of my life. There are bound to be experiences that I remember differently than others and even experiences that I don't remember at all. After all, I am now eighty-six years old.

Making Rounds originated with the remarkable, brave, and life-affirming stories of my pediatric patients and their families. Without them, there would be no story. My formative development as an academic physician resulted solely from the critical mentorship of Drs. Smith and Ryan when I was growing up and then my pediatric mentors, Dr. Jerry Lucy at UVM's College of Medicine and my chair, Dr. William G. Thurman at UVA. Although I didn't initially recognize their impact, there were significant medical women. Dr. Carolyn Brunner, Dr. Ruth Weeks, Dr. Martha Carpenter, Dr. Ann Johanson, and Dr. Margaret McChesney kept me safely on the path in my early faculty years. The formative mentors about teamwork and leadership were the interdisciplinary teams at the Children and Youth Project and the Children's Rehabilitation Center, followed by Professor Alex Horniman from Darden and the Women in Medicine Program led by Janet Bickel at the Association of American Medical Colleges. I have immense gratitude for their persistence and integrity in shaping my professional self.

I am grateful to my family of blood and my family of choice. Without the women who sustained the children and me after the plane crash killed Alan Dimock in 1974, there would have been no family, no career in academic medicine, and no *Making Rounds.* Day after day, Yvonne Thurston and Beverley Butler put their arms around us at the Mill and kept us physically and psychologically safe, as did the coaches and camp counselors who helped Kaki and Dylan succeed outside the Mill.

The women of Charlottesville from AV Sullivan and Betta Stephens on the tennis courts to Maryanne Ellwood in local politics, and the women at my fortieth birthday party who declared my mourning period over—they sustained me.

Kudos to my devoted colleagues, especially Sharon Harrigan, Reg and Georgia Garrett, Peppy Linden, and Anda Webb, who patiently and obsessively read draft after draft of *Making Rounds*. Best friend Beverley Butler perused every page, red pen in hand, correcting, commenting, and criticizing until one month before her death in September 2025.

Lastly, I appreciate the love, patience, and support from Kaki and Dylan, who cheered, groaned, and happily approved the final edits. I dedicate *Making Rounds* to them.